AFRICAN MEDICAL PLURALISM

AFRICAN MEDICAL PLURALISM

Edited by William C. Olsen and
Carolyn Sargent

Indiana University Press

Bloomington and Indianapolis

This book is a publication of

Indiana University Press
Office of Scholarly Publishing
Herman B Wells Library 350
1320 East 10th Street
Bloomington, Indiana 47405 USA

iupress.indiana.edu

The paper used in this publication meets the minimum requirements of the American National Standard for Information Sciences—Permanence of Paper for Printed Library Materials, ANSI Z39.48-1992.

Manufactured in the United States of America

Library of Congress Cataloging-in-Publication Data

Names: Olsen, William C., editor, author. | Sargent,
    Carolyn F., 1947-editor, author.
Title: African medical pluralism / edited by William C. Olsen and
    Carolyn Sargent.
Description: Bloomington and Indianapolis : Indiana University
    Press, 2017. | Includes bibliographical references and index.
Identifiers: LCCN 2016045753 (print) | LCCN 2016046920 (ebook) |
    ISBN 9780253024770 (cloth : alk. paper) | ISBN 9780253024916
    (pbk. : alk. paper) | ISBN 9780253025098 (e-book)
Subjects: LCSH: Integrative medicine—Africa, Sub-Saharan. |
    Medical care—Africa, Sub-Saharan. | Traditional medicine—
    Africa, Sub-Saharan. | Medical anthropology—Africa,
    Sub-Saharan.
Classification: LCC R733 .A365 2017 (print) | LCC R733 (ebook) |
    DDC 615.0967—dc23
LC record available at https://lccn.loc.gov/2016045753

1 2 3 4 5   22 21 20 19 18 17

In memory of Madam Ama Agyemang; 192?–2015
Mother, Grandmother, Sister, Wife, Bonesetter, Midwife,
Herbalist, part-time ɔkɔmfɔ

Contents

AFRICAN MEDICAL PLURALISM

Introduction

William C. Olsen and Carolyn Sargent

How do individuals and communities make sense of disease in contemporary Africa? What medical options arise in the pursuit of health care? Where multiple healthcare options exist, patients may draw upon a therapeutic continuum, consisting of diverse medical modalities. Varied options address the same symptoms; and they may be utilized simultaneously or sequentially. These alternatives for medical intervention are not necessarily seen as contradictory; nor are they mutually exclusive. Rather, therapeutic choices represent a spectrum of valid therapeutic interventions. For example, one fourteen-year-old patient suffering from epilepsy consulted a diviner in rural Ghana in 2002. The patient's course of treatment had included repeated visits to a large urban hospital, use of pharmaceuticals prescribed by physicians, attendance at healing churches in Kumasi, self-medication, prayer camps, anointing with oil, and consultation with a diviner. His family accompanied the boy. They received direction from other sources, advising the family about alternative approaches to healing. The diviner declared that epilepsy was the result of malevolent forces sent to the boy by a group of men and women who had stayed in the boy's home some months previously. The visiting women envied the health of the boy, and they were said to have brought about the disease through their malfeasance. Doctors and hospitals were utilized to treat epilepsy; but in this case, involving mystical causation, their abilities were considered practically useless. The diviner subsequently blocked the witchcraft. He prescribed herbal remedies for the symptoms, which the family administered. They combined the herbs with all recommended pharmaceuticals from the hospital. The child's symptoms consequently abated under this regimen.

As this case illustrates, sufferers and their kin draw on diverse healing modalities in search of working therapies. This volume presents scholarly approaches to the therapeutic continuum in sub-Saharan Africa. The continuum is a sliding scale of responses to disease—a spectrum ranging from biomedicine to various nonbiomedical personal and group choices. As we note in the case above, therapeutic choices are not mutually exclusive. In this volume, each author presents data gathered from onsite field locations to demonstrate how medical pluralism and medical knowledge are experienced and applied within various African settings. We address three broad objectives:

1. to show that African populations seek medical recourse within a wide range of possible modes of therapy, including those found within local settings, as well as options such as biomedicine and Islamic healing, practices that are present due to centuries of historical contact
2. to demonstrate that a course of action taken in medical treatment reflects local cultures as well as national and global power structures
3. to use ethnography and descriptions of interpersonal dynamics to pursue these goals and also to apply them to broader concerns of global health. While theory helps to frame detail and data, we believe the biggest contribution of the volume is to document the ethnographic realities of suffering and therapy in everyday life.

African medical pluralism is the result of historic and contemporary developments.[1] These include colonial-era efforts to eradicate and manage infectious diseases, the introduction of colonial hospitals and clinics, and Muslim healing traditions dating back centuries. Since independence, in the post-1950 decades, we see a continued and expanded reliance on biomedicine and contemporary medical missions, herbalists, ritual specialists, local midwives and bonesetters, evangelical healing, and spirit possession groups. Taken together, these modes of therapy present opportunities for sufferers to seek counsel in the search for health. This therapeutic continuum offers patients an array of interpretations of causation (microbes, breach of taboo, contagion, sorcery, spirit possession, etc.) and alternative treatments (biomedical pharmaceuticals, herbal preparations, divination, Koranic verses, scarification, surgery, and other modes of healing). The postcolonial legacy of medical knowledge, practices, and practitioners has shaped the structures and dynamics of the therapeutic continuum in evidence across the continent, in particular historical, political, and economic contexts. As noted over a generation ago, "If we take individual patients as the focus of analysis, we realize that there is already considerable informal integration of scientific and traditional medical systems" (MacCormack 1986, 156). This historical interchange has involved diviners referring serious patients to an emergency room and doctors suggesting stroke patients supplement their hypertension drugs with herbal remedies, as Olsen notes in this volume.

Medical pluralism is a concept widely associated with the writings of Charles Leslie (1975, 1976, 1980), which attracted considerable scholarly interest during the 1970s and 1980s, additional writings in the 1990s, and a recent revival of inquiry: (Alex et al. 2012, Chary and Rohloff 2015, Langwick 2015, Rhine et al). An exhaustive 116-page annotated bibliography on medical pluralism published in

2012 (Alex et al.) documents the extensive literature in this domain, from classical studies of the 1970s to very recent publications.

In his discussion of the constitution of medical systems, Leslie proposed that "medical systems are pluralistic structures of different kinds of practitioners and institutional norms" (1976, 99). Evoking the importance of historical and comparative research on medical systems, he notes that biomedicine, especially since World War II, has progressively subordinated but not supplanted other forms of practice. The preeminence of biomedicine is thought to be its prestige, its expert authority, and state legitimization and support. Yet ethnographic observations indicate the global presence of multiple medical traditions within particular societies. As Leslie suggests, the division of labor between different forms of medical practice is often an ongoing negotiated compromise, in which biomedicine and diverse local systems such as herbalism, ritual healing, midwifery, and multiple other alternatives, coexist as complementary and sometimes competitive options (1980, 191). Efforts by state and global health authorities to eliminate or restrict nonbiomedical practices, intended to generate local medical systems that are extensions of an internationally standardized system, have achieved partial success at best. From a global perspective, Leslie contends that medical pluralism is not a phenomenon of social enclaves but rather a feature of every medical system, even in the United States, where biomedicine has long been presumed to hold a monopoly on medical care (cf. Eisenberg 1993, 1998; Frankenberg and Leeson 1976; Janzen 1978; Kleinman 1980; Rubel 1979; Janzen and Feierman 1979).

With reference to sub-Saharan Africa in particular, Janzen urges Africanist medical anthropologists to think of diverse medical modalities viewed via the metaphor of a kaleidoscope, by which a "subtle turns of a lens produces new and unanticipated combinations of actors, therapies, interpretations, and institutions that appear as we move across space and through time" (Rhine et al. 2014, 4). By means of this orientation, we are less likely to reify bounded systems of medical knowledge and are more likely to recognize the capacity of local healing systems and biomedicine to mutually inform and transform one another across time and space.

Biomedicine was exported from Western Europe to Africa during the colonial period, introduced by medical missionaries and private companies as well as colonial administrations. Biomedicine initially appealed to visions of modernity and development that over time have not been realized in most African states (Prince 2014, 3). The contemporary realities of biomedicine vary in relation to uncertainties associated with the quality of biomedical care available in many African medical institutions, undermined by global political and economic policies. Whereas wealthy patients have options such as private clinics or medical travel to Europe, those living in economic poverty may continue to engage in a "quest for therapy" (Janzen 1978) that includes public hospitals as one option in a flourishing array of therapeutic possibilities. Prince observes that "a thriving medical pluralism attests to the resonance of ideas about health and healing other than the biomedical. Biomedicine has had to coexist with these other epistemologies and practices, which locate health and therapy in arenas beyond the biological body, outside the clinic and the hospital and among nonbiomedical specialists" (Prince 2014, 6).

As anthropologists have shown since the early twentieth century, disease depends on culture for its "constitution as a human reality" (Good 1994, 53). Accordingly, discrete symptoms take on different meanings in diverse classificatory systems of illness. African healing systems are the product of local histories as well as global influences, both Western and non-Western. Local understandings of illness causation, healing practices, and medical institutions reflect widely shared cultural meanings that constitute the framework for diagnosis and treatment. In biomedicine, a medical diagnosis is "an interpretation that a clinician constructs by piecing together *symptoms* provided from the narrative of a suffering person during a clinical interview and *signs* from that person's physical examination and tests" (Graham 2006, 80). Hospital and clinical diagnoses in Africa represent the variation possible in biomedicine, as local meanings and interventions shape biomedical institutions and clinical practice. Alternative options for therapy acknowledge the efficacy and power of biomedicine as well as local modes of healing. As other therapeutic choices are pursued, we become aware of varying modes of understanding and treating the body. Alternative modes of explanation, in which the predictability of science and physics are diminished, may be sustained in addition to what is provided through the course of biomedical therapies. For this reason, the Senufo of Cote d'Ivoire speak of *yaama*, or varying states of sickness along with varying causes for disease. "In a well-known process, one and the same biomedical syndrome can be distributed over different *yaama*, and different symptoms can be assembled into a single nosological entity" (Sindzingre and Zempleni 1992, 317). A common cough may be seen as the result of transgression, the unkind work of a guardian spirit, or as the result of a cold wind. As in other regions of the world, alternatives in health care are often indicative of other reasons for the disease and physical suffering. It has also been noted, regarding northern India, that "whereas a CT scan or pulse reading can tell patients how an affliction occurred, a ritual specialist can tell them why it occurred and why it afflicted someone (and not someone else) at a particular moment in his or her life" (Barrett 2008, 120). This reality is recognized in the resilience of diverse therapeutic options, as illustrated later in this book in the pursuit of treatment for a child with epilepsy in Ghana. The therapy continuum recognizes the legitimacy of biomedicine, but it also sets in motion uses of multiple forms of local healing, and often in the same moment.

As the chapters in this book demonstrate, societies across Africa rely on generalists and specialists. Herbalists, for example, may provide advice for many common health concerns involving both internal medicine and topical problems. An array of other specialists may attend to broken bones, joint pains, fevers, childbirth complications, and an array of complex problems. As numerous scholars have shown, diverse forms of treatment may be viewed as complementary or competitive. For example, in one study from the 1970s, Lusaka notes that nearly 90 percent of *ng'anga* spiritualist healers were consulted due to the failure of Western medicines and hospital care to effectively treat the patient's illness (Frankenberg and Leeson 1976, 253). Generally, pragmatism (cost, transport, travel distance from home to clinic), social relations, explanatory models, and perceptions of efficacy are among the factors that influence selection of particular practitioners along the therapeutic continuum available. These issues are addressed in the chapter by Schoepf.

The pursuit of health and well-being is a process with extremely personal and interpersonal implications. How and why people can and do make healthcare choices may have broad social consequences and reveal critical social relations (Janzen 1978) that shape strategies for healing, whether biomedical or other modalities. These social connections include family and broader kin management groups, as well as relations among healers and patients; they may engage in decision-making regarding treatment initiatives, the collective management of medications, pain, and the recognition of suffering, illness, and death. The therapeutic continuum is well illustrated in the treatment of HIV/AIDS in Zanzibar, where healers "differentiate between HIV/AIDS that is 'caused by God' (*ukimwi ya mungu*)—also explained as an 'ordinary HIV infection' (*ukimwi ya kawaida*) communicated via sexual transmission (*njia ya zinaa*)—and HIV/AIDS that is not caused by a virus but by the 'environment' (*ukimwi ya mazingira*) and thus related to witchcraft (*mambo ya kichawi*). The latter is said to be treatable only by healers, as they are able to manipulate 'the devil' who has bewitched the ailing person" (Meier zu Biesen, Dilger, and Nienstedt 2012, 11).

This book presents ethnographic and theoretical foundations of an African therapeutic continuum, or the reality which provides individuals and groups with alternative and legitimate healthcare options for making sense of and treating suffering. Medical systems, as outlined by Kleinman (1980), involve ways of thinking about health care. This involves modes of perceiving sickness, including any ideas of causation and the expected modes for alleviating its effects. African medical systems represent a patterned yet flexible organization of individuals around the reality of sickness and human suffering due to disease. One key feature of African medical systems is their foundation upon intersubjective relations, or the relations among individuals when matters of health are central to human conduct. Intersubjective responses generate "constructive, destructive, and reconstructive interaction" (Jackson 1998, 8). Relations are dynamic due to the fluid conditions of disease and the pursuit of therapy, which often changes its venue and its conceptual framework. Medical intersubjective relations are found in the encounters of healers, patients, hospital and clinical staff, health escort groups, family, and medical and health policy personnel. Patients are reconstituted as persons according to the realities of their sickness, decisions of their escorts, diagnoses of doctors, and treatment of other healers. Moreover, since being (existence) in Africa "is never limited to human being, the field of inter-subjectivity includes persons, ancestors, spirits, collective representations, and material things" (9). In other words, the quality of a moral being in much of Africa might invoke "relations between people and ancestors, people and Allah, people and bush spirits, people and totemic animals, and so on" (Jackson 1989, 106). In various settings, individuals may relate to these entities with the same validity as relating to a kinsmen such as grandfather or cousin. This means that the realities of African medical systems commonly involve beings who assume some human attributes but who are otherwise mystical and (mostly) unseen in all other regards. This point is made by Grace Harris (1978, 28) for the Taita of Kenya:

> In the world as understood and lived in by Taita, the human self, the community and the physical environment were inter-connected parts of a universe both "natural" and permeated by values and feelings. In many respects, the human self functioned as a model for the understanding of society and the non-social environment. But the human person was seen in the light of his social development and relationships and as having necessary bonds with the nonhuman world. Qualities recognized in humans were read into the world at large; but qualities of the world were also read into human persons.

African medical systems may involve human use of turbulent mystical forces such as sent sickness via witchcraft. Resolutions to such unwanted problems often reveal the very fabric of plural resources. Intersubjective relations of African medical system thus sustain a dynamic sense of self and its relationship to others in therapy management groups (TMGs), which "implicates ever-shifting pluralities and combinations of persons" (Jackson 1998, 10). Chapters in this volume sustain this approach to intersubjective relations as individuals experience disease in changing models of therapeutic choice.

In Africa, biomedicine has been present for decades. Notwithstanding its unequal access, the impact of colonial and postcolonial health policy has forged a lasting impact on livelihood and on populations. Generations of Africans have experienced a proliferation of hospitals, clinics, biomedical practitioners, drugs, community health programs. These factors facilitated colonialism, and they have been regarded as symbols of modernity. Human anatomy as a scientific truth is taught in elementary schools, and concepts of the body as a biological organism are well understood. Biomedical models of health and medicine are widely known to be practically useful, and they are verified in experience. Public and private hospitals are used by increasingly large numbers of sick in urban and rural populations. The culture of medical science is enduring and pervasive. Nevertheless, many Africans also make use of herbal medicines, local forms of health care, healers, midwives, religious specialists, and men and women of therapeutic renown, even though these may not be recognized by their Western counterparts. Research has demonstrated the reality of medical pluralism in sub-Saharan Africa. It shows that medical decisions there are not an either/or process. Local remedies were not abandoned due to the introduction of biomedicine or any other regional or international health scheme. Pluralism is a reality in medical places even when the premise of legitimacy recognizes the impact and efficacy of biomedicine. Lock and Nguyen (2010, 63) have made this argument while speaking of the vast efficacy of biomedicine.

> Nowhere is biomedicine received into an environment devoid of ideas about illness causation and knowledge and practices relating to the body, and even when exposed to scientific knowledge people do not necessarily relinquish indigenous theories of disease causation, nor do they cease to use local "idioms of distress" to express their physical discomfort.

Pluralism is increasing throughout Africa as new therapies are created both by individuals with commercial interests and by those proposing alternative practices for old problems. For example, a growing trend in West African pharmaceuticals is an expanding market for longstanding herbal remedies that are now packaged or bottled and labeled in attempts to increase legitimacy in the products. Also notable are alternative applications of differing medical paradigms as patients and their constituencies manage therapy for the treatment of a core set of symptoms. African medical systems have become interesting test cases for the capturing of local cultural knowledge of the human body which may also be amenable to the onslaught of health products within Western capitalism.

Therapy Management Groups

One important feature of health care systems illustrated by medical anthropology is the role of the patient. The patient's own identity and personhood may be diminished during an illness episode. The transition is critical since the patient also enters into other relations by virtue of sickness. With the medical practitioner, such as a doctor or a diviner, the patient encounters a recognized source of final authority. Society legitimizes the distinction of this practitioner in such a way as to make his or her medical assessment carry the weight of authoritative determination. Judges and university professors maintain a similar mantle of conclusiveness. Other opinions may be sought, but only those given by individuals who carry a similar social position carry the same weight. In addition, a patient may submit to resolutions and paths of therapy laid down by family, friends, or other medical care professionals. Such an entourage has been identified as a therapy management group (Janzen 1978); this group is found in nearly all illness settings in sub-Saharan Africa. In the Democratic Republic of the Congo (DRC), the site of Janzen's classic study, this entourage is primarily kin, and they both facilitate a "selection of therapy" and act as an intermediary between the patient and the medical specialist.

This specialist may be a doctor; or it may be a local practitioner (Janzen 1978, 4). There is little doubt in the literature that medical care options and courses of therapy used by members of a therapy management group have been strongly influenced by the renown and effectiveness of a diviner and herbalist or a Malam or a Christian pastor. Power to heal and effectiveness of medications become part of the repertoire. Diviners become men and women of renown as word spreads of their abilities to treat various disease symptoms. Renown also affects the popularity of hospitals and clinics. For example, Sargent notes the strong influence of medical care choices made by patients because of the reputation of the care provided by a hospital in northern Benin. She suggests that pragmatic observations of biomedical benefits have contributed to the public perception of hospital efficacy. "Even a small number of cases where complications of labor were successfully resolved affects public impressions of the utility of seeking treatment at the hospital" (Sargent 1989, 51). Conversely, a series of hospital deaths may greatly damage institutional reputation.

It is also noteworthy that great successes in one sphere of medicine are not necessarily predictors of future therapeutic choices. In Africa, a course of treatment is greatly influenced by the patient's therapy entourage. As Prins says, regarding his work in Zambia, "It was immediately apparent that the afflicted individual did not make these decisions alone. He or she was supported by a group of kin, of peers and of specialists who at different moments during the illness, took over responsibility for a switch in the quest for therapy" (Prins 1989, 164).

Depending on medical options at hand, the direction of therapy may lead the patient automatically toward the clinic or hospital. Many populations in urban areas of Africa have this option. This point is made in Olsen's essay in this book, which explores a path of therapy taken over one year for patients suffering from stroke in the Asante region of Ghana. The hospital or clinic is nearly always the default first option for Asante. As symptoms progress, other kinds of therapy may be endorsed. The option of a hospital is sometimes subject to the local political situation, including structural adjustment programs, as noted by Turshen (1999) and by Schoepf in this volume. Some countries remain under restrictive measures.

Sudden or grave illnesses sometimes befall a patient. When that occurs, often TMGs assume that a human or mystical agent sent the sickness and caused the disease. Under those conditions, generally doctors may treat the symptoms to at least some degree. However, if the health of the patient is not completely restored, a further diagnosis must be given by an authority such as a diviner. Yet the default for most medical care choices is likely the hospital, the doctor's office, or self-medication through Western pharmaceuticals. Distance, travel, economy and demographics also impact healthcare choices. Herbal remedies are also often used as a first resort for treating stomach and abdominal pains, headache, skin irritations, joint and arthritic problems, and some matters of internal medicine such as malaria.

The influence of the TMG in African medical pluralism is given generous coverage in the seminal work of John Janzen (1978). He claims that in the lower DRC, therapeutic decisions are the responsibility of kinsmen of the patient. This group brokers a relationship between patient and medical specialist. The group observes the severity of symptoms, the estimated need for any hospital care, and the time of recovery, as well as a host of problems which may be apparent within the extended realm of kinship. Once a cause is determined, efforts to resolve social tensions that may have brought about the symptoms in the patient are pursued within ritual and often through mystical healing. Disagreement and challenges to authority within kin organizations may lead to schisms in the TMG, and BaKongo TMGs may involve yet deeper historic and social matters. These "court" questions correspond to the complexity of enquiries regarding the health of a person or a group. In such cases, resolution of a course of therapy happens after a litigation process that clears from responsibility or indicts certain lineage members for causing or contributing to illness symptoms. Decision-making in BaKongo illness ultimately centers on the choice between "diseases of God" and "diseases of man" although the process may be adjusted even after a medical or ritual specialist "has made his diagnosis and recommended action" (Janzen 1978, 130). Resolutions for therapy follow a familiar path. They may begin in the hospital or in the village. Decisions are made according to the course of action regarded as most effective:

> The local microcosm of social relations in this health quest extends from the village arena and its social fields of kinship, economic relations, and indigenous health practices to the realm of the state, and the field of health care provided at the district hospital level. (Hunter 2001, 166)

This process and frame of reference for disease causation has implications for nearly all other work on African medical pluralism. For example, the essay by Olsen describes therapy management in Asante, which inclines strongly toward biomedicine for all ailments except mental illness and epilepsy. Similarly, Rasmussen's essay focuses on Tuareg infertility and childlessness and the courses of action pursued over the long term, which involve local healers, clinics, and urban hospitals in Niger and Mali. Mulemi shows how the TMG emerges within the hospital organization. Patients use failure of treatments as a rationale for pursuing suggestions for alternative therapies by medical care staff who are hospital employees. Cancer patients participate in "healer shopping" as they seek to learn of alternative medicines for treating various forms of cancer.

Hospital Ethnography

How do patients orient themselves to options Western medicine provides? Do African populations utilize biomedicine as often as they use local therapies? Is medical science a consistent option for health care? Contributions to hospital ethnography made by anthropologists illustrate the complexities of plural medical systems, as seen in several chapters in this volume. Hospitals may be regarded as extensions of the West and of modern science. As such, instances of medical pluralism "tend to reflect hierarchical relations in the larger society" (Baer, Singer, and Susser 2013, 11) such as gender, ethnicity, class, and professional expertise. Germ theory, technology, drugs, and instruments are products of this model. It is also noted that variations in hospital policy and health applications point to the impact of culture, politics, and economics on the process. As argued by van der Geest and Finkler (2004, 1997):

> Even though biomedicine disperses globally it does not suggest that it is practiced homogeneously, or that hospitals function in a uniform manner. In fact, variations in biomedical practice are evident among technologically developed nations.

Studies in this volume provide illustrations of variation in policy, application, treatment, and critical variables such as the categorization of and etiologies of disease. Further, in this book, Mulemi uses a study of a cancer ward in Nairobi as a basis for claims that hospitals are not replicas of one another or of the biomedical model. Differences are mediated by social and cultural constraints. For example, the Nairobi cancer ward is itself a site of medical pluralism.

> Some patients used traditional and other therapies in the ward and at home, in between hospital treatment sessions. They drew on personal and indigenous perspectives on the aetiology of current suffering. A section of patients sough alternative medicine while in the hospital and after their discharge from the ward. (Mulemi 2010, 125)

In his important book on hospital and alternative therapies in Zanzibar, Tapio Nisula provides a useful starting point for understanding pluralistic medical care in contemporary tropical Africa. Speaking in general, the issues under consideration are closely aligned to the popularity of biomedical options and treatment as these are associated with local understanding of disease and illness. This process sustains an enthusiastic use of medical technologies, instruments, and pharmaceuticals as promoted by doctors of orthodox medicines; and it also acknowledges heterodox therapies that ascribe to diseases meanings that are understood within healthcare settings identified by local medical specialists. In Zanzibar Town, medical culture includes a host of therapy alternatives which may rival, be unequal to, be contrasting, or pose parallel or complementary options. Such options introduce medical pluralism, which enables patients and their escort(s) access to medical modalities in which one system is not necessarily dominant or privileged over any other system. It is also the case that such options have a long history of general acceptance as reliable and effective (Nisula 1999, 199). Nisula reviews the historic basis for medical options in Zanzibar Town and in Dar es Salaam, places experiencing expanding use of locally produced pharmaceuticals, as well as the creation of a medical campus, hospitals, and public health programs, some of which date back to missionary endeavors from the last quarter of the nineteenth century. Among the main conditions treated are malaria, snake bite, pneumonia, anemia, bronchitis, intestinal parasites, broken bones, and dysentery.

Nisula's study demonstrates the breakdown of the authority of biomedicine and hospitals. When hospital medicine comes to be seen as ineffective, biomedicine in general loses its perceived power to treat certain symptoms. Patients may perceive as more likely a scenario involving malevolent spirits that cause disease. As Nisula observes, "there are many afflictions in Zanzibar Town which are not even considered to be diagnosed and cured by means of biomedical treatment, such as those induced by spirits" (1999, 274). This decline in the perceived legitimacy of biomedicine corresponded also with a dramatic rise in self-medication using Western pharmaceuticals.

Alternative procedures that address disease by mystical means also exist in Zanzibar Town. These are not part of nor recognized as legitimate by orthodox medicine. Nevertheless, people in Zanzibar Town do not regard traditional healers to be outside orthodox medicine. Local healers known as *waganga* address an elaborate spirit-possession complex in which invading spirits cause symptoms. *Waganga* identify themselves as Muslims, yet they seek the unorthodox path of healing spirit possession in order to resolve their clients' medical problems. Spirit possession "is Islamized" (Nisula 1999, 99). This means the usual heresy associated with recognizing lesser deities is removed or ignored. Healers and patients also "work in a complementary relationship to biomedical institutions, while accepting the power of biomedical facts, and the afflicted Zanzibaris exploit various options in order to find answers to their conditions" (99).

According to Nisula, a majority of participants in spirit-possession cases are adult women, whose symptoms addressed in possession performances—

depression, sleeplessness, nausea, and problems with sexuality—are commonly perceived to be in the domain of women. Possession may be regarded as somewhat marginal to the experience of women; thus, men "fall back on other sources of therapies." The complex itself is activated around medicine that is widely regarded as "curative and preventive practices" and that provides a "significant conceptual framework for interpretation concerning the well-being of islanders" (159). Possession is seen as the cause of illness, but only after hospital medicines and treatments have become regarded as a failure.

Contexts of illnesses in Zanzibar Town and personal and social meanings given to symptoms are not discussed in depth by Nisula. It is possible that they might resemble those given for certain women in urban Sudan who blame spirits for such crises as lacking a suitable spouse, an unsatisfactory marriage, infertility, or lack of contentment with family and female roles (Constantinides 1985). A common gloss given to "women's medicine" in these parts of Africa is that the possession rites are a means of "coping with life within the existing social parameters of a highly Muslim society" (Lewis 1991, 5). Hospitals and Western doctors in Zanzibar Town are currently regarded as "complementary, not as contradictory or mutually exclusive separate systems, but as a practical framework" (Nisula 1999, 289).

This scenario plays out in other African populations. And diviners who have been afflicted with forms of diseases that they treat are more widely seen as credible, in contrast to hospital practitioners who have not experienced such diseases (Moerman 2002, 43). Elsewhere, hospitals have become emblems of elitism due to imposed fees of SAPs. Patients in Harare hospitals now supply their own drugs, food, and basic supplies (Simmons 2012, 170; Schoepf in this volume). In such locations, traditional healers often have expanded their practices in an attempt to fulfill medical demand. And language itself becomes a form of elitist communication in many African hospitals. Local languages and dialects may present barriers between doctor and patient or doctor and therapy management group. Medical explanations are often given in the lingua franca of the country. This point is made in a recent study of an oncology ward in Gaborone (Livingston 2012, 71).

> Where translation across languages is also an issue, as it often is in Botswana, matters are further complicated, as some objects and processes expressed and understood in English simply cannot be rendered in Setswana. Biomedicine has become the therapeutic system of global health programs—its practices rely on purportedly universal bodies, technologies, and things.

Several essays in this volume illustrate how culture produces variations in hospital practices. The chapter by Sargent and Kennell shows how in northern Benin a hospital's healing practice is dominated by specific features of biomedicine, such as psychiatry. However, at nighttime the hospital is transformed into an arena for traditional medicine, as families of patients escort in diviners and other ritual specialists whose work complements the work of the doctors. Wendland's chapter describes the authority and legitimacy of decision-making in a Malawian hospital. Obstetrical and gynecological procedures regarding birthing and pregnancy made "inside the hospital" are institutionalized and state-certified. However, the same people making decisions "outside the hospital" base their decisions upon dreams, visions, and purchased therapeutic secrets. Mulemi shows us that not all forms of cancer receive equal and adequate attention within an oncology ward in a Nairobi hospital. As a result, patients move between hospital and clinic and other kinds of healing in order to expand their healthcare options. Trovalla's extended case study in Jos, Nigeria, tells of a patient whose pursuit of health resulted in multiple engagements with hospitals and clinics as well as Muslim healers. As Schoepf notes in her essay, the diffusion of biomedicine in the world hardly means equal access to doctors, medical care, and drugs.

In almost no other African medical setting is social differentiation more manifest than in circumstances involving AIDS and HIV. Prevention campaigns are often aimed largely toward women since they are least likely to be able to control the behaviors of their partners, as Chikombero has shown for Zimbabwe (2007). Elsewhere, scholars have written of the deep social stigma that surrounds dying patients. South African AIDS patients are objects of "ostracism and abandonment" as well as "feelings of discomfort in the presence of the terminally ill" (Ashforth 2010, 54). AIDS-positive status becomes a reason for migrating for work in other parts of a country, as Smith shows for Nigeria (2014) or for shame as Dapaa shows in two Ghanaian hospitals (2012). The Asante identify such dangerous diseases as *owuo yaree*, or "sickness of death." In such cases, the stigma of the disease necessitates sequestration of the patient by the family. This may involve a hospital. Pharmaceuticals are often used to treat the pain and some symptoms, and herbal remedies are often pursued as a matter of belief in the powers of remedies made from forest plants. Other kinds of sequestered diseases are known as *ɛtwa yaree*, or "disgraced diseases." Examples of such afflictions in Akan include epilepsy (Obeng 2007).

Writers who explore ethnography within the hospital bring particular focus on inequalities in the rankings of medical institutional systems. Status differences express inequalities in power relations—doctor or nurse to patient is only one example. More common in African hospitals are inequalities deriving from gender or ethnic identity. Ethnic differences and animosities and structures of gender inequality are established within wider settings of biomedicine and of science. Differences between biomedical procedures and alternative medical practices are also infused with assumptions regarding rationality and non-rational action. These distinctions presume a hierarchy of inequality. Such conditions of unequal human identity have been poignantly noted by Street in her recent remarkable description of Madang Hospital in Papua New Guinea. Doctors, she claims, know of associations between medical science and the hierarchies of Western culture. Moreover, (Street 2014, 155–156) doctors

> See the world of global science as a space of gross inequality where some kinds of medicine are more closely aligned with truth and rationality than others, and where those superior truths always belong to European doctors. Today, those inequalities are made visible in the very different opportunities and values accorded the work of national doctors and the work of foreign medical scientists in the hospital.

Hospitals are, above all, locations where people seek resolutions to problems and where they hope to improve their physical well-being. All over the world, hospital treatment brings together individual preference, therapeutic pluralism, and scientific endeavor. In ethnographies where a plurality of human interchange takes place within the hospital, it is important to comprehend both status relations of gender and ethnicity, and it is also important to understand "assumptions that govern the scientific method" (Martin 2012, 33) and the moral high ground of rationality as they are associated with therapeutic practice in the hospital. "Such a project extends the focus in science and technology studies on how scientific facts or technological assemblages travel to and become stabilized in different places in order to explore the historically specific relationships between multiple ontologies that constitute postcolonial places of science and medicine" (Street 2014, 19).

Observation and Empiricism

How effective and how empirically tested are traditional medicines? Can African medical systems be analyzed as open systems involving empirical evidence of their reliability? Prospective patients in such systems are not unaware of theory and paradigms that are inconsistent with their own views, but they may nonetheless accept a mode of explanation which closely resembles what is inherited from ancestors and deities, especially when biomedicine fails or illness is chronic. In this perspective, disease may be attributed to upheaval in one's personal social life. In such cases, "disease and misfortune are the punishment" for the avarice and ill will of spirits and malevolent human beings (Horton 1967, 55). Horton's argument heavily cites the work on Azande by Evans-Pritchard, especially when Azande appear to be unable to "reason outside, or against their beliefs because they have no other idiom in which to express their thoughts" (Evans-Pritchard 1937, 338). By contrast, open, or modern, systems are largely found in Europe; and they are identified by "awareness of alternatives, diminished sacredness of beliefs, and diminished anxiety about threats to them" (Horton 1967, 156). Horton labels Azande beliefs about disease "non-empirical," while theories influenced strongly by science are deemed "empirical." (58) The latter is regarded by Horton as the most "efficient tool for arriving at beliefs that are successful" in treating disease.

Horton's terminologies and their logic have received adequate criticism. Feierman argues that even as science and biomedicine prevail in much of the modern world, alternative modes of therapy are often regarded as legitimate, though they may not be acknowledged within the biomedical model. This structure challenges what Horton identifies as open. Feierman (1985) also notes the multilayered realities found in African medical systems, an aspect ignored by Horton's 1967 article. Horton mentions only the logic of traditional healers such as herbalists and diviners. The structure is static and one-dimensional. It is based solely on the concept of rationality and empirical choice. Yet other factors often enter into medical decision-making. Rational choice is only one variable. Indeed, as noted for Andean systems, "the choice of one or more forms of healing within broadly pluralistic health systems reflects not degrees of rationality, but degrees of negotiation among myriad social forces" (Miles and Leatherman 2003, 9). These authors argue that pluralism has increased in the Andes as new procedures are introduced. Other forces may involve such matters as proximity, affordability, empirical failure of therapy, renown of healer, or efficacy of treatment. African plural health systems involve all of these, and examples illustrate the point of efficacy and of empiricism. Janzen's essay on the DRC challenges the duality of science versus divination as he speaks of the widespread presence of healers and patients who have advanced technical and scientific training and who are also adamant regarding the reality of nature spirits and sorcery and their ability to cause disease. Nor do Africans simply default in favor of spiritual kinds of choices in healthcare decision-making, as Horton appears to contend (Horton 1967, 53).

> If a diviner diagnoses the action of witchcraft influence or lethal medicine spirits, it is usual for him to add something about the human hatreds, jealousies, and misdeeds that have brought such agencies into play. Or, if he diagnoses the wrath of an ancestor, it is usual for him to point to the human breach of kinship morality which has called down this wrath.

In much of Africa, mystical, disease-causing agents are assumed to be real. For the Bariba of northern Benin, sickness is often thought to be "caused by malevolent agents, either human or nonhuman, who bring their power to provoke affliction to bear against the strength of the victim" (Sargent 1982, 33). Yet elsewhere this is only a portion of the story. Sakata healers in the DRC address "underlying causes of an ailment" in those instances when "biomedicine sometimes does not work." At such times, healers maintain a robust business as they apply "secret knowledge" within a society where the human body is always "lacking something" (Bekaert 2000, 281–282). For the Zulu, disease is a "natural" fact, one which is grounded in key concepts of germ theory. Conditions such as headache, hay fever, diarrhea, epilepsy, chest pains, asthma and bronchitis, skin irritations, and even madness are said to run in families, with some biological strains associated with certain lineage groups. As such, these diseases are not believed to result from malicious actions. They occur within nature; "they just happen" (Ngubane 1977, 23). Naturally occurring symptoms exist in the same community as other forms of disease that are the result of "sent" sickness, and "which Western doctors could not possibly understand" (35).

In the horn of Africa, a layered system of medical pluralism is the result of international contact over centuries. The arrangement includes local Cushitic, Oromo, and Somali remedies using plants and setting fractures, a regional mode of Arabic and Amhara components, and the cosmopolitan medical model recently imposed by the central government and by European influences (Slikkerveer 1990, 167). Therapeutic pluralism in Africa's horn is composed of local herbal healers and diviners, regional teachers and religious-medical men of learned training, Islamic healing texts, *zar*-doctors, and various levels of Western medical practices introduced by Italian and then Soviet and Cuban specialists. Components of the system are accessed according to a range of social criteria: age, gender, ethnicity, religion, vocation, class and income, education, and marital status.

The Ethiopian situation resembles that in Namibia, where healthcare choices are organized in an indisputable hierarchy. An excellent source for understanding this hierarchy is provided in the quantitative data given for Wambo and Herero populations living in Katutura, a township outside of Windhoek. These data show that 152 of the author's respondents, or 58 percent, preferred biomedicine in most cases. Only 7.6 percent opted for traditional healers as a first resort. LeBeau claims there is a decision-making hierarchy regarding health care: people self-medicate in most cases for persistent cough, recurring fever, headache, and diarrhea. Herero see a diviner for impotency, infertility, and mental problems. Medical doctors are consulted most often for sexually transmitted diseases, tuberculosis, malaria, AIDS, liver disease, and high blood pressure. The overall hierarchy of medical choice is outlined in the author's statement:

> People make clear distinctions between what types of health care they would seek based on the type of illness presented to them. Traditional healers and their patients support the contention that for most universally recognized illness symptoms patients first go to Western health care, unless the illness has a social-spiritual case, or Western medicine has been unsuccessful in treating their illness. (LeBeau 2003, 81)

The process of therapy is laid out by a Herero patient who has a lengthy history with pathologies treated by both kinds of healers.

I usually only go to a healer when the illness is not clear to the Western doctor or when it is other things like madness, craziness, or bad luck. For a Western doctor you go for any pain, flus, and sicknesses that are clear. You go to traditional healers for any . . . complicated illnesses which are not clear for the Western doctor. (81)

Elsewhere in Africa, options for alternative treatments depend on the perceived original cause of the symptoms. The Tabwa of the DRC have an elaborate classification of diseases based on the circumstances of "the illness situation," or its first occurrence; they closely monitor all physiological manifestations that tend to alter the primary symptoms. "Therapy of an illness such as *kibende* makes clear that the cause of the diarrhea is being treated as such. The diarrhea itself is only a symptom which will stop spontaneously" once the root caused is addressed (Davis 2000, 77). Tabwa pluralism arises when a patient shows "unresponsiveness" to certain medicines. New diagnoses take into account socio-historic circumstances of patients and their kin, rather than physiological manifestations of the body. Symptoms of disease are viewed as a manifestation of one kind of misfortunes (93). These include accidents, social discord, and failure in hunting. Curing the disease provides empirical evidence that the real cause of the disease has been recognized either through a clinic or by way of divination. Sargent shows that in northern Benin, choice of birth attendant therapy and practice is also altered by shared expectations as birthing mothers affiliate with those Bariba attendants whose understandings of birth as fraught with mystical risk most closely resemble their own (Sargent 1982). In both Namibia and the DRC, observation yield empirical evidence for modifying the forms of treatment received. Both examples show how African medical options are open to empirical scrutiny and to cultural interpretation. The pursuit of empirical remedies is modeled by Taylor, who argues that people in Rwanda are concerned first with relief from immediate symptoms and that only later will people try to ascertain what may be a plurality of reasons for the disease. Examples also demonstrate that science does not erase other kinds of therapeutic attention. Presence of biomedicine hardly ever results in the eradication of all other kinds of medical care. Rather, as noted for Lambok, "there is complementarity between the two sets of diagnoses and treatments. Neither impinges on the other" (Hunter 2001, 164).

Tola Pearce also makes a convincing argument for the empirical reality of truths found within Yoruba medicine. She claims that "each type of knowledge develops within a different value milieu and in pursuit of different goals" (Pearce 1986, 244). Biomedical goals are factual because they confirm the values of a scientific reality. Likewise, adequate empirical proof exists within Yoruba healing practices to demonstrate the empirical reality of ritual medical rites. This is due to the subjective nature of illness, which is part of the reality of disease as much as any objective aspects do. Beyond such subjective wisdom, African healers also possess objective forms of treatment that demonstrate objective qualities of trial and error. These include massage, bonesetting, birthing assistance, and herbal remedies. This argument is likewise taken up in the essay by Koen Stroeken, who contends that non-Western medical treatments are nevertheless empirical based on the feedback provided by family members regarding the effectiveness of any specific mode of treatment. Moreover, Elisha Renne's essay shows how, in diagnosing and treating childhood ear infections and other problems in Zaria, Nigeria employs pluralism due to circumstances of malnutrition and poverty. Janzen's essay shows how an abundance of medical specialists in the DRC and access to effective pharmaceuticals are regarded with empirically tested reliance as effective.

The effectiveness of herbs to treat diseases has been tested by several authors. A. Sofowora is a professor of pharmacology in Nigeria. He details the extensive value of African herbs as legitimate modes of treatment for a wide host of diseases (1993). Yet within some moral frameworks, these are considered insufficient treatment for certain medical cases. The rationality of this moral framework engages some BaKongo to question the presence or absence of disease in America where medicines and drugs abound. In the chapter by Olsen, a stroke patient receives abundant care in various hospitals in Kumasi. It is only one year later, as symptoms reappear, that healing by divination and herbalists is sought out by the patient and his family. Pluralism in Asante accommodates active variations in medical therapy as empirical observations alter perceptions of the cause of disease. As Prins notes for Zambia, there was "extensive evidence of empirical experimentation within herbal remedies among African healers" (Prins 1989, 174). Trovalla's chapter shows that therapeutic decision-making in Jos, Nigeria, resembles a process she considers explorative and experimental rather than calculated and certain. The static features of Horton's structure yield to the dynamics of historical change. The African therapeutic continuum is not so bounded in practice or in knowledge.

Comprehending how medical pluralism evolves within a community holds a particular value for researchers in global health. Nichter argues that the way a population assumes a particular disease is acquired will correlate with how they may respond to public health interventions. That is because local modes of healing "often interact with biomedical explanatory models, producing hybrid ideas" (Nichter 2008, 44). What results often are representations of biomedical practices created within culturally salient models of disease? Working with and altering perceptions of illness causality may increase changes in illness behaviors; and this in turn may increase the likelihood of successful health intervention. A similar premise was proposed by Good (1977), who argued that the course of treatment of disease is framed by social factors such as a "semantic illness network" that includes ways of comprehending the disease and resources for responding to the problem. The immediate value of this perspective is revealed by Iliffe's history of AIDS in Africa. He claims that late-twentieth-century public health interventions were ineffective in the continent because "medical thinking underlying international policies often conflicted with the ways in which most Africans perceived the crisis" (Iliffe 2006, 80). In contrast, Thornton shows how health programs can learn from this short-sighted perspective, as they have in the treatment of AIDS in Uganda. Thornton claims that AIDS projects have been effective in Uganda because they took sex networks to be social structures, unseen and "unimagined." Anti-AIDS projects in Kampala addressed this reality. People were advised to tether their herd, graze your animals close to home, and likewise constrain sexual activity only in domestic territory. By contrast, South African AIDS projects have been less effective because their vision did not integrate cultural premises of disease causation (Thornton 2008).

It is worth considering how health education efforts might be tailored to fit popular health culture in such a way as to facilitate better medical care (Nichter 1989, 141–142). In other words, how a community experiences the meaning of a disease and its risks will "influence how individuals within that population respond to public health interventions and courses of action they choose to adopt or ignore" (Nichter 2008, 50). Studies of plural health practices of a community serve to expand the effectiveness of global health projects. Moreover, knowledge of plural health and pharmaceutical options have also reshaped new forms of "sociality, governance, and citizenship" (Langwick, Dilger, and Kane 2012, 7) across political borders and within populations of specific nations. As anthropology accounts for shifting political and scientific frames of reference, the realities of plural medical systems are understood best as responding to the changing landscapes of nation states, para-states, and emerging nonstate collectives. Healthcare options and alternatives are themselves, in part, products of such political and scientific agendas. As recently noted, "public health science today is situated and implicated by the inherent, growing contradictions of the global political economy . . . but not coextensive within it" (Geissler 2015, 21). These networks also assume forms and relations based more on local interpersonal arrangements. Data on African medical pluralism in this volume may also serve to highlight how medical interventions and options evolve within broader contingencies of international contact, micropolitical arenas, and global assimilation (Prince and Marsland 2014).

Diseased Body and Its Meanings

Can human diseases be explained and treated by nature, society, or the mystical world? Can the human body be regarded as cultural and also biological? When

Geertz stated that "there is no such thing as a human nature independent of culture," he understood the cultural meanings given to things, events, and processes. Medical anthropology includes the human body within this meaningful design. Comparative studies of the body and disease differentiate anthropology from biomedicine, which claims that they are largely separate from society and culture. Biomedicine claims that disease is pathological, observable, and rooted within the individual body. Post-Enlightenment reasoning asserts that medical proof of disease is based upon universal and scientific laws.

Csordas argues against this framework of body as biological fixture. Recent social research, he notes, supports his assertion of the human body as an icon of movement, evolution, and passage. Because the body is used to symbolize transition, decay, frailty, as well as generative powers, the body "is transformed from object to agent" (Csordas 1994, 3). The instrumentality of the body becomes almost limitless. The body becomes "the original substance out of which the human world is shaped" (6). Medical anthropologists have long since held the premise that the "efforts to allay the debilitating effects of social disorder tend to involve exertions to treat and repair the physical body, and vice versa; the body social and the body personal always exist in a mutually constitutive relationship" (Comaroff 1985, 8). Byron Good keenly illustrates how the body and disease may be given one meaning by a patient and another meaning by the professional medical staff. The patient, a Jehovah's Witness, was in need of a transfusion due to rectal bleeding. The transfusion process was routine, necessary, and medically expedient to the doctors. For the patient, blood from another person is dangerous, "filthy," and polluting. "I would lose my life," claimed the patient, by undergoing the transfusion. The patient's meaning of body diverged from those of the doctor. In this case, doctors and patient maintained contradictory positions. Oppositional meanings were derived from the same parts of the body.

Devisch provides a striking description of the body as cultural product for the Yaka of the DRC. Yaka claim that a person's body is similar to a weave of thread in which relations with kin, marriage partners, and close non-kin resemble a woven cloth. Illness and misfortune disrupt that fabric. "They close up the body in a maze of contrarieties, or they disconnect or unthread the weave" (Devisch 1993, 132). Illness separates the person from the group and sometimes from nature or from mystical resources. Healing performances seek to gather and redeem those severed associations once again into a cohesive woven frame. Divination aims to connect "the living and their world with the original fertility of a primordial couple" (180) and with ancestors.

Meaning is given to the body and to its component features. As Good argues, "symptoms are given meaning within a cultural system relationally, by the position they occupy within complex symbolic codes" (Good 1994, 99). Good also argues that the body, as well as disease, occurs not just in a biological reality. They also are realities taking place in time, in place, in history, in the social world, in nature, and often within a particular mystical setting (133). These contexts provide other associations to the body and to disease that extend beyond the biomedical model. Because the body is a culturally active entity, sickness and frailties may provide a plurality of options for understanding the causes of disease, as well as a plurality of choices for appropriate medical therapy. Several essays in this volume support Good's argument about coded associations between body and symptoms. We also concur with Csordas that the reality of embodiment is a "valuable starting point for rethinking the nature of culture and our existential situation" as cultural beings (Csordas 1994, 6). Indeed, existential dilemmas often arise during disease episodes. For example, Asante have a view of the body largely consistent with biomedical reality. The Asante perception differs from that in China, where there is no term in classical Chinese that is synonymous with the English word *body* (Scheid 2002, 27). Likewise, in India, "situations and therapeutic trajectories" of medical science and local conceptions of health and disease are combined to produce "alternative ideologies of the body, the person, natural processes, and human agency" (Zimmerman 2014, 87). In Asante, theories of most diseases are consistent with the biomedical model. But nearly all diseases may be also reinterpreted as *sunsum yareɛ* (spiritual sickness), which is brought about by *ɔma yareɛ* (sent sickness), when normal biomedical procedures fail to bring about a cure or when the disease becomes untreatable according to biomedical procedures. At such times, the *sunsum* (spirit) of the sick becomes the suspected field of an assault from a witch or some other mystical cause. Existential questions probe a wider sphere of knowledge than germ theory and epidemiology for a cure to such problems. For Asantes, *sunsum* is strongly coded for matters of life, disease, and death.

Similar perspectives on the body are found in eastern and central Africa. Langwick's remarkable account claims that "not all bodies in southern Tanzania are bound by skin." Efforts to describe disease-related attacks by malevolent spirits remain outside the domain of biomedicine. Instead, traditional healers understand such diseases to be connected to social relations of neighbors and kinsmen. Thus, healing proceeds with medicinal baths, amulets, and medicines "drawn upon the skin." The patient's waist, ankles, wrists, and neck become bound. Healing through methods of binding is often successful. "Bodies are not essentially discrete objects; their separateness, solidity, and stability are created through the interventions of healers. In other words, bodily boundaries in southern Tanzania are created and maintained through medicine (Langwick 2011, 224). Similar arguments are advanced in Langwick's essay about Tanzania and Taylor's about Rwanda. Taylor's essay details personal stories of post-traumatic stress disorder (PTSD) following the Rwandan Hutu-on-Tutsi genocide.

He describes the emergence of patterned symptoms following trauma of violence and how these symptoms are meaningful only when considering the culture of the body in Hutu life.

In a well-known ethnographic study of Tabwa medicine, Davis asserts that "the body is not universal." Illness events break apart body integrity, exposing the body to forms of nature such as winds and insects. Sickness is evident since the healthy body, which is known to balance between hot and cold, is not out of balance. It no longer "hears" or "feels" medicines, and the body "swings from the extreme heat of high fever to the extreme cold of the circulatory failure that characterizes critical illness and, ultimately, death" (Davis 2000, 65). Davis gives a remarkable account of Tabwa perceptions of body parts most likely to be impacted by sickness. This account includes cases in which illness is explained not by generalizable disease theories but by causes specific to individual patients' personal situations. Tabwa theories follow a familiar logic of those treatable by European medicines, *dawa ya kizungu*, and those treated by traditional medicines, *dawa ya asili*. As in many parts of Africa, *dawa ya kizungu* does little to change the path of Tabwa diseases believed to have been brought about by sorcery. Such conditions are brought about by the "path of man," and they hide themselves from diagnoses within the hospital or by a doctor's testing or surgery. Doctors will be unable to discover a cause, and the symptoms will once again afflict the patient once he or she leaves the hospital. Both traditional Tabwa treatment and hospital medicines have become part of the therapeutic process. Efforts are carefully made to determine the correct course of treatment and decide on the right sources of medications. Decisions like these are the responsibility of a patient's therapy management group: spouse, siblings, parents, and extended matrilineal kin. Decisions to use the hospital are made with much care and reflection, since the trip to the hospital involves 27 hours by canoe across Lake Tanganyika. It also involves travel passes outside one's zone of residence, and it requires payment of daily room and board fee in the hospital. Patients must also supply their own bedding. Hospital care often involves mistreatment by medical staff and bribes in order to obtain adequate attention. Cases from Tanzania, the DRC, and other areas discussed in this volume demonstrate that traditional healing is better aligned with local perceptions of the body, including its physiology and anatomy. Such working models of anatomy are active on a daily basis, not just in times of illness or trauma. Many examples in this volume demonstrate the precept found in nearly all of Africa, which is that when disease is present, the whole person is ill. Perhaps others in the lineage are ill as well, and comprehensive treatment is needed to alleviate the problem. Therapies are sought on a plurality of legitimate and proven levels of health care. It is often argued that local medicines are effective more because of the continuity between healer and patient and the workings of the body, and less because of any perceived powers of medical placebo that may be activated in ritual settings (Moerman 2002; see Schoepf in this volume regarding health access).

Professionalization

Can medical diagnoses lead to treatment when there is no M.D.? Are African therapeutic systems considered legitimate in Africa today? Toward the last years of the 1930s, the government of the Gold Coast rescinded earlier series of executive orders that prohibited and criminalized witch-finding and healing through divination. For decades, practicing traditional medicine had been illegal. Grounds for prosecution, however, were never effective legally. Cases clogged the courts with individuals whose ambiguous circumstances usually required either acquittal or sentences so minimal that they were dismissed by sympathetic judges who had little time to bring such cases to trial. Instead, the British opted for political posturing, and they reversed their course of legal action just as hospitals and clinics were also becoming more accessible to the public. Licenses to practice medicine were soon granted to hundreds of diviners and other types of local healers. Healers who could pay the annual tax were legitimized by the state as health practitioners. With this bureaucratic adjustment, health practitioners changed from criminals to professionals. Professionalization of health care in Africa thus employed pluralistic modes of therapy. In such historical developments, we agree with Last, who argued for a "convergence of the scientific with the traditional: no longer can a facile contrast be made between primitive and scientific" (Last 1986, 8).

Langwick's essay provides an extraordinary glimpse into the professional lives of healers in Tanzania. Knowledge of specialty forms of healing encourages professional secrecy consistent with Western ideas of intellectual property. Professional medical applications involve elements from both Western biomedicine and more traditional practices. The essay by Trovalla demonstrates the medical applications made by a Hausa doctor, living in Jos, whose healing skills and knowledge gained greater precision as he developed increased harmony and awareness of patients' lives and living conditions.

We argue that this convergence is an ethnographic reality today in both medical knowledge and in practice. For example, one may find today in Ghana, Togo, Nigeria, and Cote d'Ivoire dozens of Islamic pharmaceutical shops known as "Amen Scientific Herbal Clinic." Different herbal remedies treat and cure afflictions such as infertility, stroke, hypertension, diabetes, impotence, and high blood pressure. Treatment is scientific because "when you first come in you are given a blood pressure and other tests with a doctor's gauge. You are also asked about your medical history." Prescription drugs are remedies because "it is through the grace of God that you are healed." On each bottle, one can read

"God is the Healer." This means that "God revealed the knowledge of the herbs and how to work them for healing." It may also be a practical necessity, given the limited number of medical doctors and the wider presence of local healers. Limited ratios of doctors, particularly in rural areas, increase reliance on traditional healers for treatment of HIV/AIDS in Tanzania and elsewhere (Kayombo, Uiso, and Mahunnah 2012).

Because medical modalities are perceived as legitimate within their sphere of prestige and acceptance, one mode of therapy need not exclude another. One mode may, indeed, serve to engage another mode. The engagement depends entirely upon the culture of healing at hand. Just as in the individual devotion to Christianity or Islam, attendance in formal religious worship in a chapel or mosque does not preclude visiting a diviner or Malam for personal problems and for therapeutic resolutions. Indeed, if one model for a medical remedy is good, then two are even better. Thus, Langwick demonstrates the value of healers' knowledge as medical intellectual property and shows how this information transforms how patients in southern Uganda approach modern medicines. Likewise, several authors describe a renaissance of traditional medicine in Africa, brought about by the ministries of health in order to coordinate local political and economic agendas.

We consider the spectrum of healing modalities so widely found across sub-Saharan Africa to be a continuum of therapy. Sub-Saharan Africa is a site where local and global social transformations over centuries have generated changes at the levels of structure and lived experience. The mission of this book is to explore how individuals, families and communities create meaning in times of illness, suffering, and death; how they orient themselves to an increasingly complex and varied array of healing options; and the ways in which decisions regarding therapeutic interventions play out in everyday life.

Note

1. Medical pluralism has a rich anthropological heritage. Writers such as Leslie (1976) and Lock (1980) provide seminal examples of the topic in East Asia, as Janzen (1978) does for Africa; Adams, Schrempf, and Craig (2011) for central Asia; Connor and Samuel (2001) for South and Southeast Asia; Young (1981) for Central America; Koss-Chioino, Leatherman, and Greenway (2003) for the Andes; Frankel and Lewis (1989) for Papua New Guinea; Baer for the U.S. (Baer: 2001); and Moore and McClean for the UK (2010).

Bibliography

Adams, Vincanne, Mona Schrempf, and Sienna Craig, eds. 2011. *Medicine Between Science and Religion*. Oxford: Berghahn.

Alex, Gabriele, Kristine Krause, David Parkin, and Stephanie Stocker. 2012. *Medical Pluralism—Bibliography*. Gottingen: Max Planck Institute for the Study of Religious and Ethnic Diversity.

Ashforth, Adam. 2010. "Spiritual Insecurity and AIDS in South Africa." In *Morality, Hope and Grief: Anthropologies of AIDS in Africa*, edited by Hansjorg Dilger and Ute Luig. 43–60. New York: Berghahn.

Baer, Hans. 2010. *Biomedicine and Alternative Healing Systems in America*. Madison: University of Wisconsin Press.

Baer, Hans, Merrill Singer, and Ida Susser. 2013. *Medical Anthropology and the World System*. Santa Barbara: Praeger.

Barrett, Ron. 2008. *Aghor Medicine*. Berkeley: University of California Press.

Bekaert, Stefan. 2000. *System and Repertoire in Sakata Medicine*. Uppsala: Uppsala University.

Chary, Anita, and Peter Rohloff, eds. 2015. *Privatization and the New Medical Pluralism*. Lanham: Lexington Books.

Chikombero, Mandi. 2007. "Confusion, Anger, and Denial." In *HIV/AIDS, Illness, and African Well-Being*, edited by Toyin Falola and Matthew Heaton, 352–385. Rochester: University of Rochester Press.

Comaroff, Jean. 1985. *Body of Power Spirit of Resistance*. Chicago: University of Chicago Press.

Connor, Linda, and Geoffrey Samuel, eds. 2001. *Healing Powers and Modernity*. London: Bergin & Garvey.

Constantinides, P. M. 1985. "Women Heal Women." *Social Science and Medicine*. 21: 685–692.

Csordas, Thomas. 1994. "Introduction." In *Embodiment and Experience*, edited by Thomas Csordas, 1–26. Cambridge: Cambridge University Press.

Dapaa, Jonathan. 2012. *HIV/AIDS Treatment in Two Ghanaian Hospitals*. Leiden: African Studies Center.

Davis, Christopher. 2000. *Death in Abeyance*. Edinburgh: Edinburgh University Press.

Devisch, Rene. 1993. *Weaving the Threads of Life*. Chicago: University of Chicago Press.

Dilger, Hansjorg; Abdoulaye Kane, and Stacey Langwick. 2012. "Introduction." In *Medicine, Mobility and Power in Global Africa*, edited by Dilger, Kane, and Langwick, 1–30. Bloomington: Indiana University Press.

E. E. Evans-Pritchard. 1937. *Witchcraft, Oracles and Magic in Azande*. Oxford: Oxford University Press.

Feierman, Steven. 1985. "The Social Roots of Health and Healing in Modern Africa." *African Studies Review* 28: 73–148.

Frankel, Stephen, and Gilbert Lewis, eds. 1989. *A Continuing Trial of Treatment*. Boston: Kluwer.

Frankenberg, Ronald, and Joyce Leeson. 1976. "Disease, Illness and Sickness: Social Aspects of the Choice of Health in a Lusaka Suburb. In *Social Anthropology and Medicine*, edited by J. B. Loudon. London: Academic Press.

Geissler, P. Wenzel. 2015. "Introduction." In *Para-States and Medical Science*, edited by P. Wenzel Geissler, 1–44. Durham: Duke University Press.

Good, Byron. 1977. "The Heart of What's the Matter." *Culture, Medicine and Psychiatry* 1: 25–58.

———. 1994. *Medicine, Rationality and Experience*. Cambridge: Cambridge University Press.

Graham, Janice. 2006. "Diagnosing Dementia." In *Thinking about Dementia*, edited by Annette Leibing and Lawrence Cohen, 80–105. New Brunswick: Rutgers University Press.

Harris, Grace. 1978. *Casting Out Anger*. Cambridge: Cambridge University Press.

Horton, Robin. 1967. "African Traditional Thought and Western Science." *Africa* 37: 50–72, 155–187.

Hunter, Cynthia. 2001. "Sorcery and Science as Competing Models of Explanation in a Sasak Village." In *Healing Powers and Modernity*, edited by Linda Connor and Geoffrey Samuel, 152–170. London: Bergin and Garvey.

Iliffe, John. 2006. *The African AIDS Epidemic: A History*. Oxford: James Currey.

Jackson, Michael. 1989. *Paths Toward a Clearing*. Bloomington: Indiana University Press.

———. 1994. *Minima Ethnographica*. Chicago: University of Chicago Press.

Janzen, John M. 1978. *Quest for Therapy*. Berkeley: University of California Press.

———. 2014. "Imagining the Whole." In *Medical Anthropology in Global Africa*, edited by Kathryn A. Rhine, John M. Janzen, Glenn Adams, and Heather Aldersey, 19–27. Lawrence, KS: University of Kansas Publications in Anthropology.

Janzen, John M., and Steven Feierman, eds. 1979. "Social History of Disease and Medicine in Africa." *Social Science and Medicine* 13B(4): 239–243.

Kayombo, E. J., F. C. Uiso, and R. Mahunnah. 2012. "Experience on Healthcare Utilization in Seven Administrative Regions of Tanzania." *Journal of Ethnobiology and Ethnomedicine* 8: 1–9.

Kleinman, Arthur. 1980. *Patients and Healers in the Context of Culture*. Berkeley: University of California Press.

Koss-Chioino, Joan, Thomas Leatherman, Christine Greenway, eds. 2003. *Medical Pluralism in the Andes*. New York: Routledge.

Langwick, Stacey. 2011. *Bodies, Politics, and African Healing*. Bloomington: Indiana University Press.

———. 2015. "Partial Publics." *Current Anthropology* 56: 493–515.

Last, Murray. 1986. "Introduction." In *The Professionalisation of African Medicine*, edited by Murray Last and G. L. Chavunduka, 1–28. Edinburgh: Edinburgh University Press.

LeBeau, Debie. 2003. *Dealing with Disorder*. Koln: Koppe.

Leslie, Charles. 1975. "Pluralism and Integration in the Indian and Chinese Medical Systems." In *Medicine in Chinese Cultures*, edited by Arthur Kleinman, 401–417. Washington, DC: US Government Publishing Office.

———. 1980. "Introduction." In *Asian Medical Systems*, edited by Charles Leslie, 1–18. Berkeley: University of California Press.

———, ed. 1976. *Asian Medical Systems*. Berkeley: University of California Press.

———. 1980. "Medical Pluralism in World Perspective." *Social Science and Medicine B: Medical Anthropology* 191–195.

Lewis, I. M. 1991. "Zar in Context." In *Women's Medicine*, edited by I. M. Lewis, Ahmed Al-Safi, and Sayyid Hurreiz, 1–17. Edinburgh: Edinburgh University Press.

Livingston, Julie. 2012. *Improvising Medicine*. Duke: Duke University Press.

Lock, Margaret. 1980. *East Asian Medicine in Urban Japan*. Berkeley: University of California Press.

Lock, Margaret, and Vinh-Kim Nguyen. 2010. *Anthropology of Biomedicine*. Oxford: Wiley-Blackwell.

MacCormack, Carol. 1986. "The Articulation of Western and Traditional Systems of Health Care." In *The Professionalization of African Medicine*, edited by Murray Last and G. L. Chavunduka, 151–164. Manchester: Manchester University Press.

Martin, Emily. 2012. "Grafting Together Medical Anthropology, Feminism, and Technoscience." In *Medical Anthropology at the Intersections*, edited by Marcia Inhorn and Emily Wentzell, 23–40. Durham: Duke University Press.

Meier zu Biesen, Caroline, Hansjorg Dilger, and Tanja Nienstedt. 2012. *Bridging Gaps in Health Care and Healing*. Berlin: Freie Universitat.

Miles, Ann, and Thomas Leatherman. 2003. "Perspectives on Medical Anthropology in the Andes." In *Medical Pluralism in the Andes*, edited by J. Koss-Chioino, Thomas Leatherman, and C. Greenway, 3–15. London: Routledge.

Moerman, Daniel. 2002. *Meaning, Medicine and the Placebo Effect*. Cambridge: Cambridge University Press.

Moore, Ronnie, and Stuart McClean, eds. 2010. *Folk Healing and Health Care Practices in Britain and Ireland*. Oxford: Berghahn.

Mulemi, Benson A. 2010. *Coping with Cancer and Adversity*. Leiden: African Studies Centre.

Ngubane, Harriet. 1977. *Body and Mind in Zulu Medicine*. New York: Academic Press.

Nichter, Mark. 1989. *Anthropology and International Health: South Asian Case Studies*. Dordrecht: Kluwer.

———. 2008. *Global Health*. Tucson: University of Arizona Press.

Nisula, Tapio. 1999. *Everyday Spirits and Medical Interventions*. Helsinki: Suomen Antropologinen Seura.

Obeng, Cecilia. 2007. "Perceptions of Epilepsy in a Traditional Society." In *HIV/AIDS, Illness, and African Well-Being*, edited by Toyin Falola and Matthew Heaton, 95–115. Rochester: University of Rochester Press.

Packard, Randall. 1992. "Industrialization, Rural Poverty, and Tuberculosis in South Africa, 1850–1950." In *Social Basis of Health and Healing in Africa*, edited by Steven Feierman and John M. Janzen, 104–130. Berkeley: University of California Press.

Pearce, Tola. 1986. "Professional Interests and the Creation of Medical Knowledge in Nigeria." In *The Professionalisation of African Medicine*, edited by Murray Last and G.L. Chavunduka, 237–258. Manchester: Manchester University Press.

Prince, Ruth, and Rebecca Marsland, eds. 2014. *Making and Unmaking Public Health in Africa*. Athens, OH: Ohio University Press.

Prins, Gwyn. 1989. "But What Was the Disease? The Present State of Health and Healing in African Studies." *Past and Present* 124: 159–179.

Rhine, Kathryn, John M. Janzen, Glenn Adams, and Heather Aldersey eds. 2014. *Medical Anthropology in Global Africa*. Lawrence, KS: University of Kansas Publications in Anthropology.

Rubel, Arthur. 1979. "Parallel Medical Systems." *Social Science and Medicine* 13 (1): 1–84.

Scheid, Volker. 2002. *Chinese Medicine in Contemporary China*. Durham: Duke University Press.

Sargent, Carolyn. 1982. *Cultural Context of Therapeutic Choice*. Boston: Kluwer.

———. 1989. *Maternity, Medicine, and Power*. Berkeley: University of California Press.

Simmons, David. 2012. *Modernizing Medicine in Zimbabwe*. Nashville: Vanderbilt University Press.

Sindzingre, Nicole, and Andras Zempleni. 1992. "Causality of Disease among the Senufo." In *The Social Basis of Health and Healing in Africa*, edited by Steven Feierman and John M. Janzen, 315–338. Berkeley: University of California Press.

Slikkerveer, L. J. 1990. *Plural Medical Systems in the Horn of Africa*. New York: Kegan Paul International.

Smith, Daniel Jordan. 2014. *AIDS Doesn't Show Its Face*. Chicago: University of Chicago Press.

Sofowora, Abayomi. 1993. *Medicinal Plants and Traditional Medicine in Africa*. Ibadan, Spectrum.

Street, Alice. 2014. *Biomedicine in an Unstable Place*. Durham: Duke University Press.

Thornton, Robert. 2008. *Unimagined Community*. Berkeley: University of California Press.

Turshen, Meredith. 1999. *Privatizing Health Services in Africa*. New Brunswick: Rutgers University Press.

Young, James. 1981. *Medical Choice in a Mexican Village*. Rutgers: Rutgers University Press.

Zimmermann, Francis. 2014. "Medical Individualism and the Dividual Person." In *Asymmetrical Conversations*, edited by Harish Naraindas, Johannes Quack, and William Sax, 85–117. New York: Berghahn.

BIOMEDICINE AND AFRICAN HEALING

1 The Value of Secrets

Pragmatic Healers and Proprietary Knowledge

Stacey Langwick

OVER THE PAST TWO DECADES, tense debates about traditional medicine, herbal resources, and African science have circled around secrets again and again. Scientists argue that healer's secrets are an obstacle to meaningful collaboration. Bureaucrats assert that healer's secrets prevent the development of national resources. Healers claim simultaneously that they have no secrets and that it is their right to defend their secrets. Each statement positions the speaker in a complex landscape of science, law, and capital. This essay contemplates the value of secrets. It does not consider particular healing secrets but rather how secrecy is emerging as both a problem and a right.

In the process I unpack what a secret is in this field, when leveled as an accusation and when implemented as a strategy. While the uneven movement of healing knowledge in Africa has long been linked to the production of gender, age, and labor hierarchies, the problem of healers' secrets as it is constituted today emerged as healing became entangled with property regimes, both those that shape the institutional labor of scientists and those that structure the legal maneuvers to protect traditional knowledge.

The scientific investigation of traditional medicine in many African countries was institutionalized in the 1970s as newly independent governments struggled to find the hard currency needed to purchase pharmaceuticals critical to any national healthcare system. These efforts dovetailed with regionalist, Pan-Africanist dreams to support an indigenous pharmaceutical industry in Africa. At times, they also became entangled with international efforts promoted by the World Health Organization to mobilize traditional healers as a solution to the shortage of workers in the healthcare sector of developing countries. At other times, the scientific development of traditional medicine has been promoted as a first step in the manufacturing of African pharmaceuticals and has had a force of its own. Therapeutic plants, it seemed, offered more political and economic possibilities if they could be separated from the relations critical to healers and their healing knowledge. From its emergence as a postcolonial category of knowledge and practice, then, traditional medicine has been a reaction to international private property regimes—with attempts both to circumvent those regimes and to participate in them.

The global "harmonization" of intellectual property laws, more recently, has raised the stakes of disclosing healing knowledge. This research was collected during the initial grace period for compliance with the World Trade Organization's agreement Trade-Related Aspects of Intellectual Property Rights (TRIPS) for Least Developed Countries (LDCs). All sub-Saharan African nations were feeling particular pressure to make progress toward the incorporation of the WTO's minimum standards for intellectual property into their national laws. Under the current extension of the grace period for LDCs, debates about the value of healers' secrets continue, as do debates about the globalization of intellectual property and how it will affect therapeutic regimes and cultures in Africa.

Therapeutic knowledge in East Africa has long unfolded among healers called to serve ancestors, spirits, devils, gods, and other nonhuman actors (Feierman, Langwick 2011a, Livingston 2005, Luedke and West 2006). The sensitivities and capacities of healers are forged in efforts to manage their own afflictions and to seek a context in which they might heal (Feierman 1974; Janzen 1982, 1992). These efforts involve learning to act in relation to plants, ancestors, and spirits; that is, coming to know their potency, needs, desires, frustrations, and quirks (Giles 1999, Langwick 2007, Stoller 1995). The passing on of therapeutic knowledge through generations is, in essence, the extension of these relationships (Geissler and Prince 2009). Before human and nonhuman guides entrust initiates with new therapeutic knowledge, they gauge whether these healers-to-be have not only the intellectual capacity to know how, but also the moral fortitude and equipoise to discern when it is wise, to use knowledge that has the power to kill as well as to heal. When responsibilities to nonhuman worlds cause friction during initiatives to "develop" traditional medicine, they are often glossed as healers' secrets. As a result, healers who are interested in exploring collaborations with scientists are finding themselves in the slightly awkward position of asserting their right to "keep secrets." Such defenses of secrets remember precolonial forms of life and arenas of collective action in ways that interrupt contemporary relations between therapeutic knowledge, political authority, and property regimes.

Attributions or accusations of secrecy gloss deep dissonances. They obscure the extension of healing knowledge through carefully cultivated (and at times unpredictable) relationships with ancestors, spirits, gods, and other nonhuman actors. And they index failures in translation. Part of what has consistently muddled collaborations between African healers and both scientists and legal advocates who are interested in their therapeutic knowledge is that African medicine is an extension of relationship, not an object of property (Langwick 2011b). It is a set of obligations, not a right. Furthermore, African therapeutics generate innovation through engagement, not single authorship. Such epistemic practices and the ontological realities that inhere in them do not (always) sit easily with those of modern science or law.

The first part of this essay considers the productive frictions involved in framing the limitations and boundaries of relationship as "healers' secrets." I attend to the ways that healers' own efforts to defend their secrets have come to challenge the political work that traditional medicine is being asked to do in national and international development initiatives, which cast it as a raw material—a resource for medical science, economic growth, and health development. These defenses point to the deeper transformation required. The second part of the essay examines the experimentation in organizational forms and social relations around contemporary traditional medicine. I focus most closely on one relatively unique project to develop a school for traditional healers, which highlights many of the demands this historical moment is making on healing.

In Defense of Secrets

In 2003, a group of regional scholars and bureaucrats formed the East African Network on Medicinal Plants and Traditional Medicine (International Development Research Centre [IDRC] 2003). Putatively, this forum provides the opportunity for research agendas, priorities, and methods, as well as legal frameworks, to be developed, debated, shared, and coordinated on national, regional, and global levels. The network held the first regional Workshop on the Sustainable, Safe, and Effective Use of Medicinal Plants in Eastern Africa the first year of its founding. The organizers of the workshop engaged healers as a group of stakeholders. In the representational politics of this regional gathering, healers embodied one set of interests in evidence-based traditional medicine. Healers' claims stood as equivalent to the claims of researchers, policy makers, private entrepreneurs, and journalists. Rather than treating healers as mediums through which ancestral shades, Islamic and Christian spirits, and various mischievous nonhuman agents work to shape afflictions and their cures—rather than treating them as embodiments of the complex relations through which expertise and efficacy are constituted—the structure of the workshop strove to reduce healers to people with "stakes" in medicinal plants. The excess created by their designation as "stakeholders" simmered, leaked, and at times exploded into proceedings. In particular, through conversations about secrets, healers at the workshop illuminated the connections between these bureaucratic moves to position them as stakeholders in efforts "enterprising-up"[1] traditional medicine and current political investments in what knowledge and knowing are.

A tension ran through the 2003 stakeholders workshop between members who wanted to open the discussion to issues of secrecy and those who moved to close them down via appeals to intellectual property rights. At times some participants would explicitly identify the secrets or opacities that inhere in the ways that intellectual property is used. But even more significant, I would argue, were the moments in which secrets bubbled up, refusing to be captured under the rubric of intellectual property. These moments provide a glimpse of the limits—the contingent boundaries—of the representational politics being built up through traditional medicine and a glimpse of the exclusions—the realms of unrepresentability—that will be a fundamental challenge to the maintenance of this representational politics. Below, I quote one segment of the meeting transcript at some length as it captures one of these moments.[2]

> Mr. Kariuki (HERBALM, Kenya) asked why *there is so much secrecy*. He added that there are institutions that are willing to come forward such as Kenya Association of Manufacturers to assist in commercialization of herbal products. . . . In Africa, we are shelving our indigenous knowledge while allowing the outside world to come and take this knowledge and our medicinal plants. To alleviate poverty, we should market our medicinal plants and promote their propagation across the region, and we also need to identify those who can commercialize them.
>
> Dr. Orwa responded that *there is secrecy in commercialization*. So far on IPR [intellectual property rights] issues we still do not know how to go about it. However, with formulation patenting can be done. For scientific papers botanical names are given. Dr. Orwa believes that several people who have come up with different processes can patent one medicinal plant. There is a lot of plant material of interest. The setback is that people work in isolation; hence there is lack of coordination and linkages.
>
> Dr. Sekagya pointed out that *secrecy is important in traditional knowledge* and that secrecy is environmentally friendly. If knowledge is exposed, there is danger of overexploitation.
>
> Dr. Malecela-Lazaro [National Institute for Medical Research, Tanzania] emphasized that *secrecy creates monopoly*, which is a vital criteria [sic] for commercialization. For example, some plants that were brought in by missionaries and are growing in our countries are exported to Europe. But since there are no intellectual property rights in place, we have no hand in these issues.
>
> Dr. Sekagya commented that he has *no problem with secrecy*. He continued by saying that he started his work with 15 plants but has now more than 50 plants. *The problem is how the plants are used.*
>
> Prof. Mahunnah re-stressed that Intellectual Property Rights is [sic] not a country level issue; rather *it is a subject of international interest, controlled most by the industrialized world*. Hence, there is a need as a region to have a common regional position where IPR issues can be presented to the global arena. Developing countries have been asked to develop a *sui generis* system to handle IPR issues under the TRIPS [Trade-Related Aspects of Intellectual

Property Rights] Agreement, but not many countries have implemented this. In addition, these agreements are often being revised and have deadlines to the detriment of the developing world. Some African countries have signed and ratified these protocols, and hence are party to the decision made by the parties to these agreements [*emphasis added*].

While some condemned the secrecy of healers, others acknowledged that research into the medicinal qualities of plant, animal, and mineral products brings with it new restrictions on information, which are built into organizational structures, forms of expertise, collaborative agreements, patents, and other forms of protection. "[T]here is secrecy in commercialization." "Secrecy is important to traditional knowledge." When read as intellectual property, secrecy "is a subject of international interest, controlled most by the industrialized world." The tension is over who will disclose what, to whom, and with what consequences. As Hayden (2003) has shown in her examination of bioprospecting projects in Mexico, secrecy is not the sole purview of traditional healers. Nor is 'openness' the unqualified stance of the market. Rather the channels through which information flows—who is able to know what—constitute relationships, spaces, and even scales of activity (e.g., local, national, regional, global).[3]

Advocating for the limited exposure of particular knowledge, Dr. Sekagya's comments raise these questions about the self-evident understandings of secrecy and transparency. The secrecy for which he argues is important to the existence and to the distribution of traditional knowledge. This is a secrecy that facilitated the growth of his personal repertoire of plants (from 15 to 50). Clearly, secrecy here does not mean a lack of information or a total refusal to transmit knowledge. Secrecy marks the movements of specialized knowledge and the making of particular forms of expertise.

Through the language of the secret, Dr. Sekagya draws into this debate the workings of an emergent or relational knowledge (see also Langwick 2011a, 2011b; Geissler and Prince 2009). His secrets enact and acknowledge relationships; they are about the specificity of inclusions, not the boundaries of exclusions. He strives to hold open the possibility that knowledge is not trapped in plants, minds, or communities, but, rather, healing knowledge lives in the dynamic relations between them. In so doing, he challenges the forms of knowledge constituted through current articulations of intellectual property law, with its insistence on disclosure and enablement in exchange for an exclusive right for limited time.

In calling for "a mechanism to safeguard and reinforce secrecy," Dr. Sekagya seeks a way to resist the forms of representation and appropriation embedded in efforts to treat and protect medicinal knowledge as property. Dr. Orwa also refers to the generative power of information sharing when he states "The setback is that people work in isolation; hence there is lack of coordination and linkages." Yet who works in isolation? Not healers who actively embody their relationships with ancestral shades, a range of otherworldly entities (some with religious affiliations and some without), patients, words, books, plants, and a host of other things too numerous to name. Not scientists with their institutional affiliations, funding relationships, collegial interactions, technology, equipment, theories, and a host of other things too numerous to name. The call for "coordination and linkages" is a call to reconfigure the relationships among the human and nonhuman entities critical to the development of a particular form of traditional medicine. The question, therefore, is not whether there are "coordination and linkages," but, rather, who thinks that they should be changed and how? When Professor Muhannah insists that the group develops their strategy in the context of international property regimes, he quiets the discussion for a moment. But he does not resolve the issue. Similar defenses of secrets unexpectedly interrupted discussions throughout the regional meeting.

Contemporary struggles for control over therapeutic plants and healing knowledge in Africa are generating new forms of organization and community that embody what Schoenbrun (2006) has called a "heterotemporal modern Africa beyond the hybrid or the alternative forms of modernity" (1403, see also Feierman 1999 and Kodesh 2007). Secrets train our attentions on the frictions caused by the refusal of particular subjects and objects of healing to be confined to a particular era.

An Institutional Home for Healers' Secrets

Interested in the tactics of his interventions in the Workshop on the Sustainable, Safe, and Effective Use of Medicinal Plants in Eastern Africa, I contacted Dr. Sekagya to talk in more detail about the tensions between communal, public, and private domains of knowledge and the ways that secrets might reframe discussions about intellectual property. In response, he invited me to his Institution of Traditional Medicine, known to insiders as the Buyijja forest school for traditional healers [Figure 1]. Dr. Sekagya's forest school, which is about an hour's drive directly west from Kampala, Uganda, is a complicated answer to the questions I posed. It strives to (re)compose African therapeutics through a set of propositions related to the role of plants in traditional therapies, the constitution of communities with stakes in traditional medicine, the creation of contemporary therapeutic expertise, the kinds of collaborations possible between healers and scientists and the forms of politics these collaborations might support.[4] He does not turn away from engagements with science. In fact, the school promises to establish mechanisms that support African healers' work with scientists and biomedical clinicians. It strives to be a ground for the mutual interrogation of traditional healing and medical science. It is an experiment in an institutional structure and pedagogical technique that can interface with scientific practice but not rely on it for validation. In this relatively early phase of the forest school's development, scientific validation of therapeutic plants or practices is a vaguely defined vision. The focus of current efforts is on the built environment of the school, organizational relations to support its growth, and, most importantly for my argument here, the development of a pedagogy through which the knowledge of healing might be transmitted, expertise might be crafted, and experts elicited.

Dr. Sekagya himself exemplifies the emergence of new kind of healer-intellectual[5] in Africa, who is forged by the relationship between science, law, and capital.[6] Sekagya is a trained dental surgeon[7], an experienced healer, the founder and current president of PROMETRA-Uganda, which is the East African branch of an international organization that advocates for the restoration of traditional medicine, and the founding director of Dr. Sekagya's Institute of Traditional Medicine at Buyijja. Sekayga attends international conferences and has been the subject of international magazine articles, online blogs, and a documentary film. He can be found online commenting on various articles about health and healing in Africa. By hosting learning exchanges, directing internships for international students, mentoring promising young African students, publishing with a former employee who is now an anthropology graduate student in the United States, welcoming foreign researchers to work with his school, and inviting foreign doctors to give lectures in his classes, he not only raises the profile of this forest school, but also finds multiple ways to integrate it into international conversations about traditional medicine. He participates in and works to shape international discussions on the value of African healing. In each intervention, he argues that African therapeutics cannot be ontologically subsumed by biomedical articulations of the body and illness.

The school, which meets each Wednesday, is perhaps Dr. Sekagya's most substantial intervention. In this, he is assisted by a team of young university graduates. Kato Bernard accepted a job supporting the organizational aspects of PROMETRA-Uganda after completing an undergraduate degree in forestry and environmental conservation because of his interest in the protection of plant species and the conservation of regional biodiversity. Many of these young staff members also attend classes in the forest school. Through them I grew attuned to the way that the knowledge about traditional medicine in the forest school was co-emergent with the material realities of the forest school. Its pedagogical innovations are part of a social-material assemblage that both require and structure the space of the school and its epistemological and ontological commitments.

At the entrance of the forest school sit three well-maintained round mud-and-wattle buildings. One is a room for the director, Dr. Sekagya, the second is used as a storeroom, and the third is reserved for students training as "spiritualists" in the forest school. On the knoll behind these building stands the much larger round brick shell of a future treatment center [Figure 2]. Although in 2008 its construction stalled for lack of funds, the outer wall already sports a plaque announcing the support of the president of the Ford Foundation. Sekagya and his staff dream of a day that a medical doctor will assess patients in this building and the traditional healers will treat them. The hoped-for treatment center holds out a vision of both collaboration with clinical medicine and of coordination with international development. It flags the social relations and accountabilities central to modern power as well as the spatial and organizational translations necessary for the production of therapeutic knowledge that might find partial connections[8] with medical science.[9]

A short distance beyond the entrance stands a newly completed building for meetings and conferences. Outside sits a bank of solar panels. A bit farther on is a substantial guesthouse used for residential programs. From here one sees a narrow but well-worn path entering the dense green forest. On many days a walker is greeted with the sound of music and drumming that grows louder as she winds her way through the forest on this path. After about half a mile, the path opens into a sunny area where a performance group of twenty or so students practices dance routines to be performed in surrounding villages to advocate for traditional medicine and to teach about current health issues. The ground across the path from where the performance group practices is covered with raised garden beds [Figure 3]. Each of the more advanced students at the school is given a 5' × 5' patch and encouraged to cultivate some of the medicinal plants they use to treat patients.

Plants form the foundation of the of Buyijja forest school's curriculum. The first two years of classes teach students to identify plants and their uses. Subsequent years require students to specialize. Each course of study has a semistructured curriculum that lasts one year. Students sit for exams at the end of the course. When they pass, they go on to the next level.

The *banda* for the first-year class is the largest. Students sit in long rows on wooden benches. Two or three people cofacilitate this class. Instructors standing in the front of the class take turns holding up pieces of plants. They start with the name of the plant and then with the things that they know it can treat. Then they open the floor to the students to add other remedies they know that were connected to the plant under scrutiny. Students raise their hands to suggest other possible treatments. Another instructor writes all this down on a blackboard, which sits on a bench and leans against one of the posts of the *banda*. Students lean over school notebooks on their laps and carefully copy each reference.

One morning in 2008, as I sat on one of the long wooden benches with a Rwandan woman who translated the Luganda lesson into Kiswahili for me, a female instructor, wearing a badge indicating that she had successfully passed through the first-year curriculum, stood up from the bench in the front of the group of students. She held up a twig that she identified as *lumana*. Another instructor offered that it could be used for women who are about to give birth. It is mixed with a particular type of green vegetable that Habiba who was sitting next to me described as "those ones that turn red when boiled." A student, an older woman, raised her hand and said that when you are married and you do not want to divorce with your husband, you can plant *lumana* near your doorway. This comment drew many murmurs. Another student then added that it could be used for stomach pains. For stomach pains, a juice is made from its leaves and yellow bananas and then drunk. A third student noted that some people combined it with two other plant species and then bury the resulting concoction in their banana plantations to protect the plantations from thieves. Last, someone offered that men who are weak or impotent use it. Throughout this exchange the seventy or eighty students in the class were writing diligently in their notebooks.

In this first-year foundational class, knowledge about plants is built up through interaction. This format acknowledges that students often arrived knowing some therapeutic uses for some plants and that this knowing may carry with it its own responsibilities and obligations. Participation does not require or even compel full disclosure of a plant's uses or of any given healer's knowledge. The goal is a shared repertoire of plants, not exhaustive knowledge of the plant world. Several hundred plants and trees compose a core body of knowledge that grounds expertise in the school. While facilitators offer some possible uses of the plants, students grow more familiar with the specimens as their peers elaborate on these uses. The value of each plant grows through the discussion. This is an inclusive exchange. Students are not corrected. Plants become the sites of layered recollections of the group. This form of recollecting and the noncorrecting nature of the interaction allows knowing and (some kinds of) not-knowing to sit together.[10] In addition, there is a pedagogical refusal to make ontological difference a matter of concern[11] (that is, to separate the herbs' potentially biological effects on birth or stomach pains from its efficacy in bewitching husbands and thieves). As a result, the articulation of (in)commensurability does not emerge as a salient epistemological project.

This first year of training stands in stark contrast to the early days and months that forged other healers with whom I have worked in East Africa. Neither an illness experience nor a profound and powerful relationship with invisible realms is central to this first-year class at the forest school. Some, but certainly not all, of the students are cultivating relationships with ancestral shades or the spirits so foundational to healing knowledge elsewhere. In addition to traditional healers, the forest school attracts a range of others, including the children of healers, those who see the training as potentially helpful in earning a livelihood, and mothers caring for children or other kin who are ill. A man, holding tightly to his notebook, told me how he takes his notes back to his home each Wednesday and reads them to his children and family, telling them all about what he has learned.

Students at the forest school write in notebooks; they read plaques on trees well known for their therapeutic value; they offer their experiences up to the class and to be written down on the blackboard. These are bodies and minds disciplined by repetition and memorization. Expertise is demonstrated through successful recall during exams. Weekly lessons and exams represent plants' therapeutic value as stable; medicines did not emerge for each person as the result of immediate relations between healer, his or her familiars and ancestors, and the patient. The body or hands of the healer were not taken as a factor in transforming plants into medicines. The forest school is the experimental ground for another sort of subject. To reclaim a social basis for healing, Dr. Sekagya's Institution for Traditional Medicine poses the question *What sorts of bodies and selves are necessary to make feasible a conversation with scientific medicine and the bureaucratic entities that invest in it while still holding open the possibility of disrupting, or more precisely of refiguring, political relations, liabilities, and accountabilities?*

The second-year class gathers in a slightly smaller *banda*. The students sit on benches behind long, roughly hewn desks. A blackboard is propped up against a car parked along the side of the *banda*. Students continue to increase the number of plants with which they are familiar and their understanding of the plants' medicinal qualities. They study some basic human anatomy and learn to identify a range of common biomedical diseases. Perhaps most importantly, however, in this second year knowledge is linked with commercialization. Students learn techniques for preparing herbal products and are eager to display their medicinal soaps and powders. Collective study holds the potential to support private livelihoods.

The curriculum in Dr. Sekagya's forest school is explicitly designed to encourage students to capitalize on their knowledge. Knowledge about the 320 plants that form the core of the curriculum is generated collectively and then treated as communal in that it can be tapped by students with other skills, such as soap-making. Some argue that knowledge of traditional plants is held widely or communally in Africa, and therefore healers have no proprietary right to therapeutic plants or medicinal knowledge. The forest school's curriculum establishes a core set of plants that constitute "communal knowledge" and generates a community to which this knowledge might be said to belong.

The question is whether this process will establish both a pedagogical structure to think strategically about the constitution of the public domain and an institutional structure to articulate an effective notion of communal property rights in relation to traditional medicine. In some cases, written evidence of the widespread use of herbal medicines has been used to overturn patents—upholding their use as "prior art" and therefore "existing" rather than "novel" knowledge (World Health Organization 2001). Such defenses elsewhere in the world have rested on proof in a historical written record. In Africa, however, therapeutics have been transmitted over time through oral and drumming traditions, not through written traditions. The fixation of therapeutic knowledge about these 320 plants within the curriculum means that the curriculum itself might be able to be used to support prior-art defenses against the patenting of this knowledge by others.

Indigenous right activists, however, have argued that casting traditional knowledge of plants' therapeutic value as public domain exposes it to scientific appropriation (IWA and IMN 2005). Public domain is not the opposite of patentable knowledge; it is open to innovation, transformation, and privatization. The public domain is the necessary companion to patentable knowledge. Interestingly, Sekagya noted as early as 2003 at the International Symposium on Biodiversity and Health in Ottawa, Canada, that PROMETRA had already filed five patent applications (Stanley). In addition, PROMETRA International has spun off a for-profit organization called Medicines and Traditions of Africa (METRAF), which holds the intellectual property generated through the PROMETRA International research network. Sekagya, himself, as president of the East African branch, travels back and forth between Kampala and Nairobi to collaborate on a project funded by the Canadian IDRC, which is investigating the chemical efficacy of medicinal plants. What sorts of private collectives might emerge through these efforts?

After passing the exam that concludes the second year of coursework, each student selects one of five possible specialties for further study. In the language of the school, these specialties include herbalism, traditional birth attendance, mental health, bonesetting, and spiritualism. The staff describe a sort of hierarchy within the school that privileges spiritualism—precisely because one must be called or chosen, because knowledge comes from channeling disembodied forces—over learning achieved solely through memorization and craft. Sekagya himself is a spiritualist, and his story of being called to the forest and of wandering with the spirits is central to the history of the emergence of the school and his legitimacy as its founder and leader. Specialties are distinguished by both the amount of knowledge about plants required and the kind of knowledge the experts embody. The contrast of the effects of the foundational program of the first two years with the hierarchy of specialties is the simultaneous centering and decentering of plants and a particular relationship of mastery over them that is central to modern scientific knowledge (Fox Keller 1985).

The third-year groups spread out under the trees throughout the forest, sitting on tarps or *kanga*. Movement deeper into the forest brings one closer to the spiritualists. At this level the teaching is even less didactic, and less systematic. Students who held extensive knowledge in a particular area led lessons on the topic. At other times, they called in a "technical expert," a respected healer or professor with a particular expertise. The size of the groups varied widely, from the herbalists who had to press themselves together to make room on their tarp for us to the two women sitting with their heads together over a well-worn school notebook, studying treatments for mental-health conditions.

A small stream delineated the edge of the spiritualists' area and separated the spiritualists from the others working for PROMETRA. Those who were studying herbalism or traditional birth attendance were not ritually clean, nor had they been called into the entanglements that constitute the spiritualists' specialty. My entry into this area was facilitated by a young man called Omari. Under Omari's care, the spiritualists welcomed me to take my shoes off and cross the small bridge to their site. About a dozen people sat on grass mats that had been laid down on the forest floor. Each was wrapped in a large piece of bark cloth. Some women shared a pipe. A fire smoldered off to one side. Each of us chewed seeds to harmonize with the group.

Omari at twenty-five years old looked to be one of the youngest members of the group. The Wednesday he introduced me to the spiritualists he was acting as the "voice of the director" because Dr. Sekagya was in Nairobi. Sekagya refers to himself as a student of the spiritualists. On that sunny afternoon, a notebook lay open in front of Omari. A photocopied page in English about HIV/AIDS had been tucked into the book at this point and now lay available for a lesson or discussion. Drumming soon started.

A man in a blue shirt began shaking and his eyes rolled toward the back of his head. Omari went to greet the spirit and find out his name. This greeting involved one kneeling in front of the spirit and holding out both hands, palms up. The spirit grabbed both hands. I was introduced and was told that I too had powers with spirits, that I had some psychic ability. Omari explained to me on the side that for 120 years this spirit did not climb on anyone. Only a couple of years ago he picked this man. The spirit had had to wait a long time to find someone in the lineage who could carry out his work.

Next, a spirit from the sea who liked to eat fire took Omari. He went to the fire and started eating the charcoal. A couple of women made it their job to break up any of the pieces that he grabbed that were still red, to rub them in the dirt, ensuring that he did not burn his mouth. A spirit of a stubborn king who had been burned to death possessed another man. He took his shirt off, grabbed a handful of straw, set it on fire, and rubbed it over his head and body while dancing to the drum. After a few minutes he sat down, allowing people to approach him. This was a joyful gathering of spirits and mediums breaking up what had probably been a dry lecture on HIV.

Secrets in the forest school are silent omissions in the first- and second-year group—when students decline to speak up and contribute a technique or medicinal use of a plant under discussion. They are also the boundaries created by the demands of ritual purification. And they are those pieces of knowledge that a spirit holds—sometimes for many years—before it identifies an appropriate person to serve as a medium.

At the end of this afternoon's gathering, as we were waiting for the flatbed truck to return and take the last group of student-healers back to their homes, I was invited to the fire in front of the three round huts at the entrance to the forest school's grounds. Omari came out of the round *banda* reserved for the spiritualist students, to cleanse me by the fire. As we stood by the fire, I asked Omari about himself. He said that when he was growing up, his mother feared him. He was sent to live with his maternal grandmother. While living there, he predicted an accident his grandmother would be in and the death of this grandfather. This grandmother then kicked him out, so he went to live with his paternal grandfather. This grandfather sent him to school. When Omari arrived, he saw everyone dressed in white. He told his grandfather that he did not want to go to school, that everyone dressed in white. The next morning his grandfather woke him up and took him into the forest. He prayed, asking the spirits to let Omari go to school first. He explained to Omari that a spirit had chosen him but that it would be better to study first. Despite the fact that the spirits interrupted Omari's education periodically, he did manage to finish college with a degree in adult education.

Back in the *banda* as the sun was setting, Omari took his role among these student mediums. He did not simply witness as others were taken by a spirit; he supported, encouraged, coaxed, and pushed people to let the spirits in. We were visited by a range of ancestral spirits before the last lorry returned, including a spirit of the forest, a spirit of those who are unknown, a spirit who made his medium climb high into the rafters and hang from the ceiling beams, and once again Omari's fire-eating spirit. At one point a woman who Omari said had never been possessed before started swaying. A few of the other mediums came over to her with the rattles and started singing. She moved. Omari went over to her. He shook her. He encouraged her. She put her head down on the ground and stuck her buttocks up in the air. Her arms fell limp at her sides. Moving her shoulders back and forth, shaking her buttocks, she moved to the music, and made her way toward the drums. By this time Omari had come to sit between the drums and me. She swayed and inched forward in this bent-over fashion until she reached Omari. After a few moments bowing in front of him, the spirit left, and she blinked, stood up, rubbed her eyes, and left the room.

PROMETRA's motto is "PROMETRA one finger." Traditional medicine, the PROMETRA-Uganda staff explain, is like a pot which has been shot through with holes by colonialism, religion, and other historical transitions. The goal of advocacy, of teaching traditional medicine, of the work of PROMETRA is to plug those holes. "Traditional medicine will not be a whole system until all the holes are plugged." In practice, however, the forest school does not offer a vision of a complete African system of healing that must be fixed. What does seem clear from the forest school is that this metaphorical pot is one that is fired in the kiln of international political demands. The healers and the administrators at the forest school seemed to me to be very comfortable with outside visitors. The university educated assistants and the forest school students not only skillfully incorporated me, but they also welcomed Africans from a range of other countries and deftly drew foreign students and development personnel into their project. They managed their secrets as levels of inclusion.

Dr. Sekagya elaborates a traditional medicine that exceeds its history as a product of colonialism, missionization, nationalism, and postindependence development projects. Traditional medicine, as it is emerging in the forest school, resists modernist divides between Western vs. non-Western, scientific vs. cultural, objective vs. subjective, factual vs. experiential, physical vs. metaphysical, and ontological vs. epistemological.[12] It does this by refusing to confine the subjects and objects of traditional healing and modern medicine to different eras. The staff and students strive to embody a wide range of tools, postures, approaches, and languages developed though precolonial, colonial and postcolonial experiences that shape their contemporary political and social worlds.

An Opening

Anthropologies of the body have extended postcolonial critiques by illustrating that narratives of science and capital, like those of colony and nation, are "indispensable and inadequate in helping us to think through the various life practices that constitute the political and the historical" (Chakrabarty 2000).[13] Accounting for the body in Africa requires tracking the development and the marginalization of particular formations of healing and fields of expertise, as well as describing the institutional structures that facilitate the creation of knowledge about, and interventions into, the body. These new formations of health, born of the tension between the "indispensable and the inadequate," forge subjects that are both constituted in narratives of science, capital, and nation and yet have resources elsewhere.

The Institution of Traditional Medicine in the Buyijja forest organizes the transmission of healing knowledge in ways that draw on the longstanding relationship between healing and prosperity in African therapeutics, experiment with ideas of efficacy and therapeutic power, and transform notions of knowledge and health in ways that cut across histories of science and capital even as they reveal their profound impact. For these reasons it is offers a response (if not an answer) to my question about secrets and intellectual property with the dynamic social and material life of this forest school.

When the young woman described above successfully received her spirit for the first time, Omari said to me over the din, "You open things up. Just be open. Do you feel it? You brought all these people here. This is why she could open to the spirit for the first time." My skepticism kept me silent at the time. Yet now I see his call as a challenge: what things might ethnography open up in the face of the ever more intractable enclosure of healing knowledge by contemporary relations among science, law, and capital?

The forest school is not a manifestation of a point of view or the guardian of an alternative system. Dr. Sekagya is experimenting with a social-material assemblage that will enable argument and advocacy. The forest school is an attempt to create a place (an institutional, technical, legal, and pedagogical configuration) from which African healers can articulate substantial and substantiated positions. Part of the difficulty of this project—including the suspicion it generates— stems from the fact that it refuses to be fully incorporated into either of the two discursive projects that seem to most easily substantiate positions on and in Africa today: advancing a humanitarian instrumentality or an ethnic authenticity.

Perhaps attending to secrets ethnographically can open up these overdetermined frames—by drawing attention to spaces that maintain disjunctures, tensions that highlight the ways in which political modernity is being reconfigured, relations where science and capital are themselves being transformed as part of other spheres of social life. Secrets are about enclosure and disclosure, about exclusions and inclusions. They are about mediation. I find myself drawn into the complicated new relationship between secrets and publicity this forest school poses in its efforts to find "common cause"[14] between medical science and African healing. Secrets and publicity do not stand in opposition here. In fact, the defense of secrets arises as a strategic move to reformulate political as well as healing publics.

East African countries, as member states in the WTO, will soon have to comply with the TRIPs agreement. Which forms of medicinal knowledge might be transformed into what sort of property are both technical *and* political questions. The answers, like the questions themselves, emerge from the frictions of different epistemologies and ontologies of the body (and bodily threats) in Africa. Healers have had little space to debate the effects of this compliance. The long historical process of divesting healers from their social basis of power has left them for the most part without the language or relations to contribute to these conversations. Dr. Sekagya's defense of secrets and his pedagogical work through the Institution of Traditional Medicine in the Buyijja forest, however, work to (among other things) establish this space. His project is uncertain. Any effort to build an institution, to elicit healers, and to formulate a traditional medicine that is sufficiently comprehensible to biomedical and scientific forms that they might interact meaningfully, is tenuous. Yet such translations hold out the ambivalent promise of relations that might interrupt the configurations of science, law, and capital at the heart of intellectual property rights agreements. Most immediately, such work evokes a community that complicates simple categorization of healers as "stakeholders," even as it demands a place at the table for them. More broadly, the forest school embodies an epistemological project in an effort to innovate new political ontologies that might take root in something that could still claim kinship with modernity.

Notes

1. Phrase borrowed from Strathern (1992).
2. For examination of another time that secrets interrupted the meeting, see Langwick (2011b).
3. For more on the production of these scales, see Langwick (2012).
4. I draw on Latour's (1999) notion of propositions, which he developed through his reading of Whitehead.
5. This approach is inspired by Feierman's (1990) work on peasant intellectuals.
6. For another example of a healer working at this intersection, although through a very different set of engagements, see Fullwiley (2011).
7. He holds a bachelor's degree in dental surgery from Makarere University School of Medicine, Kampala.
8. See Strathern (1991), accounting for ontological complexities through attention to partial connections.
9. Such a space for the biomedical translation of healer's diagnoses and treatments is consonant with observational studies (Langwick 2011b). The Tanzanian National Institute of Medical Research's Ngongongare research station has also stated as a strategic goal the construction of a clinic very similar to that imagined by Sekagya.
10. See Last (1981) for more on not-knowing.
11. See Latour (2004) on matters of concern.
12. In this way, Sekagya's project joins scholarly efforts, as well as the work of practitioners of nonbiomedical therapeutic traditions elsewhere, that strive to work through these divides (Brockway 2002, Farquhar 1996, Langford 2002, Langwick 2011a, Lock 1993b, Latour 1993, Scheid 2002).
13. Efforts to excavate the historicity of the body (Farquhar 2002), to describe local biologies (Lock 1993a), to trace everyday practices of care and nurturing (Lock 1993b), and to situate experiential narratives of illness and affliction (Lock 2002, Scheper-Hughes and Lock 1987) reveal the entanglement of a range of relations that constitute the matter and meaning of bodies and bodily senses.
14. See also Farquhar (1994) on building common cause.

Bibliography

Brockway, Lucile. 2002. *Science and the Colonial Expansion: The Role of British Royal Botanic Gardens*. New Haven: Yale University.

Chakrabarty, Dipesh. 2000. *Provincializing Europe: Postcolonial Thought and Historical Difference.* Princeton: Princeton University.

Farquhar, Judith. 1994. "Political Economies of Knowledge: Comment on Harding." *Configurations* 2 (2): 331–35.

———. 1996. *Knowing Practice: The Clinical Encounter of Chinese Medicine.* Boulder: Westview.

———. 2002. *Appetites: Food and Sex in Post-socialist China.* Durham: Duke University Press.

Feierman, Steven. 1974. *The Shambaa Kingdom: A History.* Madison: University of Wisconsin.

———. 1985. "Struggles for Control: The Social Roots of Health and Healing in Modern Africa," *African Studies Review* 28 (2/3): 73–147.

———. 1990. *Peasant Intellectuals: Anthropology and History in Tanzania.* Madison: University of Wisconsin.

———. 1999. "Colonizers, Scholars, and the Creation of Invisible Histories." In *Beyond the Cultural Turn: New Directions in the Study of Society and Culture,* edited by Victoria Bonnell and Lynn Hunt, 182–216. Berkeley: University of California.

———. 2000. "Explanation and Uncertainty in the Medical World of Ghaambo," *Bulletin of the History of Medicine.* 74 (2): 317–44.

Feierman, Steven and John Janzen. 1992. *The Social Basis of Healing in Africa.* Berkeley: University of California.

Fox Keller, Evelyn. 1985. *Reflections on Gender and Science.* New Haven: Yale University.

Fullwiley, Duana. 2011. *Enculturated Gene: Sickle Cell Health Politics and Biological Difference in West Africa.* Durham: Duke University.

Geissler, P. Wenzel and Ruth Prince. 2009. "Active Compounds and Atoms of Society: Plants, Bodies, Minds and Cultures in the Work of Ethnobotanical Knowledge." *Social Studies of Science* 39 (4): 599–634.

Giles, Linda. 1999. "Spirit Possession and the Symbolic Construction of Swahili Society," In *Spirit Possession, Modernity, and Power in Africa,* edited by Behrend and Luig, 142–164. Oxford: James Currey.

Hayden, Cori. 2003. *When Nature Goes Public: The Making and the Unmaking of Bioprospecting in Mexico.* Princeton: Princeton University.

IWA (Indigenous World Association) and IMN (Indigenous Media Network), joint statement. 2005. "Review of Developments Pertaining to the Promotion and Protection of the Rights of Indigenous Peoples, Including Their Human Rights and Fundamental Freedoms." (Principal theme: "Indigenous peoples and the international and domestic protection of traditional knowledge.") The United Nations Commission on Human Rights, twenty-third session. July 18–22. E/CN.4/Sub.2/AC.4/2005/CRP.3

International Development Research Center (IDRC). 2003. Proceedings of the Stakeholder Workshop on the Sustainable, Safe, and Effective Use of Medicinal Plants in Eastern Africa. Arusha, Tanzania, November 24–27.

Janzen, John. 1982. *The Quest for Therapy: Medical Pluralism in Lower Zaire.* Berkeley: University of California.

———. 1992. *Ngoma: Discourses of Healing in Central and Southern Africa.* Berkeley: University of California.

Kodesh, Neil. 2007. "History from the Healer's Shrine: Genre, Historical Imagination, and Early Ganda History," *Comparative Studies in Society and History* 49 (3): 527–52.

———. 2010. *Beyond the Royal Gaze: Clanship and Public Healing in Buganda.* Charlottesville: University of Virginia.

Langford, Jean. 2002. *Fluent Bodies: Ayurvedic Remedies for Postcolonial Imbalance*. Durham: Duke University.

Langwick, Stacey. 2007. "Devils, Parasites and Fierce Needles: Healing and the Politics of Translation in Southeastern Tanzania," *Science, Technology and Human Values* 32 (1): 88–117.

———. 2008. "Articulate(d) Bodies: Traditional Medicine in a Tanzanian Hospital," *American Ethnologist* 35 (3): 428–39.

———. 2011a. *Bodies, Politics and African Healing: The Matter of Maladies in Tanzania*. Bloomington: Indiana University.

———. 2011b. "Healers and Scientists: The Epistemological Politics of Research about Medicinal Plants in Tanzania, or 'Moving Away from Traditional Medicine.'" In *Evidence, Ethos and Experiment: The Anthropology and History of Medical Research in Africa*, edited by P. Wenzel Geissler and Catherine Molyneux, 263–295. New York: Berghahn.

———. 2012. "The Choreography of Global Subjection: The Traditional Birth Attendant in Contemporary Configurations of World Health." In *Medicine Mobility and Power: Transnational Health and Healing*, edited by Hansjörg Dilger, Abdoulaye Kane, and Stacey A. Langwick. Bloomington: Indiana University.

Last, Murray. 1981. "The Importance of Knowing about Not Knowing," *Social Science and Medicine* 15 (3): 387–92.

Latour, Bruno. 1993. *We Have Never Been Modern*. Boston: Harvard University Press.

———. 1999. *Pandora's Hope: Essays on the Reality of Science Studies*. Boston: Harvard University.

———. 2004. "Why Has Critique Run out of Steam? From Matters of Fact to Matters of Concern," *Critical Inquiry* 30: 225–47.

Livingston, Julie. 2005. *Debility and the Moral Imagination in Botswana* (African Systems of Thought Series). Bloomington: Indiana University.

Lock, Margaret. 1993a. "The Politics of Mid-Life and Menopause: Ideologies for the Second Sex in North America and Japan," in *Knowledge, Power and Practice: The Anthropology of Medicine and Everyday Life*, edited by Shirley Lindenbaum and Margaret Lock, 330–63. Berkeley: University of California.

———. 1993b. *Encounters with Aging: Mythologies of Menopause in Japan and North America*. Berkeley: University of California.

———. 2002. "Human Body Parts as Therapeutic Tools: Contradictory Discourses and Transformed Subjectivities," *Qualitative Health Research* 12 (10): 1406–18.

Lock, Margaret and Judith Farquhar, eds. 2007. *Beyond the Body Proper: Reading the Anthropology of Material Life*. Durham: Duke University.

Lock, Margaret and Vinh-Kim Nguyen, eds. 2010. *Anthropology of Biomedicine*. Sussex: Wiley-Blackwell.

Luedke, Tracy, and Harry G. West, eds. 2006. *Borders & Healers: Brokering Therapeutic Resources in Southeast Africa*. Bloomington: Indiana University.

Nguyen, Vinh-Kim. 2005. "Antiretroviral Globalism, Biopolitics, and Therapeutic Citizenship," in *Global Assemblages: Technology, Politics, and Ethics as Anthropological Problems*, edited by Aihwa Ong and Stephen J. Collier, 124–144. Malden: Blackwell.

Rheinberger, Hans-Jörg. 1997. *Toward a History of Epistemic Things: Synthesizing Proteins in the Test Tube*. Stanford: Stanford University.

Schoenbrun, David. 1998. *A Green Place, A Good Place: Agrarian Change, Gender and Social Identity in the Great Lakes Region to the 15th Century*. Oxford: James Currey.

———. 2006. "Conjuring the Modern in Africa: Durability and Rupture in Histories of Public Healing between the Great Lakes of East Africa," *The American Historical Review* 111 (5): 1403–39.

Scheper-Hughes, Nancy, and Margaret Lock. 1987. "The Mindful Body: A Prolegomenon to Future Work in Medical Anthropology," *Medical Anthropology Quarterly* 1 (1): 6–41.

Scheid, Volker. 2002. *Chinese Medicine in Contemporary China: Plurality and Synthesis*. Durham: Duke University.

Stanley, Bob. "Recognition and Respect for African Traditional Medicine" (viewed April 10, 2012). International Development Research Centre, Ottawa. www.idrc.ca/EN/Resources /Publications/Pages/ArticleDetails.aspx?PublicationID=713.

Stoller, Paul. 1995. *Embodying Colonial Memories: Spirit Possession, Power, and the Hauka in West Africa*. New York: Routledge.

Strathern, Marilyn. 1991. *Partial Connections*. Walnut Creek: Altamira.

———. 1992. *Reproducing the Future: Anthropology, Kinship, and the New Reproductive Technologies*. New York: Routledge.

Tantala, Renee Louise. 1989. "The Early History of Kitara in Western Uganda: Process Models of Religious and Political Change." Ph.D. dissertation, University of Wisconsin.

World Health Organization. 2001. *Trips, CBD, and Traditional Medicines: Concepts and Questions*. Geneva: WHO.

2   Body and *Sunsum*

Stroke in Asante

William C. Olsen

STROKE IS A RAPIDLY growing medical problem among aging men and women in Ghana. During three summers of research (2004, 2005, and 2014), 63 patients suffering stroke, hypertension, and problems due to high blood pressure in Ashanti-Mampong (Ghana) told me their stories and personal medical histories. Many of the stories resembled the details of one 52-year-old woman. Her stroke from three years earlier changed her life in a radical manner by limiting her speech. Her mother gave details of her condition. This patient, Grace, also suffers from severe hypertension and is diabetic.

> The stroke caused paralysis on the right side of my body. At the time of the stroke, I became unconscious. My mother found me and brought me to Mampong Government Hospital (MGH). My mother has been my voice since the stroke. I cannot speak. At one time, I received physical therapy at the hospital, but I stopped going because of the cost. Also, I have received medication from the herbalist at Ninting; but my mother cannot make the weekly trip to Ninting. Neither I, nor my mother, consider the disease to be the result of *sunsum yaree*. However, my mother did take me to some Christian pastors for healing early in the disease. But now we have stopped doing that. The doctor at MGH suggests an ECG, but this must be done in Kumasi.

As we listen to illness narratives, it becomes possible to sort out the "experience of illness" (Kleinman 1988, 49), or what the disease symptoms mean and how the patients are given the best medical care. Narratives are stories told by the patient and by others in close social proximity. Narratives reveal core events and even symbolic codes and social processes that may further serve to communicate any meanings of the illness. Narratives often establish connections between symptoms of the sick body and the world inhabited by the patient. Associations are sometimes made to the social, natural, and mystical surroundings associated with the patient's physical, human, and supernatural horizons. For this reason, Kleinman (49) argues that over the course of the illness, narratives shape and define the life world of those who suffer.

To fully appreciate the sick person's and the family's experience, the clinician must first piece together the illness narrative as it emerges from the patient's and the family's complaints and explanatory models; then he or she must interpret it in the light of the different modes of illness meanings—symptom symbols, culturally salient illness, personal and social contexts.

In such a process, disease symptoms determine the course of the pathology and its treatment methodology. Conditions may improve as the body responds to treatment, or they may worsen as treatment fails. Symptoms are never simply natural, medical facts. They are cultural "truths" in the sense that they become conditional markers of the progress and decline of the person's health. In such cases, the body is not an isolated bioneurological and anatomical entity. Its reality is more than life or death. The body-person, rather, is "an organic part of a sacred, sociocentric world" (Kleinman 11) in which disease serves to engage social networks.

Sometimes these exchanges are with professional doctors; and sometimes the exchanges are with friends and family. Other times, they may involve deities and supernatural entities. It is not unusual in Africa for biomedical, as well as nonmedical personnel, to be involved in the therapy process. Therapy is often rendered once symptoms are identified as indicative of disease. However, therapeutic diagnoses may change according to observations from both doctors and from those who accompany the patient or therapy management group (TMG).

Why do patients seek multiple forms of medical remedies as equally valid therapeutic paths? What are the reasons that motivate such a course of action? How can a disease such as stroke be understood through anthropology? To answer these questions, I turn to case studies of stroke and hypertension, and I report narratives I heard from patients in the Mampong Government Hospital in western central Ghana and at the diviner's shrine in the village of Penteng, northwest of Mampong.

I argue that the social identity of the sufferer is closely tied to biomedical symptoms of sickness for a time and that disease symptoms are markers that interact with social processes to "produce distinctive forms of illness and illness trajectories" (Good 1994, 54). Disease conditions transform the body in both a biomedical and cultural sense. "Health and disease will not be taken for granted, in the medical conditions involved; they will be discussed as values and concerns more than as clear-cut facts." More existential diseases "affect the patient's self-image and his or her conceptions of the body and self, of birth and death, and of humans sharing and transferring vital identities to one another" (Zimmerman 2014, 87). Within narratives, the sick body becomes a mode of historical and cultural compilation and recollection. Speaking of AIDS in South Africa, Fassin claims "the true mark of history is inscribed in the materiality of the physical being," the body (Fassin 2007, 177). The body as defined by orthodox medicine and understood with its medical physiology and anatomy becomes an entity re-conditioned within Asante medicine. The sick body is remade by culture and by history. The body becomes subject to other illness-defining criteria that make sense within this context, yet they are not recognized as legitimate within ortho-dox medicine. Local modes of healing address these differences and complexities through medical and religious practices. Healing may involve divination, which is described as a kind of pluralistic medical exercise. Stroke presents an excellent test case of the therapeutic continuum because of its trajectory through biomedi-cine and sometimes into alternative options.

The course of any prolonged disease such as stroke may become subject to medical recommendations given by biomedical and nonmedical friends and family of the infirm. Extended case studies of stroke show the patients' course of therapy as directed by the TMG. Narratives integrate bodily affliction and dis-ease into wider social contexts. In those circumstances, "bodily memory, biogra-phy, and social history" merge. The diseased body thus serves to integrate "moral processes of social experience aggregated historical event, symbolic meaning, and social situations" (Kleinman and Kleinman 1994, 714–715). Disease symp-toms are truly biological manifestations and medical facts. They are also "corpo-real devices" that originate in "people's corporeal rootedness and participation in a cultural life-world" (Devisch 1993, 280). As such, they "impose meaning upon experience" (Geertz 1973, 45). Symptoms are indicative of larger belief systems, and it is these systems that engage "health care seeking choices and treatment interventions" (Kleinman 1980, 91). Disease symptoms are also social entities, and, like the body itself, are subject to diagnosis and interpretation. For example, Songhay illness symptoms are believed to precipitate closure of body "pathways" and junctions that must "be passed through by many diseases in the course of their journey" (Bisilliat 1976, 563). For Songhay, medical therapy reopens these routes. The complexity of disease treatment and diagnoses is noted for central Asia:

> Complex illnesses (those difficult to treat) seem to trigger multilayered etiolo-gies that are connected with different cosmologies (the various "medical" ones as well as various folk or institutionalized religious ones), that also pertain to different healing options. (Schrempf 2011, 165)

Complicated or prolonged illnesses in Africa often assume a set of resolu-tions that are pluralistic, or they become subject to a variety of modes of interpre-tation. Some of these emerge directly from the biomedical model. In that model, viruses, DNA, bacteria, diet, and lifestyle are causal factors of good health and of suffering. Asante know and act on this framework. For Asante, some diseases are commonly identified within this model, including malaria, diabetes, cancer,

AIDS, coronary disease, hypertension, and stroke. One study shows that 92.7 percent of the inhabitants in Ashanti-Mampong recognize the cause of malaria to be bites from the Anopheles mosquito, and 99.3 percent claim they would self-medicate with pharmaceuticals for treating malaria. If this course of action fails, 50.7 percent would consult a medical doctor (Kyei-Nimako 1999, 28). Other explanatory narratives come from beyond the biomodel and reflect local culture. This happens as narratives become altered, when the patient changes social settings, or when differential (pluralistic) understandings are associated with the illness. In those cases, the patient and his or her symptoms assume a transformation of how the body performs. They become aligned with the efficacies of different modes of healing. Thus, in prolonged diseases such as stroke, it is not unusual for an Asante patient to recall biomedical care given in a hospital as a first resort. Subsequent to this first attempt, narratives may also relate alternative options in therapy. These are often sponsored by friends and family who realign the course of therapy with local healers. Bono of Techiman, who also are Akan, understand biomedicine in ways similar to how Asante do. Western therapies provide two supporting roles to healing: "the elimination of the disease vector and the treatment of conditions resulting from the disease" (Warren 1979, 123).

As immediate attributes of disease, symptoms are also features of the self as described by Geertz. In this way, the person "produces a situation where people interact with one another in terms of categories whose meaning is almost purely positional, location in the general mosaic" (Geertz 1983, 68). Within plural networks of healing, the "ill body's communicative capacities contribute to a process of personal historization" such that narratives make reference to social and historic circumstances beyond the immediate illness. In this process, the body becomes an "opening onto agents and aspects or areas of life which, though unseen, nevertheless have been exerting a powerful effect on events" (Davis 2000, 110). As noted for Tanzania, "there are many bodies and many versions of the body at play in any given therapeutic interaction. One way to capture the entanglements of materiality and sociality is to trace the relations through which bodies as objects of therapy achieve durability" and are cured (Langwick 2011, 22-23). Symptoms given in illness narratives are the "cultural forms of lived experience. They are lived memories" (Kleinman and Kleinman 1994, 716) for sufferer and for the TMG. Because of this representation, the human body in times of sickness and trauma is often known to represent periods of social stress. In addition, the body also experiences those events as a "lived memory of transformed worlds."

It may be argued that the sick body generates social memory because illness narratives often recall past events, which are then drawn into a sequence of current conditions. Healing in African life generates the historical nature of the body in at least two ways medically: (1) interactions of traditional healing with biomedical procedures, which are brought about by way of generations of colonial and postcolonial medical care; and (2) the necessary invocation of past events in order to resolve contemporary problems as part of procedures of healing.

The town of Ashanti-Mampong is located in the Asante region of western, central Ghana. Mampong has a population of over 50,000. There are three pharmacies and ten chemist shops in town. People visit natural herbal remedy shops, and they often self-medicate for symptoms known to indicate malaria and other symptoms especially related to fever. A district hospital with 155 beds has provided care since the early 1970s. People in Mampong know of and embrace the biomedical model of disease symptoms. They communicate with doctors and medical staff for outpatient disorders, and most people in town openly speak of past medical problems in which doctors, Western drugs, or the hospital played an important role in the therapeutic treatment. Biomedicine is overwhelmingly the very first method of treatment. Credibility in biomedicine likely matches numbers of 72 percent, as found in studies of alternative medicines elsewhere in Ghana (Yegbey 2000, 27). Comments such as "the hospital is more effective; it is quicker" and "the hospital is more powerful because the medical doctor has all kinds of medicines to treat all sorts of symptoms" indicate the first-choice option to be the hospital, clinic, or pharmacy. Nevertheless, traditional medicine in its various forms continues to be employed by a large portion of people in and around town. Medical pluralism in Asante is active because of the presumed functionality of anatomy as taught in school classrooms and of scientific knowledge which sustains the reality of biomedical theories of disease causation. Such theories demonstrate how the body grows, develops, becomes sick, and dies. Because global concepts of disease have been present for decades, people in Mampong rely upon this model to analyze and treat sickness as a course of action in an overwhelming number of medical cases. This functional model resembles the same core features of health as that which may be taught in many medical courses in the U.S. and Europe.

Pluralism is also active in the lives of Asante because of culture and history, and culture imposes historic models of the constituent make-up of human existence, including the plurality of component dimensions of human life. I contend that the scientific and medical body differs from the cultural and historical body during periods of prolonged disease.

Case #1: Stroke in Kumasi / Treatment in Kumasi and Penteng

On November 16, 2004, 75-year old Maxwell Kwame Sarpong[1] was working his day shift as an accountant at the Ashfoam Mattress plant on the south side of Kumasi when he suffered a mild but debilitating stroke. Speech and 70 percent of movement on his right side were temporally disabled. Sarpong was taken to the large Komfo Anokye teaching hospital near the center of the city, where he was joined by his family. Within 24 hours, his symptoms stabilized and normal movement and speech returned. Sarpong was treated as an outpatient and given medication for the stroke, although he does not recall the names of the medicine. At home that evening, symptoms of restricted movement returned, and again his speech was garbled. As intermediaries for any decision-making, the family became Sarpong's therapy management group. They noted that he suffered more paralysis, numbing, and lack of body coordination, and also blurred vision. TMG members transported him to New Tafo Hospital on the city's north side. After being medicated as an outpatient, he again returned home. Because symptoms such as poor coordination, speech, and blurred vision persisted into the next day, the family brought Sarpong by taxi to Mosi Zongo Hospital. By the end of the third day, Sarpong had been seen by doctors and other medical staff at three hospitals in Kumasi. He received prescription medicines at each location, and he had followed the directions of the doctors and staff regarding pharmaceutical regimens, rest, diet, and supplying heat to his right leg via a heating pad. By the end of the week, the symptoms worsened, and Sarpong feared that worse symptoms would occur, perhaps during the night when it would be more difficult to find a doctor or an accessible clinic. The numbness and coordination problems diminished only slightly over the ensuing months. The persistence of symptoms and the ineffectiveness of doctors' care, hospital visits, and pharmaceutical medicines prompted the TMG to suggest a consultation with a diviner. Sarpong's sister had experience with the shrine priest at Penteng, a village roughly 90 minutes north of Kumasi.

Sarpong initially sought medical help at Komfo Anokye (KA) Teaching Hospital. Established in 1954, KA is a large urban medical facility in the Bantama suburb of Kumasi. An upgrade in 1975 allowed the facility to become part of the medical school at Kwame Nkrumah University of Science and Technology (KNUST), which is on the extreme eastern side of the city. The medical staff includes more than 1,000 doctors, nurses, and administrative staff. The hospital accepts patients from regional clinics and hospitals who have medical problems too complex for local facilities to treat. Specialty units in the hospital include gynecology; obstetrics; ear, nose, and throat; psychiatry; surgery; ophthalmology; orthopedics; pathology; infectious diseases; and casualty and accidents. There is also a large pharmacy, a department providing radiography and radiotherapy, and a unit for physical therapy and occupational health. Dapaah notes that the hospital also includes a voluntary counseling and testing unit for HIV/AIDS patients, which treated at least 1,686 HIV patients in 2009 (Dapaah 2012, 45).

Stroke in Asante

Medical literature from West Africa indicates alarming numbers of youth and adults showing trends related to rising numbers of health problems related to hypertension, high blood pressure, and stroke. Morris reports that after malaria, stroke is the second highest cause of death in Accra (Morris 2011, 1639). Agyemang and others (2008) shed light on the increasing rates of systolic and diastolic blood pressure increasing with age in rural and urban children in the Ashanti region. This increase in blood pressure "corresponds with the increasing prevalence of hypertension reported among adults" (2008, 20). Likewise, Cappuccio and others (2004) demonstrate the high statistical growth of hypertension at 28.7 percent in Asante men and women is consistent with rates found in urban areas such as Accra. In Kumasi's main hospital, Komfo Anokye, 9.1 percent of all admissions and 13.2 percent of all deaths are due to stroke. Death by stroke within 24 hours of admittance occurred in 13 percent of all stroke patients. The average age for stroke patients is 63 years, and 1054 stroke cases were reported between January 2006 and December 2007 (Agyemang et al. 2012, 13). Numbers for Mampong are lower, with hypertension and stroke listed as the sixth leading cause of death in 2008, with 110 cases (M-A AR, 47). Agyemang et al. report an alarming rise in cardiovascular disease in Ghana since the 1950s and early 60s. During this period, the cause of death by stroke went from being the tenth leading cause of death to being the first. During my own questioning about stroke, people in Mampong showed a mostly consistent understanding of causes and symptoms of stroke. Responses to formulaic questions to 55 people show that those under 45 possess a comprehension of stroke quite consistent with the biomedical construct: disruption of the brain due to blood flow, caused primarily by low exercise, poor diet, high salt intake, and excessive stress. Many were also aware of the rapid rise of hypertension and stroke in Asante over the past two decades. Genetics and family history of stroke were not specifically given as responses, yet uncontrolled blood pressure and hypertension were commonly associated with routine causes of stroke. In nearly all answers, respondents noted that the hospital or doctor and pharmaceuticals are essential to the healing regimen. Other answers that conform to biomedicine were also given. I asked over two dozen individuals to draw the parts of the human body mostly likely to be subject to disease and pain. Illustrations #1 and #2 indicate knowledge of the body consistent with someone educated in areas of basic anatomy, physiology, and elementary aspects of disease and medicine.

Alternative Treatment

As noted by Sargent, evidence for one mode of medical option and behavior— hospitals or clinics, for example—"does not predict the total range of preference in the realm of medical practice" (Sargent 1989, 46). Stroke is viewed in popular culture as being a disease which is widely explained and treated by instruments of orthodox medicine. Causes of stroke are consistent within this model: "parentage," poor diet and exercise, growing rates of alcohol use, high blood pressure, and age. High levels of sex and drug use are also mentioned as causes. Men and women suffering stroke routinely seek treatment from medical doctors as the bona fide mode of therapy. Nevertheless, any disease symptoms may ultimately yield alternative diagnoses by a person's TMG. As noted elsewhere in Ghana, "Friends, relatives or neighbors seemed to have a major influence on the form of medical treatment" (Yegby 2000, 32). Stroke is mostly a component of the bio-medical model, but prolonged circumstances of any disease may lead patients to options that are beyond this model. By the time we spoke in Penteng in May–July of 2005, Sarpong's symptoms had moderated. He continued the regimen of phar-maceuticals, but because his stroke symptoms had not fully abated, Sarpong's TMG became convinced that herbal medicines would be necessary. All Asante are aware of alternatives to European medicines. Alternative medicines address the symptoms as biological and medical realities, but circumstances may lead to an assumption of illness caused by reasons not found within the domain of biomedical treatment. Such options often involve witchcraft by means of "sent sickness." "The witch acquires (*ogye*) the sickness and gives it to you (*na ode ama wo*). The witch manipulates a host of destructive materials. Sickness is only one of them." Many Asante diviners are capable of healing those afflicted by witchcraft.

Sarpong received plant medicines and divinatory care for stroke at *bogyese* witch-catching shrine in the form of herbal remedies and from an intercession with the deities—or *abosom*—who served to disclose the spiritual reasons for the symptoms in the first place. This broad medical spectrum is regarded as entirely legitimate within Asante pluralism. After consulting at the shrine, Sarpong even-tually became clear in his speech and in his vision. Bodily movement improved, and he developed full use of his arms and legs. Sarpong, an otherwise healthy senior male, stated that the spirits—the *abosom*—of the shrine at Penteng had revealed to the priest that the illness was brought about by the causal actions of certain members of his extended family and extended lineage, his *abusua*. Sarpong claimed that the diviner's discovery from the consulting spirits was that "my people have brought this thing to me: brother, nephews, and all family mem-bers. It is because I am royal heir to the stool at my hometown Aboenteng." The causes of his symptoms of stroke could not be detected and were thus not com-prehensible within the biomedical spectrum of analysis and treatment for hy-pertension, high blood pressure, and other issues. Instead, Sarpong's symptoms were revealed through divination and disclosed in narrative. The symptoms, in fact, were results of something that was entirely beyond the analytical scope of Western medical practices.

As noted elsewhere in the study of stroke patients, "the struggle to over-come the body's limitations, to become capable and free, never fully ended, and it significantly affected their responses to medical treatment" (Kaufman 1988, 346). Sarpong's symptoms of stroke belonged to the domain of what is termed in Asante, *sunsum yareɛ*, or spiritual sickness. This option was not yet disclosed to the patient when symptoms first appeared. Disease symptoms were biological in nature. However, the genesis of symptoms is enclosed within family relations, specifically the history of a disputed claim to the chiefdom and stool in his hometown.

The explanation of Sarpong's illness is compatible with traditional Asante narratives of how disease results from causes outside the biomedical model. One shrine priest confided to Meyer Fortes in 1945 (ASSMa) that death and disease are typical results of envy in Asante:

> Ashanti people are full of jealousy. Whenever they see that someone who is below them in age or rank succeeds in doing any great thing, they become envious and wish him ill, and then find means to kill him. No one but a person's own *abusua* can kill him. A man's own sister may try to kill him in order that her son could inherit his property.

Likewise, a testimonial from 1941 provides witness of the healing powers of a *Tigare* witch-catching shrine. (N.A.G.: ADM 23/1/622):

> If anybody suffers from sickness, or if a woman fails to bring forth, the complainant lays his complaint before the fetish, after giving kola and making a payment of six pence. The priest lays the kola by the fetish, pours libation upon it, and gives it to the complainant to chew. This acts as a medicine and cures the sickness.

The ASSM archives describe medical practices from the 1930s, including forms of disease known as *yadeɛ fo*. As noted by McCaskie, (2000, 93) these include:

> diseases with physical symptoms but social and metaphysical causes. They were said to be occasioned by conflicted or antagonistic interpersonal relations and arose most commonly within the lineage or between the sexes. They were grave complaints in that they struck at the fundamentals of kinship, marriage and procreation. If untreated they might develop into *abusua yadɛ*, transmitted by and blighting descent.

Details of this narrative pivot between medical technologies, hospital diagnoses, global pharmaceuticals, physical therapy, and then to local culture and state history. While being seen by a medical doctor, stroke symptoms of altered speech, blurred sight, and limited mobility presented an interpretation of the patient's body as a "disordered agent of experience" (Good 1994, 116) within the paradigm of cosmopolitan medicine. This much was obvious to both patient and healer. However, the same symptoms evolved into something more than the span of medical options that are available to Sarpong and to all other Asante and other urban dwellers and rural inhabitants who live within the medical radius of Kumasi, those who routinely partake of the range of Western and local therapies in order to alleviate symptoms in the most practical of circumstances. In his quest, Sarpong sought continued medical relief that offered resolutions to his problems based on the most legitimate and reasonable forms of medical service. Upon a culturally recognized failure of treatment, new options identified the same symptoms as "icons of disharmonies in social relationships and in the cultural ethos" (Kleinman 1988, 12). Symptoms became meaningful objects that may be treated within both cosmopolitan and local or traditional medical systems. Both ends of this medical spectrum of therapy maintain power and legitimacy for serving the health needs of a population. They thus "demonstrate the complexity and ambiguity of relations between sociality and representations of bodies," (Johannessen 2005, 9) since Sarpong, like most Asante, was not compelled to limit therapeutic options to only one mode of diagnosis within a wider continuum of therapeutic and medical possibilities. Sarpong pursued options for therapy that linked his bodily symptoms first to the technological model of biomedicine and then to the cultural arena of economic and political realities of local history. Such an association integrated "disorders in the body/self and the body politic (from the family to the village, nation, and global system)" (Brodwin 1996, 16).

Body in Asante

As a product of western education, Sarpong understood the performance and frailty of the body. As Asante, Sarpong also knew that the makeup and functional dimensions of the body respond to other stimuli. How does the Asante body work? What features make the Asante body unique? Are Asante susceptible to diseases in ways that may not be explained and treated by orthodox medicine?

Like other African populations, Asante perceive body parts and functions in connection to social relations. Natural realities are also social facts, and the biology of the body also maintains a vibrant cultural dynamic. This dynamic becomes active in times of change, stress, transition, and decay. From this perspective, changes to the body that transpire through disease take place not in isolation from a particular sequence of events. They also are known to be related to particular historical circumstances (Good 1985, 133). For Asante, it becomes problematic to separate conditions of illness—especially if they are prolonged—from the livelihood and human environment of the patient. In this regard, "talk about the body . . . tends to be talk about the nature of society" (Lock and Scheper-Hughes 1987, 20). Understanding some of the cultural dynamics of the Asante body will help shed light on conditions of medical pluralism in times of stroke.

At birth, the infant begins to also take on social form and is recognized as a human entity whose being is constituted of the various features of Asante human existence and cultural life. These include body (*honam*), soul (*ɔkra*), spirit (*sunsum*), breath (*honhom*), blood (*mogya* or *bogya*), and a sense of destiny, or *nkrabea*. (McCaskie 1995, 167–169; Gyekye 1987; Wiredu 1980). The *ɔkra* is the "humanizing principle" of all humans, and as such, it is not identified as an essential element of life in animals or plants on in inanimate objects. "*ɔkra* is in the body; it gives you your life. Without *ɔkra*, you are dead. Sight, speech, hearing, and touch are all controlled by *ɔkra*." And it is the "presence of *mogya* that makes the child a human being" in Asante. (Twumasi 1975, 21). M. J. Field notes that a child is not seen as human until the father impresses his personality upon the baby, usually eight days after the birth (Field: n.d.a.: N.A.G.: ADM 11/1).

A child is born with the *mogya* of the mother, so he or she is a member of his mother's extended family. This maternal distinction orients the infant later in life toward the matrilineal dimensions of kinship, and it will be through the matrilineage (*abusua*) that the child will be provided with a majority of his or her social support.

Sunsum for a human is "the pivot of the whole body." It is the spiritual element of the person, and it reactivates the body in times of distress and disease. The *sunsum* is dynamic in that it may be weakened or strengthened. When weakened, the body may also become susceptible to disease or even death. Some illness symptoms are known to be *sunsum* in character. One may speak of this kind of illness as *sunsum yareε*. Such symptoms may be diagnosed, but they are not treatable by Western biomedicine. Illness symptoms are evident in someone whose *sunsum* is weak or burdened. Someone's *sunsum* may also be affected by that of another person, thereby bringing sickness. Children are most susceptible because their *sunsum* may not yet be strong or developed like that of an adult. Or a child's appearance may be made to resemble a monkey or some other animal by an adult, even a parent, who wishes to harm the child through altering his or her *sunsum*. Also, your own *sunsum* may "fight against you" and thereby bring about bad luck or even when you do something wrong or you show bad intentions toward others. When *sunsum* is "weighted" or "heavy," it serves a strong defense against disease symptoms of any kind brought on by witchcraft. Adults generally have a much stronger *sunsum* than do children, which allows adults to be more resilient to illness; but they are also more capable of using witchcraft. Historically, a strong, robust *sunsum* was effective even in wartime. It is also well known that the *sunsum* of the entire state of Asante was contained within the Golden Stool.

More Narrative

Sarpong descends from chiefly royalty. According to rules of succession, he should someday be recognized as paramount head in his hometown. He was to be the next in line to sit on the stool as headman of his town, Aboanteng. However, some years ago a fraud scheme by someone outside the town arose. An imposter currently occupied the chieftainship, though he was not of royal lineage. Through deception, this man was able to make promises to the queen mother of the town, and through lies about his past and status he persuaded members of the royal lineage to allow him to be proclaimed chief. In a move to retain political power, the imposter threatened physical violence and mystically caused illness and death to any family members who opposed him, thereby retaining for himself singular control over the chieftaincy. By 2005, the imposter had killed five members of Sarpong's lineage by witchcraft. One death was the queen mother of the lineage.

In early 2004, Maxwell Sarpong registered a formal plea of complaint and appeal with the *Mamponhene,* or regional paramount chief. His case was heard, and ultimately the chief ruled in favor of Sarpong as rightful heir to the chiefly stool. The imposter was ordered to sell or forfeit lands he had acquired by deception and return all money to the house of the chief. He was also publically rebuked for his deception. But the imposter resisted this judgment. In an act of vengeance, he initiated witchcraft to afflict the health of Sarpong and thereby impede his ability to govern. It was determined through divination that the witchcraft took effect within Sarpong's body via recognizable biomedical symptoms of stroke. The first legitimate courses of action were a doctor's diagnosis at the hospital and the application of Western pharmaceuticals and physical therapy prescribed by medical doctors to treat all bodily dysfunctions of Sarpong's stroke. Yet as the symptoms persisted, it was then apparent that illness had a broader meaning, one which required a wider cultural therapeutic path.

The cultural meanings of the body became associated by the patient and his family with a cause that was beyond the bounds of hospital regimens to treat and cure. Fassin argues, regarding the AIDS body, that it is through our experiences "that the past is embodied in our present but also, more materialistically, that individual and collective history is embodied in what we are" (Fassin 2007, 177). For several weeks, what had been viewed by the medical community as a legitimate set of biomedical symptoms of stroke developed over a longer period into symptoms with a deeper cause, and alternative medicines became even more legitimate as a source of therapy. The medicinal herbs of the shrine priest in Penteng had a positive effect. Paths of medical therapy unsuspected at the outset became apparent as indications of stroke persisted, and Sarpong's therapeutic choices allowed him to return to his town and take up his commission as paramount chief. At the Penteng shrine, all symptoms were treated with herbs. Within eight weeks of consultation and therapy at Penteng, Maxwell Sarpong returned to his village and became recognized as the legitimate chief of the town. All residual signs of stroke had diminished. By all accounts, he became asymptomatic; his health was restored.

All Asante in Mampong and in Kumasi are familiar with pluralistic options in medical treatment of diseases. Stroke is understood and is treated within the biomedical mode. However, when medicines are considered ineffective or when symptoms for any kind of suffering are not abated by hospital remedies, then responses to the symptoms evolve, and other modes of therapy come into play. Options for treatment are mandated by the patient's TMG. In all cases of *sunsum yaree*, the ultimate cause is determined through divination. Diviners are oracles of *abosom* who inhabit the body of the diviner. While in trance, clients consult and disclose their issues. Many problems are medically based. *Abosom* communicate the resolution to the diviner by speaking in ways that diviners alone can hear. Severe illness due to witchcraft requires a sick person or his or her TMG to sacrifice poultry or a goat. It may also require a confession by the aggressor, or the sickness may simply be "combatted" by the deities. At Penteng, nearly all diseases are also treated with herbs through ingestion, topical application, bathing, mixing with food, or drinking as a concoction. For example, persons who come to Penteng complaining of hypertension and stroke are given a mixture of *Nkaseenkasee* (*Alternanthera pungens*) and lemongrass in an enema. Also the roots of *Omaatwa* (*Apocynaceae Strophanthus Hispidus*) are boiled for hypertensive patients (Fifita 2003, 16).

Over the decades of researching medical issues in Kumasi and in Mampong, I have never encountered anyone who holds hospitals, orthodox medicine, and pharmaceuticals in disregard. Most diseases receive a partial to full regimen of therapy with a medical doctor. People also self-medicate common problems such as malaria. Nevertheless, the power and integrity of herbal remedies are respected among Asante of all age groups.

> Before the hospital, my father and grandfather went to the bush, found the herbs, boiledthem, and gave us the medicines we used. Pharmaceuticals and hospital medicines are not as good as herbal remedies. But they did not write down their prescriptions. Their remedies died with them. Black man's medicine is better than white man's medicine.

Some years later, a diviner made a similar point. He put medicine into a wider context of Asante state and civil society.

> In the past, the priests were able to prepare herbs to cure people; and the *abosom* taught our forefathers about everything they did: how to marry, about how to live as families, how to run the state and be king, and how to form the kingdom. But they also taught us about medicines and healing through herbal drugs.

This sense of history intertwined with the powers of medicines was strongly argued in a village council I attended in 2002 as they spoke in the village of Krobo.

The powers of herbs and the powers of the state are closely linked within alternative medical systems in Asante.

> Even Osei Tutu used herbs to be powerful. The high priest Komfo Anokye was primarily an herbalist, and he used herbs and herbal medicine to do all the great things he did. Before orthodox medicine, we used herbal medicines to heal all kinds of sickness, especially those which cause death.

When I asked what happened to *sunsum yaree* after the hospital was built, I received the following response:

> Our great grandfathers knew the herbs or some healers could see with their eyes (*wo di wani bɛhu*) the *sunsum yaree*. They would then still treat disease with herbs. If someone is identified as a victim of *sunsum yaree*, he must find someone else who knows the correct herbs to treat it. The people who cure *sunsum yaree* today are in the villages. You go to the village because it is near the bush, and the bush is more powerful to treat *sunsum yaree*.

A final comment regarding hospitals in Asante illustrates the fine distinctions made locally between orthodox medical practices and alternative therapies.

> In another hospital a woman was being treated, but she was not responding to treatment. It was known that while the medicine was being given its substance was being gathered by a witch. Thus, it would not be effective on the patient. This patient was in the hospital with illness due to witchcraft, and the witch would not allow him to improve. The patient died soon after being admitted. In other hospitals, some patients are themselves witches. These patients will not respond to medical treatment. In some of these cases, the witch has a strong desire to fly away and cause a commotion. They will thus be very loud, but their powers are limited because they are in a hospital and around doctors and nurses. The patient could not leave physically but could fly away as a witch.

Case #2: City to Village

A second episode of stroke was narrated to me in 2005. This was the case of Hannah Boateng, who had originally suffered signs of stroke at the age of 39 in 1985. Her symptoms included body weakness and pain, inability to walk, fatigue, poor eyesight, and memory loss. Doctors at Komfo Anokye Hospital concluded that the problems in motor skills were brought on by stroke. She was given insulin and other medicines (the patient did not recall what the other medications were). After one week of inpatient care, her condition improved slightly and she was discharged. Years later, problems with stroke returned. She was seen at two other hospitals in Accra: Police Hospital and also 37 Military Hospital. At both locations, she was seen in the outpatient clinic. Her prescribed medicines were Amocillin and "blood tonic." But the doctors "could not detect the [physical] cause." Thus, medical staff could not render adequate treatment. In private consultation, according to Hannah, a physician in the hospital suggested that her symptoms were not the result of natural causes and that to adequately treat her illness she should consult with a spiritualist healer. This opinion was supported by the patient's TMG. Hannah followed the doctor's advice and consulted with a number of pastors who lead spirit-filled Christian congregations in the city of Kumasi. She also consulted with a diviner in Kumasi. Nevertheless, symptoms of blurred vision, garbled speech, and high blood pressure continued. She was then directed by family members who had previously consulted at the shrine to bring the matter before the diviner at Penteng. After three weeks of herbal medicines, she became more stable. In addition, the *abosom* also revealed that "she is suffering from so many kinds of sickness and that the *abosom* can look after her" through the diviner. The *abosom* identified the person who inflicted the disease on Hannah; but they refused to identify that person to either Hannah or the diviner. Hannah said, "It is someone in my family or my husband's family—or even someone who is further away." When I spoke with her, she said she felt stronger, she could walk better, and body pains were decreasing.

Stroke is much less likely than other diseases to be suspected of resulting from sent sickness. As noted previously, in Asante diseases such as stroke, malaria, and cancer are on one end of the medical continuum. Unless extended treatment proves otherwise, such diseases are considered problems to be treated within hospitals by orthodox medical physicians. On the other hand, afflictions such as epilepsy, mental illness, and a culture-bound syndrome known as *asram* are nearly always considered result of *sunsum yaree*. Symptoms of these diseases usually generate suspicion of witchcraft, or *bayeɛ*. Reasons for suspicion of sent sickness deal with the likelihood or reasonableness of the misfortune or symptoms of disease. Explanations focus on matters of probability, suddenness, and immediate severity. As one friend notes:

> Every Asante knows and recognizes that people die of natural causes and they fall ill from natural causes. However, if someone who is otherwise healthy suddenly becomes sick, or if the symptoms persist beyond a reasonable period or degree of severity, or if the symptoms are unrecognizable for that person by his family and friends, then *sunsum yaree* may be suspected.

Suspicions also arise in the absence of extensive medical programs and specialists who can identify and treat complicated problems.

> In America and Europe there are specialists. But here we have no specialists in the hospital. There may be specialists in Komfo Anokye Hospital, but that is in Kumasi and it is expensive. So when a doctor explains the he cannot treat you it is sometimes assumed that you cannot be treated at all by a doctor. When that is the assumption, people may think that the symptoms cannot be treated

by Western medicines. If that is the case, they may take the patient to an herbalist or to the ɔkomfoɔ [diviner] because they suspect *sunsum yareε*.

Case #3: Rural Asante

Auntie Agyie of Ninting, south of Mampong, was 52 years of age in 2003. Her stroke seemed mild initially. It caused a warming feeling during her farm labors: "There was so much heat in my body, and I could not sustain it. So I found a place to sit and rest." She felt pain in her right leg, and then more pain in her right arm at the shoulder—like someone "was throwing stones" at her. She heard people speak, but she could not respond. But she was able to walk the three kilometers back to her home. The next day, her husband took her to a local hospital, where she was referred to Komfo Anokye Hospital in Kumasi. She remained at KA for two weeks in the D5 Unit, which serves those with the most serious cases of stroke. She was given medication for high blood pressure. Upon release, hospital staff suggested she see a herbalist at Ninting who specializes in botanical remedies for stroke. The man claimed that his medicines would cure the disease regardless of whether it was a "hospital disease" or if it was *sunsum yareε*.

Neither Auntie nor her husband suspected *sunsum yareε*, but soon after her dying mother made the declaration that Auntie had maintained the strength to survive the stroke due to her good, honest character. From that point forward, witchcraft was suspected. Auntie began having dreams of being shot by a gun or being hit by a car. Such violent actions are often invoked in describing witch attacks. At Pentecostal Prayer Camps, these dreams were interpreted by the pastor and by Auntie's TMG as indications of *sunsum yareε*. The pastor told her that the disease was sent to her and that the "problem is coming from your own home." At the time of the stroke, Auntie and her husband were having conflict over ownership and access rights to land with people who owned the neighboring farm. Because of this conflict, Auntie's husband and other family began to assert that the people who owned the adjoining land caused the sickness. Even with this deep suspicion of witchcraft, Auntie never sought consultation with a diviner.

Auntie continued to have a strong paralysis for one year. She returned to the herbalist at Ninting each week for botanical remedies. She began to improve and even became independently mobile. Auntie also obtains pharmaceuticals for control of hypertension each month at Mampong Government Hospital, and she receives weekly physical therapy there.

Conclusion

We are reminded by Cheryl Mattingly that "experience is not merely passively received but actively created" (Mattingly 1998, 82). Illness narratives represent a primary mode used to shape, rebuild, and define life's history and existence.

"Narratives give unity and coherence to the succession of clinical episodes." They provide a plot structure to what is otherwise an unstructured succession of events and happenings. In Asante, this process is especially the case when biomedical processes are unsuccessful or in times of prolonged illness. In such circumstances, Asante responses to illness resemble those found elsewhere in Africa and beyond. For example, Gilbert Lewis (2000, 2) writes a failure of treatment in the Sepik River basin:

> Explanations for the illness, both during it and afterwards, supplied a mixture of insights into the villagers' understanding of risk in the natural environment, dangers from people around them, enemies, and spirits. . . . To follow the course of illness was to see in practice how social ties were woven and how strong they were; how people interpreted an illness and reasoned about its causes; what credence they gave to dreams, spirit revelations, and divinations for understanding it.

Experiences with disease, regardless of the cultural setting, often connect the life of the sick person with wider social, natural, and sometimes mystical realities in order to provide adequate causal and epistemological meaning to the event. For this reason, Good states that "disease is not an entity but an explanatory model" (Good 1994, 53). Asante would concur with this assertion. Because of the prevalent regularity and likelihood of *sunsum yaree* within Asante communities, and because of the vulnerability of individual *sunsum*, disease is often more than what it is understood to be in Western hospital therapies. According to Zimmerman (2014, 94), rather, disease "is not a well-delineated complaint that can be ascertained by anatomical/pathological diagnosis, but a mixed condition produced by the superimposition of different levels of reality in the patient's body."

Asante narratives of illness symptoms and of the human body represent a continuum between biomedicine and traditional medicine. The system resembles what Janzen (1979, 208) discovered in Kongo therapeutic systems in the 1970s.

> Western medicine is recognized in Kongo thinking as a discrete system. It embraces recognizable premises such as the theory of microbes and hygiene; recognizable therapeutic techniques such as surgery and injections; recognizable therapeutic sites such as dispensaries and hospitals; recognizable medicines such as aspirins, penicillin, and so on; and a recognizable hierarchy of specialists including the doctor, the nurse, and the pharmacist.

A system similar to this is found in Mampong. When this system fails to cure, Asante do not consider Western medicine to be faulty or of no value. They do not blame the doctors, nor do they ridicule the hospital and its procedures. Rather, a separate but associated paradigm is then engaged, in which aspects of the body and illness symptoms become subject to a differing set of causes and effects. This paradigm is familiar to everyone. It engages history, and it looks at the human body and person in wider dimensions, which become familiar through narratives of illness.

Note

1. All names in this essay have been changed.

Bibliography

Primary Sources

ASSM. Asante Social Survey Materials: Cambridge: Cambridge University Library.
M-AAR. Mampong-Ashanti Annual Report: Municipal Health Administration.
NAG. National Archives of Ghana: ADM series; Accra and Kumasi.

Secondary Sources

Unpublished Theses

Fifita, Patricia. 2003. "Traditional Ghanaian Healing." Thesis. Brigham Young University.
Kyei-Nimako, E. 1999. "The Place of Self-Medication in the Management of Malaria in the Mampong-Ashanti Region." Thesis. Kwame Nkrumah University of Science and Technology.
Yegbey, Kwabla. 2000. "The Role of Traditional Medicine in the Management of Fevers in Bawku East District." Thesis. Kwame Nkrumah University of Science and Technology.

Published

Agyemang, Charles, and Ellis Owusu-Dabo. 2007. "Prehypertension in the Ashanti Region of Ghana, West Africa." *Public Health* 122 (1): 19–24.
Agyemang, Charles, G. Attah-Adjepong, and Ellis Owusu-Dabo. 2012. "Stroke in Ashanti Region of Ghana." *Ghana Medical Journal* 46: 12–17.
Bisilliat, Jeanne. 1976. "Village Diseases and Bush Diseases in Songhay." In *Social Anthropology and Medicine*, edited by J. B. Loudon, 553–94. London: Academic Press.
Brodwin, Paul. 1996. *Medicine and Morality in Haiti*. Cambridge: Cambridge University Press.
Cappuccio, Francesco. 2004. "Prevalence, Detection, Management, and Control of Hypertension in Ashanti, West Africa." *Hypertension* 43: 1017–22.
Dapaah, Jonathan. 2012. *HIV/AIDS Treatment in Two Ghanaian Hospitals*. Leiden: African Studies Centre.
Davis, Christopher. 2000. *Death in Abeyance*. London: University of Edinburgh.

Devisch, Rene. 1993. *Weaving the Threads of Life*. Chicago: University of Chicago.

Fassin, Didier. 2007. *When Bodies Remember*. Berkeley: University of California.

Field, M. J. 1960. *Search for Security*. Evanston: Northwestern University.

Geertz, Clifford. 1973. *The Interpretation of Cultures*. New York: Basic Books.

——. 1983. *Local Knowledge*. New York: Basic Books.

Good, Byron. 1994. *Medicine, Rationality, and Experience*. Cambridge: Cambridge University.

Goody, Jack. 1957. "Anomie in Ashanti?" *Africa* 27: 356–63.

Gyekye, Kwame. 1987. *An Essay on African Philosophical Thought*. Cambridge: Cambridge University.

Janzen, John. 1978. *Quest for Therapy*. Berkeley: University of California.

——. 1979. "Pluralistic Legitimation of Therapy Systems in Contemporary Zaire." In *African Therapeutic Systems*, 208–16, edited by Z. A. Ademuwagun et al. Waltham, MA: African Studies Association.

Johannessen, Helle. 2006. "Introduction." In *Multiple Medical Realities*, edited by Helle Johannessen and Imre Lazar, 1–20. New York: Berghahn.

Kaufman, Sharon. 1988. "Toward a Phenomenology of Boundaries of Medicine." *Medical Anthropology Quarterly* 2: 338–54.

Kleinman, Arthur. 1988. *The Illness Narratives*. New York: Basic Books.

Kleinman, Arthur, and Joan Kleinman. 1994. "How Bodies Remember." *New Literary History* 25: 707–23.

Langwick, Stacey. 2011. *Bodies, Politics and African Healing*. Bloomington: Indiana University.

Lewis, Gilbert. 2000. *A Failure of Treatment*. Oxford: Oxford University.

Mattingly, Cheryl. 1998. *Healing Drams and Clinical Plots*. Cambridge: Cambridge University.

McCaskie, T. C. 1981. "Anti-Witchcraft Cults in Asante." *History in Africa* 8: 125–54.

——. 1995. *State and Society in Precolonial Asante*. Cambridge: Cambridge University.

——. 2000. *Asante Identities*. London: Edinburgh University.

Morris, Kelly. 2011. "Collaboration Works to Improve Stroke Outcomes in Ghana." *Lancet* 377: 1639–40.

Sargent, Carolyn. 1989. *Maternity, Medicine, and Power*. Berkeley: University of California.

Scheper-Hughes, Nancy, and Margaret Lock. 1987. "The Mindful Body." *Medical Anthropology Quarterly* 1: 6–41.

Schrempf, Mona. 2011. "Between Mantra and Syringe." In *Medicine between Religion and Science*, edited by Vincanne Adams, Mona Schrempf, and Sienna Craig, 220-245. New York: Berghahn.

Twumasi, P. A. 1975. *Medical Systems in Ghana*. Tema: Ghana Publishing Corp.

Warren, D. M. 1979. "Bono Traditional Healers." In *African Therapeutic Systems*, edited by Z. A. Ademuwagun et al, 120–24. Waltham, MA: African Studies Association.

Wiredu, Kwasi. 1980. *Philosophy and an African Culture*. Cambridge: Cambridge University.

Zimmermann, Francis. 2014. "Medical Individualism and the Dividual Person." In *Asymmetrical Conversations*, edited by Harish Naraindas, Johannes Quack, and William Sax, 85–117. New York: Berghahn.

3 Spirits and Pills Who Are Against Children

Medico-Rituals and Assisted Reproductive Technologies in a Tuareg Couple's Quest for Parenthood

Susan J. Rasmussen

RESEARCH HAS DEMONSTRATED the reality of medical pluralism, as well as local moral worlds accompanying the spread of Western biomedical technologies (C. Good 1987, Green 1999, Kleinman 1992, Sargent 2007), whose encounters affect illness etiologies and treatments (Boddy 1989; Rasmussen 1995, 2001, 2006; Sargent in Inhorn 2007, 165–82). Local cosmologies, philosophies, and technologies are neither compartmentalized nor isolated from religion, "magic," or science— these latter now widely recognized to be Western categories (Houndtondji 1997; Rasmussen 2006, 2013; Tambiah 1990; West 2007). Moral subjectivities as well as infrastructure systems powerfully shape local concepts of reproduction, its disruptions, and responses to them (Clarke 2009; Inhorn 2007; Moore, Sanders, and Kaare 1999). This essay examines the meanings, consequences, and responses to childlessness among rural Tuareg in Niger, where human and extrahuman (bodily/organic and spiritual/cosmological) forces play important causal roles. There is an illustrative longitudinal case study of a rural Tuareg married couple's long-term quest for a child, as yet unfulfilled but still hopeful, as they navigate through local medico-ritual and biomedical etiology and treatments and ponder alternative theories of the causes of their childlessness, over an approximately thirty-year span in the Air Mountain region in northern Niger. Relevant here are prevalent local cultural concepts of gender/sexuality; childbearing; and organic, spiritual, and social causation.

Tuareg (or Kel Tamajaq) are predominantly rural, seminomadic, Muslim, traditionally stratified. They speak Tamajaq, a Berber (or Amazigh) language, and follow bilateral property inheritance, with high social prestige and economic independence for most women and much free social interaction between the sexes. My purpose here is not to generalize definitively about Tuareg culture on the basis of a case study but, rather, to show how this particular case resonates with and departs from prevalent local cultural values, specialists' knowledge, and, more broadly, medical anthropological findings on reproductive technologies and symbolic anthropological theories of pollution/contagion. The Tuareg data shows associations, but also divergences, between biomedicine and local moral systems.

Assisted reproductive technologies (ARTs), including artificial and partly artificial methods, are widely used in diverse cultural settings to achieve pregnancy. Yet as Roberts (2012) points out, with few exceptions (Inhorn 2003, 236–56; Sargent in Inhorn 2007, 170), less attention has been paid to proliferation of ARTs in poorer countries where, historically, outsiders have been more preoccupied with spacing children among the poor than with infertility. Worldwide, women's inability to bear children can be a source of intense heartache, stigma, shame, and even divorce. Also relevant here, I show, is the problem of men's sterility (admittedly a Western allopathic concept, which, while reluctantly recognized by the husband eventually in the case study here, was not seen by many in his community as a strictly somatic or bodily condition). Ways in which childlessness is socially defined for both sexes yield insights: for Tuareg men, as well, this can be a source of personal heartache, social stigma, shame, and even marital tension, if not always divorce. Thus parenthood and childlessness—as order and disorder—among Tuareg, as elsewhere (Brandes 1980, Guttman 1996, Inhorn 2003), include local understandings not solely of local femininities and concepts of motherhood, but also of masculinities and fatherhood.

Ethnographic Background and Theoretical Framework: Preliminary Overview

Among the Kel Ewey group within the Kel Air Tuareg confederation, who reside in the Air Mountain region near the Bagzan Massif in northern Niger, residents do not always blame solely the woman for a couple's childlessness but recognize that either the man or the woman, and additional causal agents beyond, may be responsible. Like most Muslims in the Middle East (Clarke 2009, 44), most Tuareg understand that the production of children requires sexual intercourse and that the man, as well as the woman, plays a role in this process. Secularly educated Tuareg know of semen or sperm, which they usually refer to in French and which can alternatively be translated approximately as "seeds" or "origins" in Tamajaq (*aghasen*). But most residents state that the man's "heat" (Tamajaq, *tarraf*) makes the woman pregnant. Sperm donation to an ovum, unlike in some other Muslim communities where it is forbidden and associated with adultery (Clarke 2009), in the Air region does not yet arise as a debated issue, since most people in Niger cannot afford such services.

The role of the woman in conception and reproduction is also important; some Tuareg colloquially compare the woman who conceives to a kind of leather sack, though others also emphasize love as the main source of conception and pregnancy. Thus, in contrast to what Delaney (1991) reports in a Turkish village, where the man is the seed and the origin of the child and the woman is the soil and a kind of container, the Tuareg meaning of "leather sack" on closer scrutiny differs slightly, for this view of the woman as a leather sack refers more to the important role of women in working hides (in leatherwork and tents) than to women as mere receptacles. The uterus is conceptualized as a "child's tent" (*ehan n barar*), not a mere container, and this alludes to married women's ownership of the tent. As in some other Muslim communities, shared milk is a female substance. A pre-Islamic matrilineal legal category distinctive to Tuareg, however, is *akh ihuderan*, "living milk herds," a property endowment passed to daughters, sisters, and nieces as an alternative to Qur'anic inheritance.

Despite the impacts of intermittent wars, displacements, labor migrations, droughts, and economic upheavals, most Tuareg women still enjoy relatively high social prestige and some degree of economic and legal independence, (Claudot-Hawad 1993, Rasmussen 2009). Rape and wife-beating are rare. Free sociability, conversation, and visiting between the sexes are accepted, even culturally valued. Local residents do not necessarily suspect any physical intimacy between a man and a woman because they visit each other or work together.

Tuareg couples do not always divorce in cases of childlessness, even if it is interpreted as caused by the wife's infertility, but the husband may become polygynous—a form of marriage permitted in Islam, but until recently opposed by most women and less prevalent than monogamy in Tuareg society (Rasmussen 2010). Yet in contrast to some other societies, a man's sterility is the source of greater social stigma and public insult. Why, exactly? Significant here are both somatic and extrasomatic forces: human, spirit, and organic—all these constitute powers that are locally recognized, at different times, as responsible for childlessness, and remedies can shift over time.

Many rural persons believe that childlessness is contagious. I analyze exactly how and why, its consequence, biomedical and medico-ritual means of coping with childlessness, and the wider implications for theories of pollution and causation in (cultural) medical anthropology and anthropology of religion. Fundamental to understanding these processes is an analytical framework integrating the medical, the moral, and the symbolic. The attribution of responsibility and blame, the Tuareg case shows, can change over time and can include both organic and moral causation—not solely one or the other, though moral causation is powerful because it can shape interpretations of organic conditions, expressed both literally and symbolically. Also illuminating here are local residents' responses to this researcher's own childlessness, in a mutual construction of ethnographic knowledge concerning pollution/contagion, viewed by many Tuareg, I argue, as absolutely central to childlessness.

As Inhorn (2007, 28) points out, moral decisions are part and parcel of gendered health experiences; hence the importance of highlighting local moralities. Many studies show the importance of official, mainstream (state-sponsored, organized) religious ideas concerning reproductive technologies. Kahn (2000) describes how male rabbis in Israel legislate on the appropriate uses of new reproductive technologies for their followers. Inhorn (2003, 2007) shows how in Egypt, Sunni Islamic religious authorities have issued *fatwas* prohibiting many new reproductive technologies found in neighboring Israel.

Clarke (2008) observes, regarding Islam, that "while the Shariah is eternal and universal (in the officially dominant Islamic scholars' view, I would add), the production and consumption of Islamic jurisprudential literature are very much local and contextual" (Clarke 2008, 8). Less understood are more "unofficial," popular local religions, sciences, and technologies concerning reproductive health and their connection to the uses of medico-ritual and reproductive technologies—these latter may be used simultaneously or sequentially, or one or the other may be delayed. Local cultural interpretations of Islam are important in etiologies and treatments of organic and nonorganic illnesses (Bernus 1969; Nicolaisen 1961; Rasmussen 1995, 2001, 2006) among most Tuareg, who converted to Sunni and Malaki Islam, with Sufi influences from North African marabouts between the eighth and eleventh centuries. Most residents oppose recently encroaching Wahabist/Salafist piety reformist movements. The uses of amulets, visits to shrines, and spirit possession rituals are common, the latter disapproved of but tolerated by most Tuareg Islamic scholars, popularly called "marabouts." Although Islamic scholars/marabouts prohibit neither pre-(popular) Islamic medico-rituals nor most biomedical ARTs in the diagnosis and treatment of childlessness, they tend to favor local medico-rituals, including their own Qur'anic healing. They do not, however, forbid couples from consulting western allopathic reproductive technologies, though as I show, some frown on contraceptive pills. In Niger thus far, primarily oral (pill) hormonal treatments are available (both to space children and to enhance reproduction), and only to those who can afford to travel to the few hospitals in major towns. This essay explores the wider implications of these attitudes and practices in relation to a therapeutic continuum, as well as therapeutic gaps in uncertain access to medical pluralism. Tuareg concepts of pollution and other notions of causality, local healing specialists, and wider health care options play important roles in diagnosing and treating childlessness.

As Moore (1999, 1) points out, in many African societies there is an abiding concern with sexual morality, the power of sex, and issues of sexual access and denial. The larger context for this concern is the relationship between body processes and social—and I would add moral—processes. Since, as noted, many Tuareg, including the married couple featured in the case study, believe that childlessness is contagious, local religious and scientific theories of causation guiding the etiology and treatment of childlessness are as important to analyze as the availability and accessibility of biomedical reproductive technologies. Masquelier (2005, 10–11) observes that dirt is a situational rather than substantive category and can only be defined in relation to a system of order, albeit not in a static sense. Purity is about the strategic capacity to project a virtuous public image. This, I show, is crucial to Tuareg concepts of gendered prestige and honor, and in local cultural interpretation, having a "normal" child affirms such prestige and honor, and not having children or having an anomalous or disabled child is evidence of not following cultural rules. In other words, one must appear to follow moral rules, and fertility or infertility are outward manifestations of doing so or not doing so. Breaking rules implies violating categorical boundaries, in Tuareg society, specifically, breaking sexual taboos or neglecting social or ritual obligations. Filth may be sin, and those who engage in morally suspect activities are considered dirty and in need of cleansing. Prevalent Tuareg concepts of fertility, infertility, sterility, parenthood, and childlessness, and local uses of plural medical treatments, I contend, have a direct relation to purity/pollution/contagion, as expressed in the order, interrupted order, and disruptions in individuals' lives and the life of their community and region more generally.

First, it is instructive to describe health care and healing alternatives in northern Niger.

Health Care and Healing Specialists in Northern Niger

A number of diagnostic and treatment alternatives in the Air region of northern Niger are available, though many are expensive, irregular, and/or hard to access geographically. As elsewhere outside the capital city, Niamey, and major towns, biomedical allopathic health care is limited. There are clinics, private practices, and hospitals in the northern towns of Agadez and Arlit, with doctors trained in western biomedicine. These institutions were state-sponsored until the IMF and World Bank restructuring policies in the 1980s but are largely privatized now. There are also biomedically trained "lay" first-aid workers (*secouristes*), nurses (*infirmiers*), and mobile immunization units. In the Air countryside, there are now also a few clinics, but supplies are erratic because of rough roads and political violence.

Attitudes toward hospitals and clinics have changed much over the past few decades: until very recently, most rural people were afraid of them as places of death or considered them lacking in sympathy (Rasmussen 2001). More rural patients now come to the Agadez hospital, usually after local healers advise antibiotics or surgery. Still, many remain ambivalent toward hospital staffs' requiring women giving birth to lie down on a table (contrary to the usual Tuareg preference, of kneeling on soft sand). Some patients conceal "shameful" illnesses (*tawarna n idwaden*) at first (for example, suspected STD's), only later seeking hospital treatments.

Traditional Tuareg healing specialists usually acquire skills through inheritance and apprenticeship and treat sometimes overlapping organic and nonorganic illnesses. Islamic scholars/marabouts (*ineslemen*) heal predominantly nonorganic illnesses with Qur'anic verses and amulets and conduct psychosocial counseling. Herbal medicine women (*tinesmegelen*) primarily diagnose and heal stomach ailments and "hot/cold" illnesses with leaves, bark, roots, and therapeutic massages; they also conduct some marital counseling (Rasmussen 2006). A few divine by dreaming (*timaswaden* or *timanai*), and some have been trained as midwives by the Agadez hospital. Non-Qur'anic diviners (*bokaye*) divine and treat with perfume, cowry shells, and mirrors. Bonesetters (*imadasen*) treat fractures, sprains, and broken bones. A trance possession exorcism ritual (*tende-n-goumaten*) with predominantly female adepts features musical and group therapy (Rasmussen 1995).

In this wider context, I follow a married couple's journey of interpreting and treating their childlessness over a thirty-year time period.

The Childlessness of a Married Couple

Adama and Atakor

Adama and Atakor (pseudonyms) were a married couple with whom I sometimes lodged during several field research trips to rural Niger. The husband, Atakor, often assisted me with transcriptions and interviews. After returning home from my earlier (doctoral) fieldwork, I had kept up contact with the couple, exchanging letters. They had married around 1986—the same year that I married back home. We congratulated each other on our marriages, and I sent them a wedding present. Around 1991, while I was lodging with them in another research project, the wife, Adama, asked me, "Do you have any medicine for having children?" I regretfully said no, I did not. Many local residents worried about my own childlessness, as well. Upon my return to Niger after an absence of some years, many were upset that I still did not have children, essential for help with work, old age support, and familial continuity.

Although Tuareg women's roles involve much more than childbearing, motherhood is highly valued. Many clans trace their descent to matrilineal female ancestors predating Islam. Loss of herds, sedentarization of nomads, and more oasis gardening have brought new pressures on women to bear more children to assist with work. Some more prosperous men are contracting polygynous marriages for prestige purposes and also in cases of a childless first wife. Since droughts and wars have devastated much livestock, an important source of women's wealth, many wives have become economically more dependent upon the male household head, and fewer can afford to opt out of a polygynous marriage (Rasmussen 2009).

Adama asked me if I knew what causes a delay in having children. I tried to help by suggesting the need for a balanced diet and rest, difficult to achieve in practice, I inwardly noted, given the arduous work and irregular food situation in her community.

By 1991, Atakor had begun settling down to oasis gardening. They were residing virilocally in Atakor's natal village, permitted following initial uxorilocal residence and completion of bridewealth and groomservice obligations.

Adama and Atakor both had some formal education. They had been among the first children in their region to complete primary school at a time when most parents opposed secular schools. In addition to their first language, Tamajaq, both also spoke Hausa and French. Adama related how she had been forcibly taken by soldiers to primary school but later enjoyed it. After graduating first in his primary school and also finishing Qur'anic school, Atakor did caravanning and herding for a time. Then he went to Lagos, Nigeria, where he worked as a security guard at an embassy. In the late 1980s, he returned home and worked for a livestock distribution and veterinary project.

Atakor, a brilliant local intellectual with insightful exegesis of Tuareg culture, was a member of a prestigious maraboutique and chiefly family of aristocratic social background. He was marginal in only one way: his childlessness. For this, a few men and women occasionally mocked him. He was also somewhat fragile physically, with intermittent health problems that compelled him to seek medical attention often, at first usually from local healers in his rural seminomadic, agropastoral village. Yet he was an active member of his community, respected by most for his intellect, resourcefulness, and accomplishments. He often held leadership positions in cooperatives and other projects.

Physical strength is widely valued in Tuareg men as it is necessary to withstand the rigors of traditional herding, caravanning, raiding, and nomadic wandering across the desert. But character traits are also valued, such as respect/reserve, religious devotion, cleverness, verbal conversational skill, and a dignified and graceful appearance in both men and women—especially in tasteful dress and in men's careful styling of the men's turban/faceveil (Loughran and Seligman 2005).

Men are expected to be respectful and protective of women, elders, and children. Since children are the external manifestation of social and moral prestige, childlessness, birth defects, and other reproductive misfortunes reveal possible violation of certain sexual and other taboos by parents, discouraging those afflicted thus from seeking medical help initially until greater social pressures compel it. Fatherhood is also highly valued, and childless men are as unhappy as childless women. Fatherhood is bound up with social prestige, virility, masculinity, and moral personhood.

By 1991, a series of droughts and the outbreak of the 1990–1995 rebellion caused massive flights and returns of refugees, most dispossessed and unemployed. Residents near Mt. Bagzan built solid mud walls around compounds, installed doors with locks on tents and houses, and used powerful amulets. Atakor placed an amulet on the door of his storehouse, which repelled thieves by reportedly causing the intruders to lose their way, and made an amulet to protect me, as well. There were no clinics yet in the villages around Mt. Bagzan in Air. But there were diverse local healers and a few first-aid workers there.

In the mid-1990s, Adama traveled to the town of Agadez to train as a first-aid *secouriste* in a program run by a French health care worker who explained basic biomedical first-aid remedies and their uses and provided her with a small first-aid kit in a metal box.

Before we knew it, it was 1995, and I returned to the field. Hoping to find advice on childbearing matters, Adama read a small book in Hausa by a marabout based in Kano, Nigeria, sold in Agadez, Niger, offering guidelines and advice for Muslim women on how to be a proper wife and mother. She kept this on a table next to her first-aid kit. She related how in the early 1990s she underwent a gynecological examination at the Agadez hospital, but the staff found no precise cause of her childlessness, and moreover, she did not like the procedure or the personnel, who she felt were "not nice to rural people," and required her to obtain a notebook and an ID card and to buy expensive medicine at the pharmacy.

Later, Adama was diagnosed by the Agadez hospital as having a stomach or ovarian cyst. In Tuareg science of the body, the stomach, uterus, and ovaries are located inside the same sack, and though herbal medicine women healers know Tamajaq terms to distinguish between stomach (*tedis*) and womb (*ehan n arraw/ barar*, literally "the child's tent"), most persons colloquially tend to gloss all these as *tedis* (stomach). As in much western science, they extend this term metaphorically to convey matrilineality, as for example in the term for womb referring obliquely to the female-owned nuptial tent, where babies are born and children are traditionally educated by mothers in local cultural knowledge. Adama reluctantly had emergency surgery in the Agadez hospital for this ailment, which she called a "stomach" problem (in Tamajaq) and Atakor called a cyst (in French). The couple blamed this as a possible cause of childlessness at that point. Adama later stopped drinking tea and underwent a medicine woman's herbal treatment with plant remedies reputed to make a woman fatter and thereby increase fertility, but to no avail.

In 1995, this couple still remained childless, and so did I. I heard several men tease Atakor, at times caustically, "You have no baby!" Once, as we ate a meal and drank tea in Adama's village, one of her sisters discovered that I had no child, and teased, "If you eat with this man [referring to her brother-in-law, Atakor, who was present], you'll never have children!"

Local symbols and rituals make analogies between saliva and sexual fluids, food and sex, and mouth and genitals. These analogies guided some local residents who attributed both my own and Atakor's childlessness to contagion/pollution from our sharing food and utensils. Some "womanizing" men are believed to have excess saliva, analogous to sperm (a Tamajaq expression says, "The [men's] faceveil and the trousers are brothers," both of these representing modesty for men). If a woman does not eat a lot, some surmise that she does not like men (Rasmussen 2010). Usually, food is an aphrodisiac that confers female fertility, but here the obstacle appeared to be the polluting counterforce from a childless male. There is also a local concept approximating microbes, *izufnen*, recognized by some specialists such as herbal medicine women, though no one diagnosed the cause of childlessness in this way.

Atakor, in the meantime, felt that some of his health problems might be at least indirectly causing his childlessness. He appeared thinner and suffered from a chipped or impacted molar tooth. He was treated by an herbal medicine woman's heated *ilaten* (a concoction combining several different medicinal plants), a biomedical painkiller, and a topical basic (nonprescription) first-aid gel I offered him. However, he attributed the cause of this toothache not to an organic condition or microbial cause but rather to economic jealousy and coveting by others. He explained, "for example, if someone with *togerchet* (evil mouth or eye) sees how many date pits you leave and then gossips about how much you eat, this can give you a toothache." Because of intermittent adversity, self-restraint and generosity to others with food are important cultural values. *Togerchet*, that pervasive motivating fear, in general a gloss for unpleasant destructive gossip, can be caused by jealousy and coveting, hoarding, greed, and guilt, often involving food. This married couple in their relative (albeit fluctuating) economic success, especially Atakor, frequently fretted about this and sought medicines and amulets to combat it, as well as its possible consequence of childlessness.

Indeed, around the same time, he and his wife grew increasingly anxious over their childlessness. For this problem, multiple organic and nonorganic forces were considered as potential culprits. For a while, Atakor vacillated between blaming forces from outside, himself, and his wife. He had a female artisanal smith make a red leather amulet to promote reproductive force. He also saw the family's Islamic scholar healer who specialized in *itran alekhustara*, a horoscope-like divining consultation. Atakor also pondered whether this childlessness was caused by an *akirkiwi*, a type of sorcerer from outside Tuareg society, whose power, "witchcraft-like," can be automatically activated, who sucked his blood while he was once at the Niamey SNTN bus station during his travels. He explained, "Around my return (home), I fell ill for one month. Men and women in certain families (*ikarkawen*, or in Hausa *sarkin mayou*) inherit this power, and sometimes use it as an aphrodisiac (*mahiba*)." Despite the importance of nomadism, caravanning, and migrant labor, travel is fraught with dangers. Some men fear they may contract illnesses from strange women while traveling; most recently, some explain contraction of HIV in this way.

Some weeks later, after a lengthy conversation in private with a very elderly herbal medicine woman, who, following this consultation, asked me why I was childless (I gave my usual reply: "I am not sure. I like children. I guess that Allah (God) did not give me any. Or maybe it is because I travel so much"), Atakor indicated with some relief that he was "in good form," and did not believe childlessness was his own fault. Perhaps there was a force around that did not like children?

Following Adama's gynecological consultation in the Agadez hospital and Atakor's additional consultations with other herbalists and a non-Qur'anic *boka* diviner/healer, he acknowledged, reluctantly, that childlessness was perhaps not his wife's fault, but his own: from his *tessmut*, a "cold" illness in the local humoral/thermal classification system (Fiore and Walet Faqqi 1993). This required a "hot" treatment to counteract it. Young Tuareg men should ideally be hot, not cold (though not too hot), and young (childbearing-age) women should be cold, not hot (though not too cold) in balanced bodily health, character, and temperament—the organic and nonorganic are not rigidly divided in local science. Most *tessmut* illnesses in men tend to be in the urinary and/or genital area. The counteractive cure requires no bathing for one week and drinking warm, not cold water, to reinforce plant medicines. But since one cannot touch the genital area during that week's treatment, Atakor was reluctant to do this cure during the hot season.

Then events took a different turn. Atakor returned to the elderly herbal medicine woman he had earlier consulted, and she referred the couple to an Islamic scholar/marabout, who conducted a ritual that, in effect, transferred the responsibility for childlessness to Adama, and on another level, subtly, that ritual also included me as a focus of concern.

This ritual, an infertility consultation, diagnosis, and treatment focusing overtly on Adama, took place in the morning. In advance, the couple gave the marabout 20,000 CFA ($50). First, the marabout calculated numbers based on the married couple's names. He spat (to conduct his *al baraka* blessing power) three times on a measuring cord. He then measured Adama's forearm length and waist with this cord, and calculated the measurements in the sand. The cord appeared to have grown in length. According to the marabout, "this means that the woman is less than fertile. The cause (of this condition) is a blocking from Western biomedical pills and spirits who are against children, and they have caused Adama to become diminished and lacking (in fertility)."

Next, the marabout sacrificed a white male goat of Adama's, its meat to be eaten by the family and the marabout. They must not dry it, for this undoes the treatment. The opposition here between wetness and dryness corresponds to the Tuareg and some other African peoples' (for example, northern Sudanese) (Boddy 1987) notions of reproductive qualities: wetness is associated with fertility and dryness with infertility. Adama was to eat the lungs of the animal, suggesting breath and life. In Tuareg cosmology/philosophy/medical science, the intestines and liver (*tessa*), which are considered a seat of strong sentiments such as love and anger, were cooked with a little fat in a pot. Significantly, the intestines and liver were not grilled, since the pot is iconic in representing the woman's stomach, which, as noted, together with the uterus, in Tuareg medical concepts, contains the child. The family ate this meat first, and later they would consume the rest of the meat in the couple's compound. In three days, the couple was to drink vegetal ink verses from the Qur'an that the marabout would prepare. Its writing must be on a fresh tablet, an allusion to newness and youth. Then the couple would eat three soft-boiled, shelled eggs with the same Qur'anic verse writing on them. This process must be repeated three more times afterward. If successful, the married couple would give the marabout 15,000 CFA more (about $45) as payment later.

Toward the conclusion of this ritual, the marabout turned to me, asked my age, and said he wanted to do a calculation (*lisafe*) for me, also, at some time in the future "to see if all is in good condition." Here, the moral and the somatic are not separated. He explained, "childlessness or (having) few children runs through women in certain families; it is inherited (*gado marawen*)." Here, the focus shifted to several means of transmitting childlessness: fictive kinship with the anthropologist/guest; and matrilineal inheritance, a kind of physical counterpart (in a woman's infertility) of diminished *akh ihuderan* livestock property, which contrasts to (and in its positive endowments, counterbalances) the more general patrilineal Islamic/Qur'anic legal and medical bias. In effect, the woman, like some herds, was diagnosed as "dried up." This exonerated Atakor and his patriline from blame. Yet at the same time, the marabout also alleviated Adama's guilt somewhat, in also mentioning the possible role of biomedical pills— possibly, birth control pills, since many Tuareg believe that these may cause problems later in conceiving (though I do not know whether or not Adama took those; it is doubtful, given her wishes for a child). Hence the recognition of the possible ill effects of technology on fertility—birth control pills disrupt a woman's (and by extension, the matriline's) reproductivity, and matrilineal spirits (prominent in trees yielding herbalists' fertility medicines) might be angry, perhaps from competition! There may also have been some fear of other humans' possible jealousy of Adama and me and our friendship, though I never heard confirmation of this.

At the ritual's *takote* (sacrificial offering) meat consumption, I was served apart in separate bowls and utensils—very unusual for me in that household. Did this have to do with my own childlessness and the common belief that if one eats with childless person, they cannot ever have children? Here, symbolic pollution and also literal contagion were simultaneously at play, as well as the organic and the inorganic, thereby blending concepts of metaphorical and figurative that are sometimes opposed in anthropology (Green 1999, West 2007). Indeed, some persons in that community felt that sharing food with a childless person might transmit childlessness through eating together and using the same utensils.

Throughout all this, both during the immediate ritual and later, over the long term, complex processes were occurring. The symbolism was embodied and stemmed from somatic/corporeal experiences but referred to social and moral concerns. Recent anthropological accounts of symbolism and ritual (Gottleib 1993, Masquelier 2005, Moore et al. 1999, West 2007) have emphasized that the sets of symbols, including purity/pollution oppositions, are part of a logic that underpins a philosophy of social and natural continuity and reproduction forged by the demands and requirements of everyday life. If the maternal body and images of a cooking pot and breath (lungs) undergird the female contribution to fertility and childbearing, and gardening and caravanning are the contribution of the male, images of livestock in the sacrificed animal underpin both sexes' contribution—an equalizing balance here that corresponds to the Tuareg ideal of both women's and men's sharing of reproductive responsibility.

Although the ritual on the surface addressed primarily Adama's presumed condition of infertility, perhaps caused by hostile spirits; there were hints that it also addressed the need to protect both women and men from possible outside contagion: the possibility of contagion/pollution from Western biomedical pills and from my own childlessness—or vice versa, contagion/pollution to me from theirs, and also perhaps some external human social malevolence polluting me, or them, and passed onto a third party. There was no hostility toward me, nor were direct statements to that effect made by either Adama or Atakor, only by others: healers and bystanders. Childlessness involves contagion and/or pollution (on a literal-figurative continuum) between childless persons that can be either reinforced or combated and may combine with other more external social and other extrasomatic forces in various times and places. Local women friends would often stare at me and muse pensively, "You do not have children. Atakor does not have any children."

Update: Later and Most Recent Developments

1998 saw late rains, scorching heat, and a malaria epidemic, and sporadic fighting—post-peace accords—persisted between the national army and some dissident rebel forces. No births took place for one entire month, a circumstance rare in that community. The couple fled attacks on Atakor's village and again resided uxorilocally near Adama's parents in their smaller seminomadic camp farther up the mountain, but more long term and indefinitely, and in a smaller compound than previously. Atakor started another garden in his wife's village but kept the compound in his natal village. He earned extra income by renting camels to tourists in the region's peaceful intervals. Adama had become skilled in tailoring and continued to practice as a *secouriste*. In moving to flee political violence, some couples' postmarital residence arrangements had been permanently altered. Atakor and some other men found themselves under greater authority of their parents-in-law later in their marriage, the opposite from usual after initial uxorilocality, when they can choose to move away for greater independence. This predicament, in addition to childlessness, threatened Atakor's male pride. Also, overcrowding of lands around Atakor's home village compelled him and other men to plant gardens farther out, and women to graze their small herds farther out to find good feed.

By 2001, Atakor's natal village had become more sedentarized, with fewer tents. Livestock had much diminished, especially the "living milk" matrilineal endowments for younger women. Adama had only seven ewes and two small sheep left; her other animals had died. The longstanding Tuareg connections between fertility of herds and humans became even more precarious. Now the fertility of women and men became more connected to that of the land and crops. Some Islamic scholars warned during droughts that Allah had withdrawn *al baraka* from the land and herds in Air because of the sins (*ibakaden*) of humans. Soon after my return, women at a baby's nameday welcomed me warmly but asked me many questions regarding my husband, my childlessness, whether I had a co-wife, and whether I feared my husband would contract a polygynous marriage while I was in the field. Perhaps this was also their way of showing empathy for the anthropologist's loneliness in separations from loved ones during intermittent visits to the field.

One afternoon, while a female artisanal smith styled Adama's hair, Atakor's cousin joked that he needed a second wife, since Adama had still not yet become pregnant or given birth after several years' marriage. Atakor joked back with his cousin that she should give him her younger sister in marriage. Later on, as we prepared dinner, Adama asked whether we have polygyny in the United States. I replied, "no, but we do have divorce." She thought for a moment, and then, mournfully, commented that, "even if the first wife divorces her husband who contracts a polygynous marriage, she eventually goes back to him because she is sad." I later learned that Atakor was in fact beginning negotiations for a second wife.

In the interim between my 2002 and 2012 field trips to Niger, I conducted two research projects in northern Mali. I wondered: would Adama and Atakor remain childless during my absence, or would they succeed in having a child? Would they consider these events—whatever occurred—to be a coincidence, a concept that in Evans-Pritchard's classic observation, is absent among the Azande (1937)? The concept of coincidence does exist among Tuareg, but the Tamajaq term (*elquisat*) is rarely mentioned.

After my return to Niger in 2012, Atakor related to me how a local man had hurtfully insulted him by saying that he was "not a man" because he still had no child. Men and women count children as important workers and capital—symbolic as well as material—in the more prevalent oasis gardening economy. In the political violence, social turmoil, and widespread unemployment in their regions, many Tuareg men face challenges to longstanding values exhorting men to protect women and children. Despite some economic success, Atakor felt unhappy because he could not completely fulfill these ideals as long as he remained childless. Thus there were external pressures on him to reaffirm his masculine pride through polygyny.

Yet the causes, diagnoses, and cures for childlessness could still be continually negotiated and reinterpreted. Cultural concepts of reproductive health and dangers to it, wider changes in their community, and this couple's "trial and error" strategies—were based on not solely medical pluralism availability, but also local religion and science—had all prompted Atakor, now in his early forties, to move Adama back to her natal village permanently, work his second garden more intensively, and contract his polygynous marriage. His second wife, Toua, who has also remained childless, resides in his natal village. Atakor now divides his time between two households, two villages, and two gardens.

Atakor and Adama, like many other residents, became aware of additional treatment options (many beyond their means) in wider communication networks and health programs. Yet Atakor still drew on local cultural models, not solely western allopathic biomedicine. Even when, around 2011, he was tested at the hospital in Zinder, a town in southern Niger, by a biomedical gynecological and urological specialist who found his sperm count to be low or, as Atakor described it, "not (sufficiently) matured," Atakor still worried about an additional possible source of childlessness: contagion/pollution. He commented to me, "People here think childlessness is the fault of the childless person; for example, they think that I work with Europeans (many of whom appear to local residents as childless during their stay in Niger, and thus polluting/contagious) on purpose, so as not to have children." Here, again, the concern was with moral/social rules of prestige, and with wider polluting forces.

The doctor in Zinder referred Atakor to another specialist in Niamey, who prescribed a western hormonal medication, which he instructed Atakor to take for the second two weeks of each month after the wife's menstrual period. This medication was very expensive, and I contributed a sum of money to help. Yet this new development raised an issue: Atakor, as noted, now has two wives, and so he is obliged to organize his schedule accordingly but faces the challenge of minimizing the jealousy of his co-wives over his residential arrangements with each and also, now, the added rivalry over the medicine and who would benefit more from this reproductive technology! Here, Western science and technology's efficacy depended upon local moral and social considerations, not vice versa. Most Tuareg polygynists ideally are supposed to alternate for two days' duration between villages of different co-wives, not several weeks' duration. Moreover, there was the psychological stress of discovering that, after all these years and polygynous marriage as a last resort, Adama and Toua were not, in fact, the causes of childlessness.

Here it is instructive to examine more generally held local theories of gender, sexuality, and reproduction that enhance understanding of this updated case.

The Wider Context

Gender, Sexuality, Reproduction, and Protecting Maternal-Child Health; and Local Integration of Philosophy/Cosmology and Science/Technology

In Tuareg society, men are supposed to protect women, and everyone is supposed to protect children. There are numerous and elaborate concepts focusing on maternal and child health. Theories of pregnancy and childbirth express a preoccupation with the vulnerability of women and children, especially to spirit and human dangers, and promote many ritual restrictions to protect them. A child born after a sibling's death is given the name of an animal such as Eggur (jackal) or called Ekli/Teklit (slave) in order to distract spirits so they do not take away this child, too. If one has children of all the same sex and then has one of the opposite sex, this child is given the name of an animal, plant, or rock so the spirits do not take him/her. Twins should be treated exactly the same. Pregnant women should avoid bitter medicines (from tree bark), potatoes, and coffee (these cause *tuksi,* hot illnesses), avoid dishes with salt, and "heavy" foods like dates, wheat, and milk because they make the stomach "dirty" (*ta jerga*) and cause a baby to grow too heavy, causing a difficult birth (Rasmussen 2006). Women should wear amulets against the Kel Essuf spirits of the wild during their period because these may take away menstruation, and childlessness and solitude ensue.

Many Tuareg, including marabouts (as shown) believe that a woman conceives with great difficulty if she has taken local contraceptive herbal plants and/ or Western biomedical birth control pills, which are believed to cause infertility later in life. This attitude, widespread in many Islamic societies (Clarke 2009), favors marriage and a husband and wife both jointly participating in reproductive matters, rather than an unmarried person managing reproduction (whether contraception or ARTs) independently, outside marriage. By contrast, in many non-Muslim African communities, the widespread valuing of a woman's fertility and reproduction encourages acceptance of a woman bearing a child outside marriage (Moore, Sanders, and Kaare 1999). Thus far, in contrast to a case in northern Nigeria, there have been no rumors in northern Niger of inoculations against polio causing infertility in women. Rather, many residents indicated to me that women have problems in pregnancy because they continue to do hard physical work.

There is much fear of childlessness and infant mortality (the latter a problem in rural Niger generally), as well as anomalies and disabilities. These are considered shameful and are widely attributed to the parents' violating protective sexual taboos. Sexual intercourse in the wrong place (e.g., outside the nuptial tent under direct moonlight or even inside a breezeway or doorframe) is thought to make children turn out crazy or deaf, though the sorcery of a parent's enemy can also do this. Several healers attributed albinism to having sex during the woman's menstrual period. Healers warn that if one does something bad to a pregnant woman, for example a husband's making his wife angry, this causes *tourgoum*, which in turn causes a birth defect (Rasmussen 2006). *Togerchet* (covetous "evil mouth/eye") may also cause muteness. Adama believed that a girl's mental disability resulted from her mother leaving her in the doorway of a compound or tent, where spirits entered the baby. Adama and many others felt it dangerous to comment that a baby looks healthy, for the latter invites *togerchet*, and may cause the baby to fall ill and die. Sometimes, a birth defect in a child is caused by spirits who have replaced the mother's child with their "changeling" child. Mostly women offer the foregoing explanations, however; men tend to insist that "only Allah does those things."

The point here is that widely held (i.e., by lay and healer interlocutors) Tuareg theories of conception, pregnancy, birth, and concepts of causation have a moral and social, as well as technological and somatic logic: they encourage actual and potential parents, including men, to practice many precautions from concerns about psychosocial and physical harm to mothers and children. Technology and science are not separate from moral obligation. These concerns have very logical bases in environmental dangers: intermittent droughts, political violence, refugee flight, and other population (and family) dispersals, uncertain and fluctuating food supplies, and social and religious tensions, and they reflect the high infant and maternal mortality rate in rural Niger. But these precautions and restrictions lead friends, kin, and rivals alike to also suspect moral, not solely physical, causes of problems with reproductive and childrearing. Even spirit-driven causes are often provoked by human social tensions, neglect of some moral obligation, or ignoring some social or moral boundary.

Although believed vulnerable during pregnancy and childbirth, women are not considered entirely weak or passive. They assert much social agency and sometimes cause misfortune or shame, and their sexuality is powerful, though not in the same sense of overall "polluting" qualities of childbearing age women, in contrast to some other societies such as Bengali India (Lamb 2000). Islamic scholars warn about the dangers of the voice and appearance of a beautiful woman and associate them with Iblis, the devil—a tempter who distracts men from prayer but who is also necessary for reproduction (Nicolaisen 1961). The Tamajaq expression "The woman is the trousers of the man," conveys the role of a wife in the husband's social prestige. Many men insist that some women are unlucky to marry because they cause a husband's herds to die and him to become poor (Rasmussen 2001). On the other hand, a few women divorced husbands with whom they had no children, suggesting active female recognition of, and measures to protect wives against, male sterility. Perhaps Atakor feared this might occur, though unlike Adama who mentioned her fear of his eventual polygyny, he did not directly state this.

Attitudes concerning sexuality and reproduction are therefore complex, and do not, in Tuareg society, feature a clear-cut double standard in which inevitably women or men are always blamed. But the bilateral descent system is nonetheless appealed to selectively in attribution of blame for the causes of childlessness. Although in some respects, as in northern Sudan (Boddy 1989), women's bodies are considered more open and vulnerable to danger, this condition varies in degree and across contexts, and women are most vulnerable to dangers during pregnancy and just following childbirth. Yet since many men tended to emphasize caution in sexual contact with outsiders—for example, contact with women in Europe during labor migration are often blamed for a Tuareg man's contracting AIDS—men and women are both vulnerable in some contexts to pollution from others—equally open to human and spirit dangers. This suggests not so much disdain for or fear of women's "impurity," but men's fear of women's sexual power, social influence, and control over men's reputations.

Discussion, Conclusion, and Broader Significance

Although ARTs have served to defamiliarize what was once understood to be the natural basis of human procreation and relatedness (Ragone 1998, 118; Clarke 2008, 31), I would add here that ARTs are not unique in this, and perhaps no human reproduction is understood as completely "natural." For the Tuareg case shows that local medico-rituals, also, can defamiliarize. Indeed, there is no un-constructed "natural" basis of human procreation anywhere or anytime, with or without biomedical ARTs. Medico-rituals, in effect, are a local science and technology, not always the "Other" in relation to ARTs, sometimes shunned, and sometimes combined with them on the therapeutic continuum by the same couple, even the same individual.

The paths taken by husband and wife were not identical, and their medical pluralism did not involve a linear sequence of abandoning one diagnostic or healing technology altogether, or replacing it with another. Etiologies and treatments for childlessness in Tuareg society are not, furthermore, reducible to neat Western biomedical or academic categories; they include overlapping symbolic (analogic/metaphorical), counteractive, "naturalistic," and "personality" systems (Kleinman 1980), often used by the same person at different times in response to wider predicaments. Medical pluralism (availability of various treatments) here is not the sole cause driving all therapy; rather, it is critically reflected upon, and is but one effect of local theories of causation. The reason is that some notions of pollution/contagion and danger in Tuareg society are situated between the organic and the inorganic, the coincidental and the intentional. Over time, this married couple's explanations and strategies derived from overlapping rather than mutually exclusive moral and organic causes. This couple (and many other persons) sometimes understood their childless predicament by referring to local and outside allopathic theories as well as their interpersonal relationships with other Tuareg and with outsiders such as travelers, guests, and "sorcerers" of different ethnicities and regions, spirits, and even this researcher—whose shared status as a nonparent—possibly both contaminated and contaminating—was the focus of much local preoccupation and commentary, despite the warm hospitality shown.

Also, importantly, in local reproductive and marital strategies intended to protect women's and children's health, masculinity is implicated. These obligations are points of honor for most men, and without the opportunity to fulfill obligations to protect women and children, a Tuareg man often feels lost, his male pride threatened, even if he is respected and successful in other contexts. Fertility and its associated taboos ensure that households are large enough for the labor required, but also more: that everything creative remains in its proper place, recalling the Beng separation of the fertility of humans and the fertility of the forest (Gottleib and Graham 1993).

Labor migration and sporadic refugee flight separate Tuareg husbands and wives for longer time periods than older subsistence travel in caravans and herding, sometimes destabilizing spousal relations and heightening concerns with maternal and child health, expressed in some taboos. In pollution and contagion, therefore, the system of order is not static, but changes according to context. There is a trial-and-error strategy of alternating between local theories and practices in response, according to local gendered concepts of social prestige and reproductive health and illness.

Atakor, until very recently, relied somewhat more than Adama on traditional medico-ritual methods; why? He may have dreaded a possible biomedical diagnosis of his low sperm count, which suggested, in local metonymy, "immature masculinity." Adama earlier on sought not only longstanding medico-ritual but also biomedical methods (e.g., at the Agadez hospital). Undoubtedly her earlier first-aid training in Agadez had exposed her more closely to Western allopathic knowledge and advice concerning gynecological matters.

But the realization of the organic/somatic basis of childlessness was still grounded in local moral concepts of causality, in that it corresponded to changes in the productivity of the land: previously dependent on the connection between fertility and herds, the Air Mountain region is now becoming more dependent on the connection between fertility and crops. At one point, this wider regional change influenced shifting of responsibility to Adama, resulting in Atakor's eventual polygyny; yet on the other hand, this trend also caused Atakor to later reflect further on his role as male household head with obligations to support wives whose herds were no longer so numerous.

These data suggest ways toward more nuanced understandings of medical pluralism in relation to pollution/contagion, from insights at the interstices of medical anthropology, symbolic anthropology, and anthropology of religion. Here, the local prognosis is complex: some things left their proper place inside the body (saliva through shared food and eating utensils) and mixed with other hosts (Masquelier 2005). Other things (sorcery and evil eye/mouth in the economic jealousy of others) improperly entered the body. Ultimately, there was an encounter between these theories and the Western biomedical diagnosis of a low sperm count or in Atakor's explanation, "immature sperm": things improperly dormant (his not yet emerged mature masculine status) in his body, and also a metaphor for a childless man's socially "childlike" status in his society.

Thus incorporating local science, philosophy/cosmology and medico-ritual into the analysis of ARTs may, one hopes, minimize the problem of slippage in anthropological endeavors to translate and compare moral systems and reproductive technologies.

Acknowledgments

In my research projects on spirit possession, aging and the life course, healing specialists and medico-ritual healing, rural and urban antisanal smiths, gender, verbal art, and youth cultures in rural and urban Tuareg communities for approximately thirty years in Niger and Mali, and briefer research among Tuareg and other Berber (Amazigh) expatriates and travelers in France and the United States, I am grateful to Fulbright-Hays, the Wenner-Gren Foundation, the Social Science Research Council, the National Geographic Society Committee for Research and Exploration, Indiana University, and the University of Houston.

Bibliography

Bernus, Edmond. 1969. "Maladies humaines et animals chez les Touaregs Saheliens." *Journal de la Societe des Africainistes* 39 (1): 111–37.

Boddy, Janice. 1987. *Wombs and Alien Spirits*. Madison: University of Wisconsin.

Brandes, Stanley. 1980. *Metaphors of Masculinity: Sex and Status in Andalusian Folklore*. Philadelphia: University of Pennsylvania.

Brett, Michael, and Elizabeth Fentress. 1997. *The Berbers*. New York: Blackwell.

Casajus, Dominique. 1995. *La Tente et l'Essuf*. Cambridge: Cambridge University.

Clarke, Morgan. 2009. *Islam and New Kinship: Reproductive Technology and the Shariah in Lebanon*. Oxford: Berghahn.

Claudot-Hawad, Helene. 1993. *Les Touaregs: Portraits en fragments*. Aix-en-Provence: Edisud.

Evans-Pritchard, E. E. 1937. *Witchcraft, Magic, and Oracles among the Azande*. Oxford: Oxford University.

Fiore, Barbara, and Fadi Wellet Faqqi. 1993. *Isefran: Maladies et soins en milieu Touareg*. Perugia, Italie et Bandiagara, Mali: Editions CRMT/PSMTM.

Good, Charles. 1987. *Ethnomedical Systems in Africa*. New York: Guilford.

Gottleib, Alma. 1993. *Under the Kapok Tree*. Chicago: University of Chicago.

Green, Edward. 1999. *Indigenous Theories of Contagious Disease*. Walnut Creek: AltaMira.

Gutmann, David. 1996. *The Meanings of Macho: Being a Man in Mexico City*. Berkeley: University of California.

Hountondji, Paulin. 1997. *Endogenous Knowledge: Research Trails*. Dakar: CODESRIA.

Inhorn, Marcia C. 2003. "The Worms Are Weak: Male Infertility and Patriarchal Paradoxes in Egypt." *Men and Masculinities* 5: 236–56.

———, ed. 2007. *Reproductive Disruptions: Gender, Technology, and Biopolitics in the New Millennium*. Oxford: Berghahn.

Kahn, S. 2000. *Reproducing Jews: A Cultural Account of Assisted Reproduction in Israel*. Durham: Duke University.

Kleinman, Arthur. 1980. *Patients and Healers in the Context of Culture*. Berkeley: University of California.

———. 1992. "Local Worlds of Suffering: An Interpersonal Focus for Ethnographies of Illness Experience." *Qualitative Health Research* 2: 127–34.

Kohl, Ines. 2009. *Beautiful Modern Nomads*. Berlin: Reimer.

Lamb, Sarah. 2000. *White Saris and Sweet Mangoes*. Berkeley: University of California.

Loughran, Kristyne, and Thomas Seligman, eds. 2005. *The Art of Being Tuareg*. Los Angeles: Iris and B. Gerald Cantor Center for Visual Arts and UCLA Fowler Museum of Cultural History.

Masquelier, Adeline, ed. 2005. *Dirt, Undress, and Difference*. Bloomington: Indiana University.

Moore, Henrietta, Todd Sanders, and Bwire Kaare, eds. 1999. *Those Who Play With Fire: Gender, Fertility and Transformation in East and Southern Africa.* London: Athlone Press. *London School of Economics Monographs on Social Anthropology* 69.

Nicolaisen, Johannes. 1961. La Magie et la religion touaregues. *Folk* 13: 113–60.

Norris, H. T. 1990. *Sufi Mystics of the Niger Desert.* Oxford: Clarendon.

Ragone, Helen. 1994. *Surrogate Motherhood: Conception in the Heart.* Boulder: Westview.

Rasmussen, Susan. 1995. *Spirit Possession and Personhood among the Kel Ewey Tuareg.* Cambridge: Cambridge University.

———. 1997. *The Poetics and Politics of Tuareg Aging: Life Course and Personal Destiny in Niger.* DeKalb: Northern Illinois University.

———. 2001. *Healing in Community: Medicine, Contested Terrains, and Cultural Encounters among the Tuareg.* Westport: Bergin & Garvey.

———. 2006. *Those Who Touch: Tuareg Medicine Women in Anthropological Perspective.* DeKalb: Northern Illinois University.

———. 2009. Do Tents and Herds Still Matter? In *Gender in Cross-Cultural Perspective*, 5th edition, edited by Caroline Brettell and Carolyn Sargent, 162–74. Saddle River: Pearson.

———. 2010. "Re-Making Body Politics." *Culture, Medicine, and Psychiatry* 34 (4): 615–32.

Roberts, Elizabeth. 2012. *Gods' Laboratory: Assisted Reproduction in the Andes.* Berkeley: University of California.

Sargent, Carolyn. 2007. "When the Personal Is Political: Contested Reproduction Strategies among West African Migrants in France." In *Reproductive Disruptions*, edited by Marcia C. Inhorn, 165–83. Oxford: Berghahn.

Tambiah, Stanley. 1990 .*Magic, Science, and Religion.* Cambridge: Cambridge University Press.

West, Harry. 2007. *Ethnographic Sorcery.* Chicago: University of Chicago Press.

4 Science in the Moral Space of Health and Healing Paradigms in Western Equatorial Africa

John M. Janzen

THIS CHAPTER EXAMINES the ongoing formulations of a moral framework among experts in scientific or technical fields relating to health, as they work with a populace that expects answers to the questions What? Why? Why me? and Who? regarding sickness and misfortune. During fieldwork in Lower Congo in 2013, hints of such a moral framework were evident in observations and in questions asked of the author, such as "Do you have poor people in America?" "Do you have mad people (*foux*) in America?" "Do you have sorcerers in America?" These questions reveal the logic and preoccupation of moral expectations about who gets trampled or marginalized economically and emotionally, and whether power is acquired licitly or illicitly. Articulating the contours of such a moral universe is becoming ever more urgent for the many people who are economically trapped in the rampant neoliberal globalized context that is the Democratic Republic of Congo today.

Health and healthcare resources in the region under study, the North Kongo "Manianga," include WHO-inspired primary health care structures and hospitals and clinics staffed by well-trained specialists with access to effective medicine. The region's caregivers also include herbalist-healers (*banganga*) and prophet-diviners (*bangunza*). This combination of health and healing resources reflects earlier findings of the continued use of Kongo medicine and healing alongside global biomedicine (Janzen 1978, 1982), all of whose practitioners are now Congolese. Clearly science-based medicine and technology have become the most prominent modes of seeking healthcare, but they do not *ipso facto* replace the older, yet ever-evolving, understandings of disease, threat, and misfortune. Interviews and participant observation reveal the widespread presence of individuals with advanced technical and scientific training who firmly believe in nature spirits, sorcerers, and the practice of people who use natural phenomena—crocodiles, lightning—to engage in mystically "eating" others to gain power and influence. These approaches often combine science-based formulations with spirit- or mysticism-based formulations operating either in concert or parallel.

This range of types of knowledge and the proliferation of alternative explanations for sicknesses and approaches to treating them may be best understood in the context of a particular disease. Malaria, the most prevalent chronic disease in the region, offers focused insight into the ways that science and other logics of explanation interdigitate or are used alternately. This essay suggests ways that a moral envelope integrates alternative kinds of knowledge, and reasons for the persistence of such a condition. These include a sense of personhood embedded in complex relations of community, divergent legitimations of power in healthcare and public services, and a weak state or government, as well as the apparent absence of a moral framework in logical empiricism in the worldviews of those who become experts in scientific or technical fields. The resulting distinctive combination of scientific thinking and practice that has emerged in western equatorial Africa offers a unique challenge to the anthropological study of culture and science.

The Shape of Knowledge in Africanist Medical Anthropology

This distinctively Kongo or Central African engagement with alternative approaches to knowledge in the world, with regard to health and healing issues, mirrors the debates that have raged and propositions that have been forwarded for several decades in medical anthropology and the history of science and medicine. Once upon a time, in the early postcolonial 1960s, most Western scholarship adhered to the sharp contrast between objective knowledge of science, the backdrop of biomedicine, and the rest of human thought, characterized either as superstition, or most generously, folk knowledge. These knowledge traditions were the result of centuries of unilinear scientific evolution that had produced the miracles of the Industrial Revolution, modern medicine, and other sciences.

However, like slowly-trickling drops of water on stone, other kinds of thought were beginning to percolate that would challenge the received wisdom on knowledge. African Studies and other disciplines such as the history of science and philosophy were confronted with the ramifications of Evans-Pritchard's seminal work (1937) on the thought world of the Azande people of northeast Congo and South Sudan. Evans-Pritchard had argued that Azande thought, epitomized by Azande beliefs in witchcraft as an explanation for misfortune, was rational, although not scientific. It was part of an alternative rationality that saw the world differently from Western science and logic. Generations of philosophers and anthropologists puzzled over this challenging evidence. Robin Horton's writing on Western science vs African thought (1967) had a very long life, as these two stereotypic constructs, although asymmetrical in the extreme, were endlessly compared with ever more local studies. Others framed their studies, policy recommendations, and proposals for research in terms of a broadly modern theoretical framework contrasting "modern medicine" to "traditional medicine" (Foster and Anderson 1978). The comparative study of medical systems, launched first by scholars of Asian medicine, yielded the notions of "medical pluralism" (Leslie 1976; Janzen 1978, 1982) and "epistemological pluralism" (Leslie and Young 1992) for the serious consideration of alternative ways of seeing the world of health and medicine. Some medical anthropologists insisted on seeing the field of all therapies in a given location as "medical culture" (Last 1992) that "imagined the whole" (Janzen 2014, 19), thereby encouraging the consideration of the possibility of commensurability between diverging logics and types of knowledge.

A radical shift in perspective on the nature of the relationship of culture to science emerged in American anthropology and the history of science and medicine, asserting that science itself was culturally constructed. Thus, one could examine the "culture of biomedicine," the values and structures of thought that expert and instrumental knowledge illustrated (Hahn and Gaines 1985; Lock and Nguyen 2010). From this point in the 1980s and 1990s, the field of medical anthropology evolved rapidly with a much different understanding of the biosciences than had reigned in the 1960s, an era when science reigned supreme as objective-empirical knowledge. The undoing of some universalist models of disease—for example, depression (Kleinman and Good, eds. 1985), Alzheimer's (Cohen 1998), and menopause (Lock 1995)—in favor of culturally or nationally distinctive syndromes opened the way to visualizing other conditions more commonly dealt with in African settings in terms of cultural variability and culturally specific constructions. The reading of disease in Africa in terms of its cultural construction was however slow to occur, especially in tropical Africa where such widespread dangerous epidemic diseases as malaria, cholera, HIV/AIDS, and Ebola ravaged communities and overwhelmed medical resources.

Still, researchers of the colonial history of science noted the transforming effect of this setting in the unique situations faced in studies of such fields as agriculture, environment, medicine and public health. The results often revealed a new and distinctive local cast (Tilley 2011). Phrases such as "endogenous knowledge," "vernacular science," and "competing epistemologies" characterize this growing attention to variability and adaptation in practical problem-solving and science (Tilley 2011, 314–328). Distinctive understandings of the cultural, social, and political contexts of health conditions in African settings made their appearance in due course with regard to the cultural and moral dimensions of disability (Ingstad and Whyte, eds., 1995; Livingston 2005), the moral and emotional-humanizing consequences of HIV/AIDS (Dilger and Luig 2010), the broader consequences of living with malaria (Fulwilley 2011), and the importance of local responses in numerous campaigns against Ebola. Within medical anthropology, an entire subfield emerged around the study of science, in which one leading scholar refined the concept of "epistemic cultures" arising out of PTSD (Young 2009) to deal with the continuities and discontinuities in specialized knowledge.

Without totally relativizing science, it is possible to see variability in knowledge and truth shaped by environment and culture, and to be open to creative applications that arise in the face of unique needs and urgencies.

These scenes from the world of health and healing in western equatorial Africa and beyond raise interesting scholarly issues having to do with science, medicine, and religion. How is authoritative knowledge produced? How is it legitimated? Particularly, how are the sometimes competing claims of spiritual and scientific modes of knowing reconciled, interdigitated, or fused? Is there perhaps an emerging and recognizably Kongo, or western equatorial African, synthesis of holistic knowledge regarding health, healing, and illness?

The Continuing Health Challenge of Malaria in Western Equatorial Africa

Malaria offers a vivid portrayal of the ways in which local practice and several types of knowledge interact in the general framework of health, disease, and healing. Malaria is pervasive, almost invisible, taken for granted, something that has been with the community as long as anyone can recall. Thus the forms of local knowledge brought to bear in dealing with it are practical, everyday considerations of how to get through a particular day, or episode, or individual crisis. Yet these mundane and routine episodes involve issues of causality, resistance, resources, and networks of support, the parameters within which "culture" is articulated. They involve the knowledge that has been learned in school biology and biochemistry classes, and which is held in more advanced form by the dozen or so physicians in the region, the hundreds of nurses and lab technicians working in hospitals and clinics, and by the populace. A basic outline of the extent and impact of malaria in the Manianga (more or less coterminous with the Territory of Luozi) and western equatorial Africa is helpful to the general reader of this chapter.

The Luozi Health Zone reports in the past decade that annually 20 percent of the population have experienced episodes of infection severe enough to require visiting a recording health post, center, or hospital; up to 100 deaths (in a population of 80,000) are reported annually to be directly due to malaria infection (Luozi Health Zone). The numbers of unreported episodes and deaths are likely far greater, due to other reported causes that are symptomatic of generalized malaria infection. But malaria affects everyone. Indeed, most of our acquaintances during four months in Luozi were "down" at least once with malaria or "fever." My wife Reinhild, despite dutiful taking of the prophylaxes, came down with a serious case that was successfully diagnosed and treated by Doctor Rose and her staff at the Luozi Catholic Hospital.

Malaria, named after "mal-aire," bad air, was for centuries thought to be caused by a combination of swamps, muggy air near to swamps, or spirits lurking in various kinds of bad air. The link between mosquitoes, the spirochete, and the disease's symptoms was only established in the early twentieth century. Lower Congo residents' preferred habitations were atop the hills that prominently figure in the landscape, because they were considered healthier than the lowlands near the rivers. Breezes kept the insects to a minimum, and with the help of shade trees, the air was coolly comfortable. The exploration team lead by Henry Stanley in 1884 thought that his near fatal bout with fever and chills at Manyanga station on the Congo River (near an old slave market by the same name) was caused by the sudden chilling winds that came through the river canyon after a hot day.

A century of medical research and education has advanced local knowledge to include the most sophisticated understanding of what causes the disease and its periodic flare-ups, and how individuals should deal with the agents and conditions that cause it. These details will demonstrate to what extent popular actions taken against malaria infection, or treatments and protocols arranged by experts, are effective or merely maintain the status quo. Transmitted by several subspecies of the Anopheles mosquito, "the sporozoite (the parasite form inoculated by the female mosquito) of *Plasmodium falciparum* invades a liver cell, the parasite matures in 6 days and produces 30,000–40,000 daughter cells (merozoites), which are released into the blood when the liver cell ruptures. In the blood, after a single merozoite invades a red blood cell, the parasite grows in 48 hours and produces 8–24 daughter cells, which are released into the blood when the red blood cell ruptures" (CDC). Infected individuals develop fever and chills that occur in waves lasting several hours and continue to recur with increasing severity. In children, this can lead to severe anemia and death. In youth and adults, it contributes to chronic weakness and inability to perform intellectual or physical tasks, and is overall very debilitating.

The red blood cell "ruptures" produce the fever and generate a more rapid replacement of the cells. When the *Plasmodium falciparum* became endemic about the time of the beginning of food cultivation in West Africa four to five thousand years ago, the condition that came to be known as "sickling" of the red blood cell conferred an adaptive advantage on populations living in the emerging malaria zones. The genetic mutation that developed created three types of predispositions in offspring in relation to malaria: a resistance to malaria through a kind of normal sickling behavior (seen in offspring of heterozygous parents), extreme sickling, resulting in anemia attacks (seen in offspring of homozygous parents), and no resistance or anemia, thus no resistance and susceptibility to malaria attacks. Sickle cell anemia is a fairly common condition in the Manianga; its presence is made known when a series of children in a family die early in childhood. Such a condition is extremely hard on women in a pro-natalist society, resulting often in divorce.

Maniangans use a range of local traditional products and methods to deter malaria. Some people rub themselves with a poultice of several plants before they go off into the bush, or they chew the leaves and swallow the juice. They say that the aroma of the plant repels mosquitoes. About a third of the households in our survey mentioned keeping the yard around the house free of grass and sweeping it daily to keep mosquitoes and other insects away; indeed, these households reported fewer incidents of malaria than those not mentioning this technique. However, no one seemed to take charge of dealing with large water-filled pot-holes in streets and pools of water in ditches close to human traffic.

Methods of treatment have taken several directions, each with only partial and temporary success. Generally, Congolese do not take commercial prophylaxes. As a cure, quinine was and continues to be a regular treatment. But it does not confer immunity, and if taken in too large doses for too long, causes ringing in the ears and may result in temporary mental dissociation. Generations of other drugs have come and gone, with some degree of efficacy and usually with side effects if taken for long periods of time. Yet most physicians, public health officials, and many local inhabitants are aware of the negative long-term effects of several chemicals that were used in combatting malaria, particularly the ability of mosquitoes to develop resistance to chemicals used to eradicate them. DDT became a favorite method of mosquito eradication in the 1950s and 1960s. Tropical cities such as Kinshasa were saturation-sprayed from airplanes. But this chemical proved disastrous. It was highly toxic for all wildlife and humans, especially affecting their reproductive capacities. Furthermore, a few surviving mosquitoes developed resistance to the chemical. Thus, extensive spraying produced a superior bug. Drug treatments and prophylaxes were plagued by the same phenomenon: genetic adaptation and resistance by the mosquitoes and the spirochetes.

Awareness of the evolutionary and adaptive tendencies of the Anopheles mosquito and the malaria spirochete has thus become part of the consciousness of the Congolese professional medical, pharmaceutical, and academic classes. The medicated mosquito nets that everyone in our survey used, courtesy of the WHO, Ministry of Health, and the Health Zone, has reportedly reduced malaria incidents somewhat, without appearing to cause resistant forms of spirochetes to develop. But many people are still bitten in early twilight or morning hours before mosquitoes withdraw for the hot sunlight. Thus, although the overall infection rate of malaria has only somewhat diminished, the consciousness of evolutionary processes in malaria infection has had other consequences.

Pharmaceutical experimenters have discovered that synthetic drugs designed around a single chemical property or process are more easily resisted than chemicals with complex structures, such as natural products like quinine.

Manianga pharmacist and drug manufacturer Batangu Mpesa, founder of the Centre de Recherche Pharmaceutique de Luozi, has conducted extensive experiments with approximately 100 medicinal plants known to have been used by healers as anti-malarials. Out of these, he has identified a dozen that when used alternatively and in combination produce a treatment that has not produced resistance thus far. His company currently serves about a million clients annually (his estimate of households supplied) with Manadiar, a prophylaxis, and Manalaria, a treatment especially for infants that relieves the fever and calms the diarrhea that often accompanies malaria outbreaks (Batangu-Mpesa 2009). Below, I will explicate Batangu-Mpesa's worldview as a Kongo-African scientist.

Sickle Cell Anemia and Coping with Multiple Death Syndrome

Even if a cure or effective prophylaxis is discovered or developed in the fight against malaria, the most difficult challenge of the disease is sickle cell anemia, or Drepanocytose (French usage). This affects many people in the Congo and in western equatorial Africa, even without their being bitten by spirochete-carrying mosquitoes. As a chronic condition understood by experts and academics, it has many cultural overtones and implications. But what is it in biomedical terms? Sickle cell anemia is a hereditary condition transmitted by the heterozygous-gene-carrying father and mother (both with A/S) to some of their children. The statistical chances of such parents transmitting the gene and the condition to their offspring is 25 percent for A/A (noncarrier, nonsickler), 50 percent A/S (carrier, and potential transmitter, but with a sickling condition that gives some immunity against malaria), and 25 percent S/S (full-blown sickler, susceptible to anemia and other crises, usually early death if not carefully managed; no cure available). Thus the offspring have a one in four chance of being S/S. In the Lower Congo (DRC), fully 30 percent of the population is A/S (Mbaku 2013).

Dr. Joswe Mbaku of the Free University of Luozi faculty, professor of psychology, specializes in public health awareness raising about sickle cell anemia (Drepanocytose). In a pamphlet that he distributes to any and all persons in his entourage and classes, he explains the symptoms and the life chances of those affected. The first signs of the sickness may manifest themselves as early as six months, in swelling of the feet and hands, bone or head deformities, and yellowing of the eye whites. Often severe physical pain accompanies the condition, due to the deformation of red blood cells (the hemoglobin "S") that clog blood vessels preventing good circulation and oxygenation. Anemia and infections follow. The immune system is weakened and organisms become sensitive to all kinds of infections: malaria, retarding of growth, cerebrovascular conditions (AVC), and so on. Sickling cannot be cured. It may be treated, or better, attacks may be avoided. But without care or attention, early death is very common.

Dr. Mbaku's tract offers the following treatment: At home, the pain of attacks may be diminished by staying in well ventilated areas, with stable temperature; frequent drinking of water; eating a good and varied diet; and avoiding strenuous exercise. Medical treatments include very expensive drugs; blood transfusions may be necessary in certain cases.

The tract concludes by emphasizing that a long life is possible for S/S sicklers and that their parents should be encouraged to put and keep them in school. They have a future in occupations that do not require strenuous physical activity, such as some professions, for example. Psychological counseling and moral support are very important elements of leading a reasonably normal life as a sickler.

Not surprisingly, a number of our 105 Intensive Sample households showed the pattern of couples who had parented sicklers. The women were in their 50s and 60s, at the close of their childbearing years. One had borne eight children of whom six had died; another had borne nine of whom six had died, three survived; a third had borne six children of whom five had died, one survived. This pattern of the majority of children dying produces an enormous burden, especially upon the woman, who is expected to bear children and is blamed for a string of child deaths. In the first-mentioned case, the woman was divorced by her first husband and remarried. Her second husband divorced her after the deaths of several more children. Her third husband had died. When interviewed, she was living in a modest house in Luozi with her fourth husband. Both had been widowed. She said of him that "he agreed to take care of me, so we married" and he, a healer, seemed to favor this opportunity. The woman's only daughter, in her 20s, lived with them and was pursuing university studies.

Manianga historian Kimpianga Mahaniah (2001, 54–56) has written a history in Kikongo of his own lineage with heavy S/S frequency, which was formerly accused of harboring witchcraft, occasioning anger, estrangement, and poison ordeals. In an entire chapter devoted to this, he seeks to explain the genetics of sickling to a KiKongo readership.

Several of our acquaintances with whom I discussed sickle-cell anemia said that before there was any consciousness of it as a hereditary condition, the children's deaths were usually thought to be caused by an unfinished, inadequately paid-up bride price. The importance of the alliance bond between families was so great that failure to complete the transaction adequately brought to the fore undercurrents of miserliness and jealousy that were thought to cause sterility or child deaths. Deaths of children were usually diagnosed as "deaths caused by man" (*lufwa lua muuntu*) as opposed to "deaths of God" (*lufwa lua Nzambi*, "natural"). As awareness grew of the nature of the condition through public

Table 4.1 Household Sample: Offspring/adult woman

Reproduction figures among women aged 50 to 70 in Luozi and Manianga region, showing the number of persons in the household, each woman's age, years of education, number of children born, those surviving, and those having died. Shaded cases are those whose children may have suffered sickle cell anemia. From intensive sample of 105 households, J. M. Janzen, 2013.

Age group	HH#	Age	Yrs school	Births	Youngest	# Deaths	Living	Offspring/ woman	
50-70								all	living
	1	67	5	11		1	10		
	8	58	9	7	9	0	7		
	10	58	8	8	21	6	2		
	11	52	15	6	17	0	6		
	13	67	0	12	15	2	10		
	15	52	7	7	13	1	6		
	19	54	8	7	15	0	7		
	27	54	8	7	13	1	6		
	29	51	3	8	2	4	4		
	34	51	10	1	?	0	1		
	40	53	8	9	3	6	3		
	44	50	?	10	13	3	7		
	56	71	5	8	18	1	7		
	57	51	2	7	12	0	7		
	67	61	10	8	13	3	5		
	68	61	6	9	4	2	7		
	80	54	6	6	?	5	1		
	89	67	3	6	18	1	5		
	91	61	14	6	18	1	5		
	92	53	8	10	17	3	7		
	104	50	9	5	12	0	5		
Totals	22		6.5	158		40	118	7.18	5.36
						25%			

health education, it took the form of a vague sense that something was amiss in the biological makeup of the parents. But without an adequate understanding of genetics, this awareness was limited to identifying certain families or kin groups as somehow flawed, resulting in their children dying.

With more schooling, especially in the biological sciences, and with the training of many lab technicians and the advent of numerous Congolese medical doctors and nurses, a fuller comprehension of sickle cell anemia has emerged in Manianga society, and in this wider region of Africa so heavily affected by malaria. Today genetic testing is becoming a prerequisite for marriage among educated young adults. If both are determined to be A/S carriers, or have somehow survived to marriageable age as S/S, the dominant strain of the disease, medical counselors and psychologists as well as clan elders routinely advise them to break off their engagement and find other partners. This introduces a whole new source of tensions. Those who refuse to break off their engagement are asked to sign a document informing them of the likely consequences and that they fully understand what they are confronting.

The emergence into public consciousness of a genetically transmitted condition as severe and life changing as the S gene introduces new issues of identity, life choices, and moral considerations. Tampering with God-created nature or having to break off a cherished relationship may require a new kind of moral framework, one informed by evolutionary bioscience. Furthermore, to complicate matters even more, medical specialists suggest that there are multiple alleles in the genetic picture, and that more refined testing can demonstrate gradations of severity in sickling ranging from extremely likely problems to less severe problems. The consciousness of a sickling propensity introduces the kinds of ambiguities that have been confronted in genetic testing for fetal birth defects.

Science and spirit are so intertwined here that a sophisticated moral and emotional compass is required to cope with each stage of this complex condition. The logic of family and clan reproductive politics imposes itself upon the purely science-minded individual or couple. Such logic dictates that social sensibilities be taken into account, even though the reading of the pathology is done with a detached scientific lens. Other considerations enter in to the reasons why multiple knowledge paradigms persist in western equatorial African understanding of health, disease and healing.

Personhood, Social Legitimation, and 'Epistemological Pluralism"

Many people in the Manianga and in Western Equatorial Africa express the desire for some kind of divination (*mfiedulu*) when dealing with misfortune. That is, they search for a deeper understanding of the questions that arise when individuals and families suffer sickness, accidents, economic setbacks, or inability to advance in the ways to which they aspire. As already seen, within the broad cultural field of misfortunes, a distinction is made in Kongo society, and much more widely in central and western Africa, between those misfortunes that are "of God," and those that are "of man." The first is in the natural order of things, or just happens; the second is caused by human affairs—such as human ignorance, an unfortunate verbal assault made in a fit of anger, or in the worst case, intentionally caused physical or mystical harm to do deliberate injury through misfortune or sickness. In the first sort of causal attribution, there is no hint of a post-Reformation divine retribution. The second attribution corresponds geographically to the very widely distributed proto-Bantu word *kuloka*, or *lok*, the power of words, or *dok*, the one from whom such words emanate. Clearly, the nature of the intervention will differ depending on which of the causes or combination of causes cited here is considered to have been in play. If an individual suffers a malaria attack with no attending suspected human cause, a visit to the hospital or clinic is in order, and the straightforward theory of the spirochete carried by the anopheles mosquito will apply. If the episode passes with treatment, then the case was confirmed to be "God-caused." If, however, there is a human dimension surrounding the case, either suspected or confirmed by evidence or divination, then the clinic treatment may be complemented by a further investigation—*mfiedulu*—of possible human issues in the life of the afflicted. As research on extended cases in the Manianga revealed years ago, there may be a shifting etiological understanding within the therapy-managing group or network, including the individual sufferer, or among a group of common sufferers. That is, a case that at one phase may be agreed to be "of God" may at another point come to be seen as "human-caused" if such evidence emerges (Janzen 1978, 1982).

Clinical, theological, and cultural explanations have been given for this causal logic that entertains a wider field than the individual and invisible agents as well as scientific empiricism (Masamba ma Mpolo 1981). My scholarly interest in personhood in Kongo therapeutic logic was aroused first when I tried to make sense of nganga nkisi Nzoamambu's medical cosmology. The diagnostic gloss "kimbevo kia muuntu" (sickness of man) corresponded in his dynamic scheme to a sequence of ever more severe reactions of the heart: palpitations, wild beating, "fear in the heart," and "madness." Such signs in a sufferer, especially if demonstrated sequentially over time, were evidence of "something else going on." This entire model I called Nzoamambu's "theory of the person" (Janzen 1978, 169). But this theory of the person is more widespread than one clever twentieth century *nganga nkisi*. It resonates in writing and practice in Central Africa and beyond. In Kongo history, MacGaffey has summed up his understanding of the power of *min'kisi* as "the personhood of objects" (1990, 2000, 78). The *nkisi* mirrors the entire scope of relations of the *nganga*, the client, and the "other" of threatened aggression, society and nature. These relations combine metonymic and metaphoric allusions, as well as artistry in the harnessing of unique styles and surprises. In any event, the person in Kongo thought and life is often more expansive and complex than the post-Enlightenment Cartesian Christian bounded autonomous individual of current Western psychological and medical construction (Janzen 2002, 137–148).

The contours of this unique Kongo–western equatorial African personhood include a number of aspects of identity, rights, and believed associations. There are the rights at birth to one's mother's lineage land and other privileges and obligations focused on the relationship to one's *nkazi*, maternal uncle, who holds proprietary rights over his sister's children. An individual also is held to have deep ties to father and father's kindred that are often associated with intellectual and spiritual powers. A kind of bilateral identity ensues that has within it networks with other individuals and roles. Yet the individual is still in some sense original and autonomous. Naming, for example, is independent of these other lineage/clan associations. Individual names may be changed by lifecourse transitions or personal whim (Janzen 2002, 141). But it is this wider fan of kin that is usually invoked when suspicions of "something else going on" are raised in connection with sickness or other misfortune.

We must also add to the fan of influences upon this expanded personhood, in Kongo and western equatorial Africa, the impact of the state and other public power relations. Modern individuals are not only members of clans and their alliances, they are also church members, workers for employers, neighbors in towns, businessmen and women in markets and wider commercial networks, officials in government and operatives and bosses in political parties, subscribers to internet services, and users of cellphones. Each of these arenas or networks becomes part of the persona of the individual. Because these arenas are not necessarily hierarchical, they proliferate as segments of self or alternative dimensions of personhood (Janzen 2015). This segmentation of self is all the more acute in western equatorial African society because of the weakness of the state, particularly in the Democratic Republic of Congo. It is there in an embryonic, shadow-like quality (Ferguson 2006). Recent authors addressing the impact of the state on identity have invoked the writing of Michel Foucault, in which the state's endorsement and use of medicine (biopower) exerts control over its subjects, who internalize the whims and dictates of the state in their subjectivity. This conceptualization of the state's power over its subjects through medicine may have been forceful in centralized nineteenth-century France, and in some contemporary societies. But in twenty-first-century west central Africa, the state is a vacuous, often nefast presence. The main phrases I heard in expressions of the state's role in the wellbeing of citizens in the Congo were "abandonment," "betrayal," and "loss of hope." If anything of the state gets internalized, it is the anxiety over chaos created by the absence of order, services, and consistency. In such a setting, the occasional emergence of witchcraft suspicions and accusations, and fear of the illicit exercise of power in causing disease and distress, are hardly surprising (Geschiere 1997, Ashworth 2005).

The epistemic pluralism of healing, medicine, and wellbeing in western equatorial Africa is also amplified by the absence of moral precepts in scientific theory and practice. A university student who takes courses in chemistry, biology, and mathematics will hardly develop a working appreciation of the history of science, philosophy, and religion that situates this knowledge within a morally discerning framework. Post-Enlightenment science teaching is premised on the assumption that there is no vested interest in such a framework. The normative scientific method does not allow for such a system to even exist. This means that our scientifically-trained Congolese medical practitioners and school-educated citizens continue all the more to bring a range of other moral logics to their encounters with sickness and misfortune.

The broader, more inclusive, more widely connected personhood of Kongo thought and society, in which the etiological suppositions "of God" and "human-caused" about the fates and fortunes coexist, also explains the manner in which God, the ancestors, nature spirits, and other individuals taking the form of animal familiars, may occupy the same space as narrowly defined scientific theorems. Scientific understanding has the effect of shifting the focus of specific etiology of disease, but does not apparently obviate the general breadth of personhood and the accompanying epistemic pluralism.

Situating Scientific and Medical Understanding Within a Moral Universe

Given the existential context of plural epistemologies, how does the moral umbrella already alluded to and heralded in the title of this chapter make itself manifest? The questions mentioned at the outset of this chapter—"Do you have poor ... mad people ... witches ... in America?"—hint at the outlines of such a moral framework that anticipates the nature of power—who is in and who is out, and how one gets there. Several illustrations of a more explicit approach to situating science or knowledge within such a framework are offered here. The first kind of evidence comes from three of many university thesis invocations by students who situate their scientific learning within a wider framework. The second and lengthier portrayal is of the moral universe of pharmacist/politician/educator Batangu-Mpesa, already introduced.

In 2008–2009, a nursing graduate at the Free University of Luozi produced a master's thesis on "Evaluation of Care in Gastro-Enteritis Fever in Children from 0–5 Years: Case Study in the Catholic Hospital of Luozi." The title page carried the epigraph: "The Lord is my light and my salvation; whom should I fear? The Lord is the refuge of my life; of whom then should I go in dread? (Psalm 27:1) Take life as it comes, without regret, nor surprise, nor being upset, for the essential thing is that which remains for you to do." The thesis was dedicated "to the Eternal, my God, the Almighty who protected me and upheld me during all the years of my studies until today."

Another research thesis at the Free University of Luozi , Faculty of Health Sciences, entitled "The Evaluation of the Nurse's Contribution in the Care of a

Case of Microscopic Positive Pulmonary Tuberculosis: Case Study at the State Hospital Centre of Kisenso," carried the epigraph "In thee, O Lord, I have taken refuge; never let me be put to shame. As thou art righteous rescue me and save my life; hear me and set me free . . . (Psalm 71:1–2). Holy Father, bless me in my life so that I will acknowledge my father, my mother, and all those who have helped me surmount the many obstacles encountered during the three years of study at the Free University of Luozi."

A third example was a thesis on "The Contribution of the Nurse in the Care of Infected Operating Wounds," at the Catholic Health Center of Luozi, 2004–2005. It carried this epigraph: "Blessed be the Eternal, for He hears my voice, my supplications and He lends his ear toward me during the period of my studies; may my cry reach thee, O Eternal; give me the intelligence and the wisdom according to your promise; may my supplication reach Thee; deliver me according to your promise. May each work with his hands to have something to give he who is in need (Saint Paul)."

These are three of the many university theses at the Free University of Luozi that situate the student's first original research project in the context of a sacred space, often defined by a scripture passage and an invocation or wish. Many times gratitude is expressed to parents, siblings, and other kinsfolk, even elders and ancestors, for their support and for having modeled for the student the wisdom and intelligence needed to complete a course of studies. Some observers of this pattern of situating scientific research findings within a spiritual framework may explain this as youthful enthusiasm, perhaps an attempt to impress the examiners with diligence and piety.

The manner in which pharmacist, politician, and academic Batangu-Mpesa moralizes and legitimizes his research on malaria offers an illuminating example of how science and other types of knowledge are situated within a moral framework. In a 2009 lecture to a national colloquium on scientific research on malaria in the Democratic Republic of Congo, he situates his work within the overall program of and priorities of the World Health Organization. This includes taking note of the WHO's recommendations for medicines that are combined into cocktails—Coarsucam, made up of Artesunate-Amodaquine and Co-bister (Batangu-Mpesa 2009, 12)—to offer a better chance of resisting resistance on the part of *Plasmodium falciparum*, the leading variant of malaria spirochete in tropical Africa. Despite an earlier flurry of interest of pharmaceutical prospectors in African medicinal plants, the likely lack of a lucrative market for malaria meant that there was little research and development of better drugs among the big pharmaceutical companies of the northern world (Janzen 2012). Noting the lack of research on new malaria drugs in relation to overall global output of drugs, he lays out the WHO's program for research into new medicines, primarily from the existing work of herbalist-healers. Such healers are identified as practicing

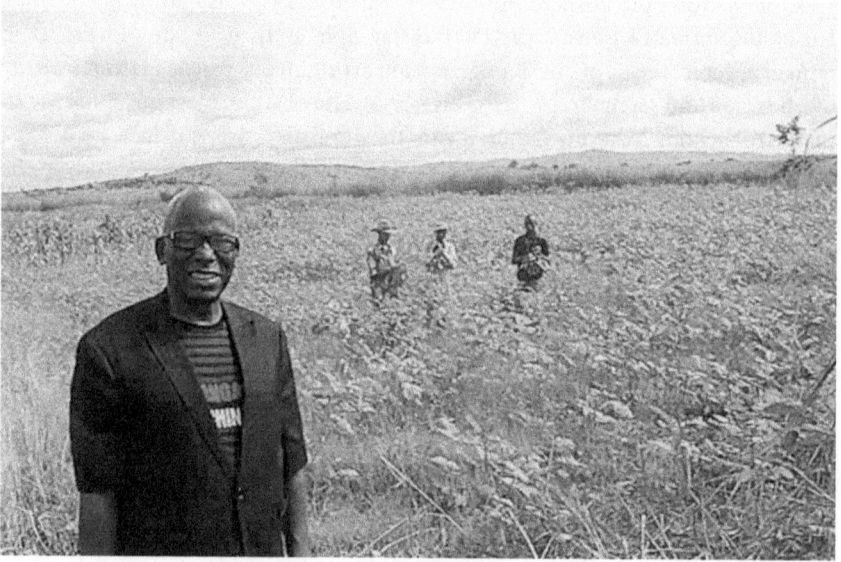

Batangu Mpesa in Artemisia plantation, outside Luozi, Lower Congo, Democratic Republic of Congo. Photo by J. M. Janzen, 2013.

therapies of spiritual healing, manual techniques, and using materials of plant, animal or mineral substances. The researcher's goals are to identify and extract active principles of these substances; to produce the most promising plants directly in his own plantations; to study their toxicity on experimental animals; to stage clinical trials of medicines that show promise, within an ethical review framework; to request market authorization; and then to make the new drugs available.

Against the backdrop of this WHO framework, Batangu-Mpesa sketches his own research and development program. Malaria is at crisis levels, the leading cause of morbidity and mortality across the DRC, especially in poor sectors of the population. His own motivation for his thirty-year research program rests on his care for himself, his family, his immediate community, and others. With such a track record, for all to see, he has obviously not poisoned his family and those others who benefit from his medicine, including the million or so households per year who buy Manalaria (2009, 31–32). This is an intriguing comment and postulate that suggests the fear in the community of exactly such a practice, and the relative absence of the rule of law that would deal with powerful, unethical persons with drugs. Then follows the passage where he lays out the moral foundations of his project (2009, 32).

- I am a native of the Luozi region;
- I am a pharmacist-analyst;
- I am a political person;
- I believe in God.

These four anchors assert his identification with the region, his scientific expertise, political acumen recalling his days as national parliamentarian, and finally, invocation of the supreme being. These claims encourage everyone to identify Batangu as their researcher/ citizen/ leader/ believer. They encourage trust in his skill as a pharmacist, confidence that as a former national deputy, he will take care of you, and finally, that he is in touch with the true source of power and the natural world.

This cosmological manifesto is presented in visual form in a large mural extending across an entire end wall of a large plant drying shed/theater in Batangu-Mpesa's Luozi compound, not far from a plantation of medicinal herbs. The landscape scene, reminiscent of the Manianga with the Congo river flowing

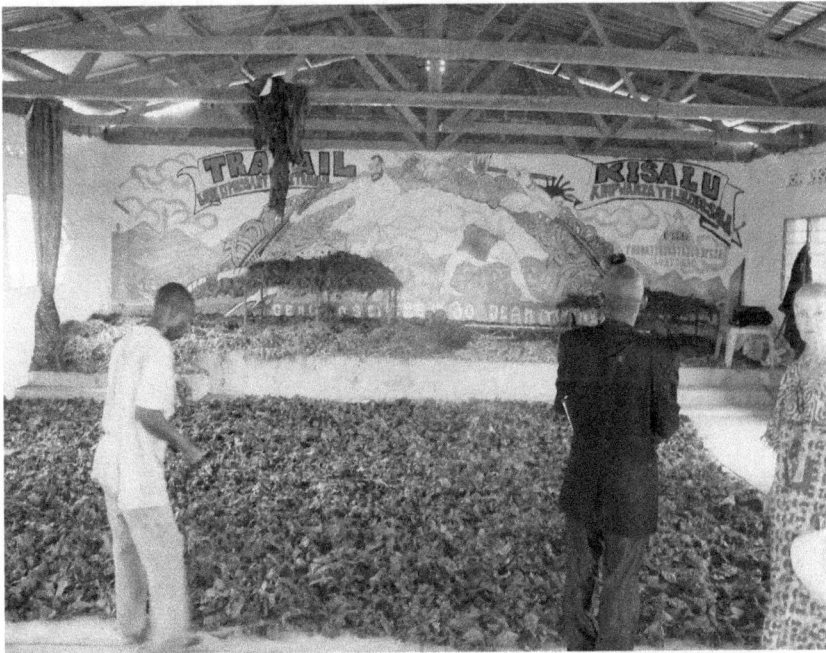

Batangu Mpesa's cosmic panorama, Luozi, Lower Congo, Democratic Republic of Congo. Bantangu, back turned to camera, tablet under left arm, examines the mural in his combined theater and plant-drying shed; far right, Reinhild Kauenhoven Janzen; far left, plant tender. Photo by J. M. Janzen, 2013.

through it, features Prometheus-like male and female figures engaged in role characteristic productive activity. The male figure is hauling in fish with a net. Nearby in the water is a severely wounded crocodile that has just been attacked by the fisherman. This detail, partially obscured by a leaf drying rack, alludes to the fearsome crocodile attacks of the 1970s and 1980s upon fishermen and women and children washing clothes and drawing water from the river. It also reminds the viewer of Batangu's decisive action in1986 as parliamentarian to take on the crocodile crisis by organizing nighttime searchlight hunters to go after as many crocodiles as possible in the region where the attacks took place. The woman holds a hoe in her raised hand ready to cultivate her garden plot before her. Banners spell out "Work makes free and powerful" in French and KiKongo. Smaller detail scenes in the landscape depict industrial and communications technology, showing the high power lines that run parallel to the east bank of the Congo River bringing electricity from the Inga Dam downstream to the large cities upstream like Kinshasa, Mbanza Ngungu, and Kisantu. The transmitting tower with waves spreading from it alludes to Batangu's own radio station, Yenge, "Joy," and the pervasive use of cellphones across the DRC. Centrally placed in the mural, a dove hovers, suggesting peace that prevails in this utopian world. Two Biblical text references offer further detail to spiritually anchor this social realist depiction of the Kongo world of tomorrow. Beneath the male figure in big letters is Genesis

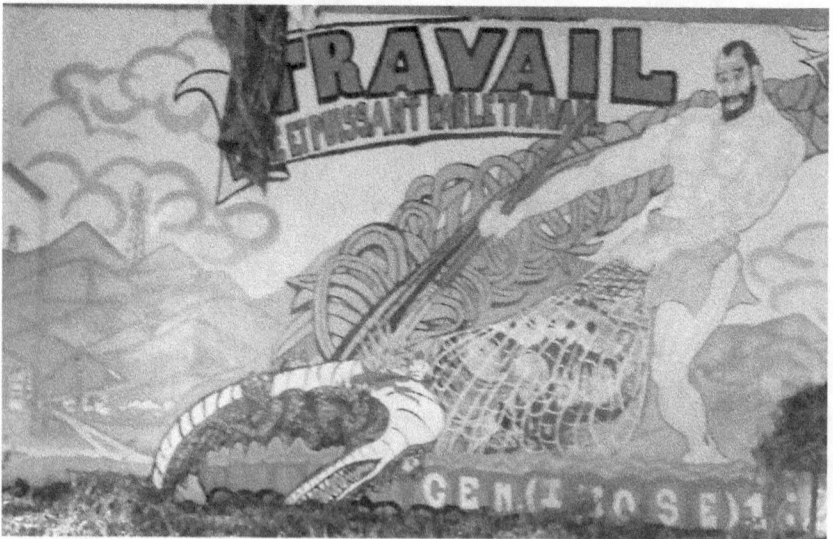

Details of Batangu's mural: Male figure as fisherman, pulling in net full of fish and wounded crocodile; industrial installations bottom left of scene; high-power line tower top left. Road to Congo River ferry on distant shore. Photo by J. M. Janzen, 2013.

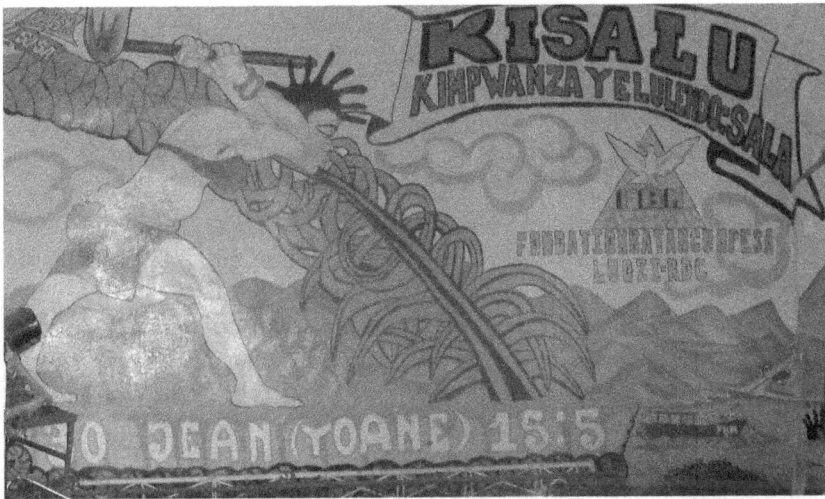

Details of Batangu's mural: Female figure hoeing garden; fishing boat lower right on Congo River, road receding between hills in distance. Insignia with dove of peace and prosperity announces the Batangu Mpesa Foundation. Photo by J. M. Janzen, 2013.

1:26–30, the passage in which God declares his creation good, and gives Adam dominion over it. Beneath the female figure is John 15:5, the passage in which Jesus declares himself the vine, and his disciples the branches; with Him you will be fruitful. The gender complementarity of the two human figures, although situated above the scripture verses about God's good creation and fertility, echo classic Kongo themes of cosmic dualism that undergirds life. Many *min'kisi* have a male and a female aspect, as well as referents to domestic and wild realms. In the Western Kongo or Mayombe altars of the historic Nkimba initiation rites, the male and female figures in the scepter represent the two complementary heads of the cosmic serpent. Batangu's mural, commissioned from a Kinshasa artist, synthesizes historic and contemporary themes into one epic visual panorama. The large hall and stage before the mural are intended to serve as a backdrop for performances. In a bow to the practical needs of pharmaceutical manufacturing, the mural displays its remarkable themes to drying Artemisia leaves that will be turned into malaria medication.

Knowledge, Practice, Politics, and Legitimacy

What are the implications of this contextualization of expert knowledge within a transcendent canopy or legitimation framework? First, there is less of a clear-cut distinction between what we in the West call "science" and what we call "religion." Just how this is done may vary from era to era, from case to case; or rather, "science" is framed by or subsumed within transcendent order and power. Second, knowledge and technique are portrayed as conventional and practical, as in fishing, gardening, transmitting electricity and telephonic communications. These are in the natural order of things. Third, the advent of crises such as sicknesses, accidents, and brushes with death, such as crocodile attacks, illustrate the need to transform the context into a moral universe. This process of ordering the universe of knowledge within a transcendent order is similar to the way *minkisi*, consecrated medicines and techniques, were historically anchored in Kongo society in a pedigree leading to a founding *nganga* and inspiring spirit.

Such integration of different kinds of knowledge into one framework as we have seen here appears to be a fairly widespread historic and contemporary African phenomenon, found in such realms as metallurgy, agriculture, warfare, political office, family relations, and especially approaches to sickness and healing. Steven Feierman and I recently reviewed a number of historic and contemporary examples from eastern and western equatorial Africa of this embedding of technical, specialized knowledge within a sacred canopy. We suggest that "the moral and humanistic envelope of knowledge that integrates science and religion may well be a genuine contribution of African tradition to the world community" (Feierman and Janzen 2011, 248).

Bibliography

Ashworth, Adam. 2005. *Witchcraft, Violence and Democracy in South Africa*. Chicago: University of Chicago.

Batangu-Mpesa, E. F. 2009. "Polyphytothérapie combinatoire et alternative du Paludisme. [Combinational and alternative polyphyto-therapy for malaria.]" *Exposé aux 1eres Journées Scientifiques sur le Paludisme en RDC, sur le thème: Paludisme, Récherches et Perspectives en RDCongo*. Faculté de Medecine, Université de Kinshasa. 10: 22–23.

Centers for Disease Control and Prevention. "Malaria Facts." Last modified April 15, 2016. http://www.cdc.gov/malaria/about/facts.html.

Cohen, Lawrence. 1998. *No Aging in India: Alzheimer's, the Bad Family, and Other Modern Things*. Berkeley: University of California.

Dilger, Hansjorg, and Ute Luig, eds. 2010. *Morality, Hope and Grief: Anthropologies of AIDS in Africa*. Oxford: Berghahn.

Evans-Pritchard, E. E. 1937. *Witchcraft, Oracles, and Magic among the Azande*. Oxford University.

Feierman, Steven, and John M. Janzen. 2011. "African Religion [and Science]," in *Science and Religion around the World*, edited by John Hedley Brooke and Ronald L. Numbers, 229–51. Oxford: Oxford University.

Ferguson, James. 2006. *Global Shadows: Africa in the Neoliberal World Order*. Durham, NC: Duke University.

Foster, George, and Barbara Anderson. 1978. *Medical Anthropology*. New York: John Wiley & Sons.

Fulwilley, Duana. 2011. *The Enculturated Gene: Sickle Cell Health Politics and Biological Difference in West Africa*. Princeton: Princeton University.

Geschiere, Peter. 1997. *The Modernity of Witchcraft: Politics and the Occult in Postcolonial Africa.* Charlotte: University of Virginia.

Hahn, Robert, and Atwood Gaines. 1985. *Physicians of Western Medicine.* Dordrecht: Reidel.

Horton, Robin. 1967. "African Traditional Thought and Western Science." *Africa* 37: 50–72, 155–87.

Ingstad, Benedicte, and Susan Reynolds Whyte, eds. 1995. *Disability and Culture.* Berkeley: University of California.

Janzen, John M. 1978. *The Quest for Therapy in Lower Zaire.* Berkeley, Los Angeles, London: University of California.

———. 1982. *The Quest for Therapy: Medical Pluralism in Lower Zaire.* Berkeley: University of California Press (paperback edition).

———. 2002. *The Social Fabric of Health: An Introduction to Medical Anthropology.* New York: McGraw-Hill.

———. 2012. "Afri-global Medicine: New Perspectives on Epidemics, Drugs, Wars, Migrations, and Healing Rituals," in Hansjorg Dilger, Abdoulaye Kane, and Stacey Langwick, *Medicine, Mobility, and Power in Global Africa,* 115–37. Bloomington: Indiana University.

———. 2014. "Imagining the Whole: Local Medicine and Global Health," in *Medical Anthropology in Global Africa,* edited by Kathryn Rhine, John M. Janzen, Glenn Adams, Heather Aldersey, 19–26. Lawrence, KS: University of Kansas Publications in Anthropology.

———. 2015. "Divergent Legitimations of Post-State Health Institutions in Western Equatorial Africa." Working Paper #14 of the Priority Programme 1448 of the German Research Foundation Adaptation and Creativity in Africa. Leipzig & Halle, 2015. www.spp1448.de.

Kimpianga Mahaniah. 2001. *Kikulu kia chefferie Luangu.* Luozi: Presses de l'Université Libre de Luozi.

Kleinman, Arthur and Byron Good, eds. 1985. *Culture and Depression: Studies in the Anthropology and Cross-Cultural Psychiatry of Affect and Disorder.* Berkeley: University of California.

Last, Murray. 1992. "The Importance of Knowing about Not Knowing: Observations from Hausaland," in *The Social Basis of Health and Healing in Africa,* edited by Steven Feierman and John M. Janzen, 393–406. Berkeley: University of California.

Leslie, Charles, ed. 1976. *Asian Medical Systems.* Berkeley: University of California.

Leslie, Charles, and Allan Young, eds. 1992. *Paths to Asian Medical Knowledge.* Berkeley: University of California.

Livingston, Julie. 2005. *Debility and the Moral Imagination in Botswana.* Bloomington: Indiana University.

Lock, Margaret. 1995. *Encounters with Aging: Mythologies of Menopause in Japan and North America.* Berkeley: University of California.

Lock, Margaret & Vinh-Kim Nguyen. 2010. *An Anthropology of Biomedicine.* New York: Wiley.

Luozi Health Zone. *Principal Diseases, 2002–2013.* Unpublished record.

MacGaffey, Wyatt. 1990. "The Personhood of Ritual Objects: Kongo *Minkisi.*" *Etnofoor* 3: 1, 45–61.

———. 2000. *Kongo Political Culture.* Bloomington: Indiana University.

Masamba ma Mpolo. 1981. "Kindoki as diagnosis and therapy." *Social Science and Medicine* 15B (3), 405–14.

Mbaku, Joswe. 2013. "Qu'est-ce-que la Drepanocytose? [What Is Sickle Cell Anemia ?]" Printed tract. Université Libre de Luozi.

Tilley, Helen. 2011. *Africa as a Living Laboratory: Empire, Development, and the Problem of Scientific Knowledge 1870–1950.* Chicago: University of Chicago.

Young, Allan. 2009. "When Anthropology meets Science." Vincent Ducles' interview of Allan Young in "Somatosphere—Science, Medicine, and Anthropology—Collaborative Website;" first published in *Altérités* 6 (1), 110–18.

5 Medical Pluralism Revisited

A Memoir

Brooke Grundfest Schoepf

THIS VOLUME on medical pluralism raises an important question in an era when biomedicine is present in some form across most of sub-Saharan Africa, and formal schooling, including biology and human anatomy, is also widespread. Some may wonder why so many Africans continue to consult traditional healers.[1] My first response is that most African children do not complete elementary school and are not taught biological science, and that most people do not have access to biomedicine of a reasonable standard. Sufferers' social locations, and those of the people who assist them, greatly influence their trajectories as they review their options (Janzen 1978; Schoepf 1986; Colvin, Smith, Schwartz et al. 2013). Two factors encourage medical pluralism. First, consider the precarious state of education and health services available to the poor rural and urban majorities in most African countries. Although traditional healers' therapies are seldom cheap and prices have risen in recent decades, many offer credit and delayed payment schemes, which biomedical services do not. Second, consider the cosmology involved in the diagnosis and explanation of the causes of sickness. These will be discussed in turn. First, a digression that may suggest a parallel.

My first experience with folk practitioners came in 1957, during village fieldwork in southern France, where Professor Mircea Eliade urged me to study the survival of traditional medicine in a rural community. When I consulted the elders, they laughed and pointed to the sole folk practitioner, a *rebouteuse* or bonesetter, an unkempt woman who lived up in the terraced hills at some remove from the village. They said that formerly she had set broken bones, attended births and treated many in the community for minor ills. At that time, the doctor was far away and transport uncertain. But now there was National Health Insurance, a pharmacist with a telephone down the hill, a *sage-femme* (midwife) in the next village, and the doctor who came regularly in her car from Toulon. I spent many hours perched on a stool in the back room of the pharmacy as people came to discuss their complaints with *Monsieur le Pharmacien* to decide whether to consult a doctor or to try an over-the-counter remedy first.

Sitting on a bench near the fountain in the main square, seventy-year-old Madame Grisolle, a retired small farmer, confided, sotto voce: "When I was a girl, *La Rebouteuse* was reputed to cast spells and work protective magic against the evil eye, but the young do not believe in *tout ça*." I studied the interface of local and national politics in the village, instead.

African folk practitioners, too, may act to ward off misfortune or to bring good fortune to clients. Moreover, African treatments and explanations of disease have not remained frozen in a timeless ethnographic present, but have changed and adapted over the years. Amazing bricolages, inventively hybrid combinations of divination, herbal medicines, and spirit mediumship are buttressed by paraphernalia, disease categories, terminology and medications derived from biomedicine (Schoepf 1976a, 1986, 2001, 2014; Feierman 1979; Geschiere 1995; Symonds and Schoepf 2000; Marsland 2007). In the 1970s and 1980s, paraphernalia used by healers in Zaire included homemade facsimiles of the stethoscope, microscope, X-ray machine and other biomedical diagnostic tools, and a cat skin used in French folk medicine at least into the 1950s. Given the changes anthropologists have observed, healers are no longer "traditional." Therefore, I prefer the term "folk practitioners" rather than "traditional healers" or the French *tradipraticiens* (Schoepf 1976a, 1986).

The search for health is a social process in which navigation of the therapeutic itinerary takes place in a shifting social field (Buakasa 1998; Parkin 2013). Janzen (1978), who charted the course of people's "Quest for Therapy" in Kinshasa and the rural Lower Congo region in the 1970s, found that people rarely faced their afflictions alone. Family members most involved in the sufferer's quest came to constitute what he called the therapy managing group. Often it was they, rather than sufferers themselves, who chose among the therapeutic modalities and personnel available. Few readers appear to have noticed that Janzen and his physician collaborator parted ways before the end of the research. As a consequence, no biomedical data on diagnosis or treatment efficacy of the folk practitioners were included (Schoepf 1976b). Since that time, the activities of folk practitioners have become enshrined in global health policy as part of the campaign for "Health for all" (WHO 1978a).

Which Medicine? Who Decides?

In the city of Lubumbashi in the late 1970s, women whose husbands worked for the two largest employers, the copper mining company, Gécamines (GCM),[2] and the national railway, SNCZ, lived as nuclear families in company housing. They were issued health cards and took their children to employer-provided health clinics without the need for their husbands to supply money. Able to take responsibility for their own and their children's illnesses, they preferred to bring them to biomedical health services. Women married into patrilineal, patriarchal ethnic groups, such as the Luba-Kasai, feared that if mothers-in-law mixed in, they would take the children to consult a folk practitioner. Mothers explicitly wished to avoid such interventions. They worried that folk practitioner interventions would lead to "complications," that is, conflict, in the family, and that they, the mothers, would be blamed for causing misfortune.

Poor women living in the *cités,* or popular quarters, that were home to other working class families, especially feared folk interventions in the case of vaginal discharge suggestive of sexually transmitted infections, as healers' framework of "pollution" beliefs assumed the women's infidelity. They sought care at church-supported neighborhood clinics staffed by nurses, and at the public hospital. The latter's many deficiencies included, for example, patients with suspected tuberculosis paraded before a defunct X-ray machine. Some physicians came from Eastern Europe and were unable to communicate with patients. When unable to cure or explain disease, such as sickle cell anemia, in terms that patients and their families could understand, African physicians might tell them to "go and settle things among your family," which patients interpreted as an instruction to call on a folk practitioner to search for a culprit (unpublished field data 1976–1979).

Even in Katanga Village, a rural community of 3,000 people eighty miles from the city that I studied with Claude Schoepf and students from 1975, women sought biomedical services routinely when home remedies failed to resolve their own or their children's perceived problems. Indeed, the UMHK had funded a clinic there, staffed by a diploma nurse, as part compensation for their expropriation of village lands (Schoepf 1987). A mission health center, some five kilometers distant, staffed by Belgian nuns, provided much-appreciated maternity services. In this matrilineal, matrilocal Lemba community, there was no question of blaming women for misfortune, except at the death of Chief Katanga in 1977, when his much-disliked and envied widow was suspected. Her elderly parents, the father a respected retired pastor, walked five kilometers from their farm to defend her. The palaver lasted long into the night; in the end, no charges were brought (unpublished field notes July, 1977).

In Zaire, as elsewhere, infant mortality and child health vary with the availability of biomedical health services and quality of nutrition. From the late colonial period, the best infant survival and growth statistics were among urban children in Elisabethville/Lubumbashi with access to the UMHK/Gécamines clinic and family rations; the next best were in the *cités;* the worst were in the rural area around Lubumbashi (Parent 1961; Cassiers 1973). In the 1970s, sex workers' children were the most at risk in the city for severe malnutrition (Dr. Daniel Talleyrand, pers. comm. 1977).

Folk practitioners often answered clients' questions of "Why me?" by attributing blame for sickness and misfortune to an intimate. Witchcraft was a serious matter in Katanga Village. One elderly "healer" lived in isolation near the highway, about a mile from the village. Tolerated by the chief, he apparently was not consulted by local people during our research. Rather, his clients came from afar. A woman in her thirties performed trance dances and channeled the voices of ancestors when consulted on family matters, but avoided making accusations. Once, a *muganga* (practitioner) from a distant town was called on by local authorities to "smell out a witch." Claude Schoepf, who witnessed the performance, termed it an exercise in suggestion (unpublished field data 1978).

Following our departure for the United States, an elderly man whose children had migrated to the city was accused of witchcraft. He was banished to live in a hut in the bush at some distance from the village. Informed by the young chief on the occasion of a one-day visit in 1981, I was unable to get the full story, and sadly, had no time to visit him. I suspect that as he no longer had relatives to help care for him, he may have become a burden on neighbors. Still, illnesses perceived to be curable by biomedicine, or even merely treatable, such as leprosy, were brought to biomedical practitioners.

A recent review of research on response to childhood illness across Africa finds consultation in extended family networks. Nevertheless, urban residence, wealth, and mothers' education and independent control of resources hastened consultation of biomedical health services when home remedies failed (Colvin, Smith, Schwartz, et al. 2013). If an illness persists or worsens, even rural poor mothers may make all efforts to reach a biomedical facility. Late arrival to care often compromises such treatment as is available, most of it very poor. Both transport costs and user fees keep the poorest mothers in Tanzania and elsewhere away (Schellenberg, Victoria, Mushi, et al. 2002; Say and Rayne 2007; Spangler 2011). Even where users prefer biomedicine, general deterioration of public health services, consequent upon Structural Adjustment and AIDS, has increased resort to folk practitioners. In Zanzibar, the rising prices of both biomedical and "traditional" medicine have resulted in what Beckmann (2010) characterizes as "the commodification of misery." It was not always this way, as the following case from Zimbabwe will illustrate.

Soon after independence from white minority rule, the government of Zimbabwe sought to provide primary health care services close to home for the majority rural population. Both public and mission clinics expanded their reach. In Masvingo District, I visited a Catholic mission that held a well-baby clinic each week in a different rural site, rotating on a monthly basis. Mothers walked several miles with their infants, all dressed in their finest, to have the children weighed and vaccinated, and talk over problems. I asked sixty women about their choice of healers. Shona, all, they lived in viripatrilocal hamlets under the watchful eyes of their migrant husbands' mothers, who often preferred to consult folk practitioners for children's illnesses. But since the clinic was free, with a good reputation, the women could strike out on their own, and many dared to do so. They feared folk practitioners for their frequent imputation of responsibility to mothers for their children's illnesses (field notes 1983). Yet Structural Adjustment (ESAP in Zimbabwe) put paid to the advancing biomedical health care system (Bjilmakers, Bassett and Sanders 1996; Schoepf, Schoepf and Millen 2000).

Why Do Folk Practitioners Sometimes Succeed?

Much non-biomedical therapy uses ritual rather than pharmacologically active ingredients. In Africa, as elsewhere, intensively practiced prayer and other religious rituals may ease suffering (Corin 1979; Kopytoff 1980; Devisch 1985; Janzen 1992; Dilger and Luig 2010; Luhrman 2012). Anthropology professor Buakasa describes how his mission-educated schoolteacher father became a noted Kongo healer (both ngang'a-nkisi [healing priest], and ngang'a-ngombo [diviner]) following successful ritual treatment for his own health problems, which the nganga ascribed to family conflict. The father served an apprenticeship, learning to make nkisi (sometimes translated as a fetish, or more properly, spirit) of various kinds that he would call upon to accomplish sacred healing rituals (Buakasa 1998).

Healers' rituals that prescribe remedial action may be reassuring—or, as Malinowski noted many decades ago with respect to belief in magic, they may raise anxiety and so mobilize people to search for solutions. As Dr. Albert Schweitzer of Lamboréné fame noted, many conditions experienced as ill-health are benign, self-limiting conditions which will fade away without treatment of any kind. Others are psychogenic in whole or in part. These Schweitzer believed could safely be left to the "witch doctor." He persuaded many African practitioners to refer patients with conditions requiring surgery or treatment with pharmaceuticals to his clinic (recounted in Offit 2013, 253–255).

Freud is, of course, the high priest of psychogenic healing, but many physicians recognize the value of the doctor-patient relationship in curing. In the 1950s, a British physician estimated that the illnesses of 75 percent of people who consulted his London general practice involved self-limiting or psychogenically induced symptoms (Bailint 1957). My "Raging Hormones" paper of 1971 pointed to interconnections between brain and experience in regulating hormonal expression via the hypothalamus (Schoepf 1971), a trajectory which my neurophysiologist father pioneered (Grundfest 1959). Recent imaging studies of processes underlying placebo responses and the medical rituals of laying on of hands implicate various aspects of neurochemistry in areas of the brain that modulate pain reception, memory, anxiety, pleasure and reward (Kradin 2008; Benedetti 2012; Offit 2013). In particular, both the hypothalamus and the pituitary gland produce an endogenous morphine released in response to pain, spicy foods, exercise, excitement, and orgasm. Hence the name "endorphins" coined in the 1970s

by discoverers of the process by which endorphin release mediates placebo anal-
gesia (Levine, Gordon and Fields 1978, cited by Offit 2013, 224). However, "neither
placebos nor rituals can cure AIDS or brain tumors or improve healing following
reconstructive breast surgery" (Offit 2013, 97).

A demonstration of the placebo reaction in treatment for symptom relief
of migraine headaches compared the effect of a widely used drug with that of
a dummy pill. When told the placebo would work, patients in the United States
reported that it reduced their pain by nearly half as much as those who were
given the real medication. "The information provided to patients and the ritual of
pill-taking are important components of care" (Kam-Hansen, Jakubowski, Kelley, et al. 2014). Ted Kaptuchk, who led the research team, hypothesized that the
placebo effect, based on patients' expectation of efficacy, would enter into play in
other painful conditions that involve subjective components, such as intestinal
cramps, backaches and asthma.[3] A recent experiment found that an expensive
placebo was more effective than a cheap one among twelve patients with Parkin-
son's disease (Espay et al. 2015, cited by Bernstein 2015). There was no follow-up to
discover how long reported improvement in function lasted in this small sample
of patients because they were soon put back on levodopa, their regular medication.[4] I suggest that African folk practitioners' rituals, remedies, and laying on of
hands may trigger placebo effects.

What About Plant Remedies?

Herbalists and diviners both provide highly valued healing interventions. Many
herbalists are indeed skilled in the use of local vegetal resources, and some work
with ethnopharmacologists who seek to identify active ingredients. Others prefer
to keep their ingredients secret. Ethnobotanical literature from Africa includes
studies that analyze plants and other substances used by local practitioners in
order to identify active ingredients, but I could find no randomized clinical trials
of safety or efficacy published.[5] For example, of the more than 700 plants identified by Rwandan practitioners, 25 were tested by pharmacologists for evidence of
anti-microbial activity. They found sixteen to contain ingredients active against
Nesseria gonorrhea and *N. meningitis*; six against *Streptococcus pyogenes* and five
against *Staphylococcus aureus* (van Puyvelde, Geiser, Rwangabo, et al. 1983). Many
preparations contained salicylate from willow bark and other plants, the active
ingredient of aspirin. The painkiller may help to mask symptoms and reduce fever. Later, Rwangabo (1993) provided a list of plants used by healers against syphi-
lis. The quantities employed and their clinical effects were not tested, however.

Biomedical evaluation can provide assessments of efficacy and safety, as
happened long ago with *Rawulfia*, a vine from the Congo forests. Despite some
healers' extensive herbal knowledge, and the placebo effect of both assumed

remedies and accompanying ritual, the claims of many folk practitioners to heal disease are suspect. In particular, the extent to which their treatments are efficacious against infectious diseases, neoplasms, and genetic biochemical and metabolic errors remains to be demonstrated. Methods of administration may be without biological effect. For example, plants supposed to cure children's respiratory ailments were administered by means of smoke inhalation, warming the child's buttocks over a fire in which herbs were burned, liana strings tied around the neck or waist, and infusions in bath water that was later spread on a crossroads (Disengomoka, Delaveau, and Sengele 1983).[6] Moreover, some preparations include animal parts, spider webs, anthill soil, insect nests, bones and other substances which I, for one, would not like to see administered to humans unless proven harmless.

Some "healers" are expert poisoners (Mudimbe 1981). Certainly, dangerous alkaloids were used in the poison ordeal at dosages known to be fatal. Kin with stigmatized diseases, including infants considered abnormal, might be dispatched by such means. Knowledge of plants such as the ubiquitously growing white trumpet flower or thorn apple, *Datura stramonium*, all parts of which are toxic (Patterson 1983), may be called upon to speed release from suffering, convulsions, and madness. A common ingredient of healers' preparations in Lubumbashi in the 1970s, *Datura* can have a narcotic effect when used in minute quantities, but it is easy to overdose, especially in the case of children, for whom it was used to treat *ndegedege* (literally "bird," meaning convulsions), which might be due to a high fever or to epilepsy. We found it growing in our Lubumbashi city garden in 1974. Other common toxic plants such as *Euphorbia candalabrum* and *Lantana trifolia* also grew there. In 1977, a university student died, poisoned by an abortifacient supplied by a folk practitioner, which physicians were unable to identify. An autopsy study in South Africa found cases of fatal hepatitis caused by a toxic plant remedy—apparently dose-dependent—commonly prescribed especially for young children (Popat, Shear, Malkiewicz, et al. 2001). These authors cite literature on other toxic plants, sometimes given in fatal doses by African folk practitioners.

Efficacy trials of alternative medicines used against other infectious and chronic diseases such as hypertension and diabetes are far from encouraging. Pharmacologists worry about drug interactions between herbal preparations and between these and prescription drugs, especially possible concurrent pharmacodynamic effects of traditional medicines on bodies dependent on antiretroviral drugs (ARVs) for survival. Several herbs widely used in the US,[7] such as St. John's Wort, increase the likelihood of ARVs' therapeutic failure (Lee, Andrade, and Flexner 2006).

The means by which folk practitioners acquire what they claim as knowledge vary. Some serve apprenticeships with an experienced *nganga* as did

Professor Buakasa's father (1998). Others dream their remedies. Lloyd Swantz (1990), who studied the practices of 83 Zaramo *waganga* and nine Muslim clerics in Dar es Salaam in the 1970s, discovered that some had inherited a medicine bag (*mfuko*) entitling them to practice from a grandfather, without any special training; some learned from a dream or from possession by a spirit (*pepo*, also meaning wind). A significant number said they had acquired their skills "here and there" (*hivi hivi*), but some served apprenticeships of varying length, running errands and observing a *mganga* at work. The *waganga* Swantz studied closely observed patients' behavior but made no attempt to examine patients' bodies to arrive at diagnosis. Patients in Dar were most frequently treated by Muslim "healers" who used water in which Koranic verses had been soaked, or given amulets containing verses, or made to inhale smoke or vapors of magical substances. Divination using the *bao* game board with its two rows of holes was another popular method. Most healers used herbs, and about half accepted mental patients. Patients rarely expressed dissatisfaction to Swantz or his research assistants. "Healing" was good business in the popular quarters of Dar, as it was in Lubumbashi during the same years: "For the present, public opinion, tradition and demand assure the successful *mganga* a place in Zaramo urban society . . . the majority of *waganga* keep at their occupation only so long as people come to them and are willing to pay their high fees" (Swantz 1990, 21). Nowadays, Muslims in Dar may travel to consult *waganga* in the interior, while people from the interior travel to the coast to consult Koranic healers (Parkin 2013), testimony to the itinerancy of the quest for therapy.

Calls for collaboration with folk practitioners with respect to HIV/AIDS continue in governments and development agencies. While many practitioners claim to cure AIDS, whether herbal preparations are effective in treating opportunistic infections is an empirical question to be answered through research using laboratory studies and controlled clinical trials of their safety and efficacy. In the mid-1980s, the World Health Organization (WHO/GPA) announced that they were evaluating medicines used by traditional healers as potential antiviral agents, but no results have been published to date. WHO also was interested in "the utilization of traditional healers in the provision of social/medical support to AIDS patients" (Dr. Jose Esparza personal communication, May 1989).[8]

Treatment of psychogenic disorders by charismatic ritual specialists is probably the least controversial of their interventions, although some rituals may involve physical and psychological abuse. Moreover, given what we know about neurological disorders, ritual treatment is not always indicated. Closely associated with these activities is the use of charisma and power for social control (Schoepf 1981, 1982; Janzen 1982; Feierman 1985). I am hardly alone in my skepticism. Wyatt MacGaffey, a long-term student of Kongo religion, was unimpressed by claims to medical efficacy by traditional healers: "Most of what is known as healing in contemporary Kongo consists of little besides the claim by one wishing to be known as a healer that healing has taken place, and acceptance of that claim by others in accordance with the distinction of ends and effects" (MacGaffey 1980, 303).

Health Services: Who Gets What?

Decolonization brought a weakening of colonial ideology and a search for authentic African ways of life. While they expanded biomedical services following independence, many governments also sought to rehabilitate African medicine that had been denigrated and suppressed by the colonizers. Political leaders and academics discovered medical pluralism.[9] The concept assumes that people have a choice. This is true only to a point, however. In much of Africa today, biomedicine of reasonable standard, with well-trained physicians, sophisticated diagnostic tests, cogent explanations, quality pharmaceuticals and supplies, and skilled, respectful nursing care, is unavailable to most rural and many urban poor populations. High government officials and wealthy businesspeople may travel abroad for biomedical treatment. Many other people have not got a choice. For many, health services were and are too costly and too far away, and transport, especially in the rainy season, is too onerous or simply unavailable.

In the 1970s, international policy-makers discovered that many Africans relied upon a congeries of "traditional practitioners" for health care and asserted (without citation of research) that these actors provided primary care to 80 percent of people in developing countries, not just in Africa (WHO 1978a, b). Bibeau (1979) noted that WHO's idea of collaboration between African and biomedicine amounted to little more than reliance on folk practitioners for primary care.[10] This could hardly meet the goals of WHO's (1978b) Alma Ata Declaration which proposed to achieve "Health Care for All by the Year 2000," with health understood as "a complete state of physical, mental and social well-being." Yet the assertion that people prefer medical pluralism and the 80 percent figure continue to appear in policy documents.

The main problem, of course, was not belief, but money. In the 1980s most African governments succumbed to pressure from the Washington Consensus of the Regan and Thatcher governments, along with the Institutions of International Finance (IFIs), to carry out Structural Adjustment (SAPs) and other measures in aid of debt reimbursement, reducing millions to dire poverty. Stringent budget cuts made many public health workers and teachers redundant and froze the wages of those remaining. By imposing user fees for services and encouraging private care provision, SAPs narrowed access not only to curative, but to preventive services (Lurie, Hintzen and Loew 1995; Turshen 1999; Schoepf, Schoepf and Millen 2000). Urban as well as rural care deteriorated, just as AIDS spread across the continent (Schellenberg, Victoria, Mushi, et al. 2003; Say and Rayne 2007; Beckmann 2010; Dilger 2010; to cite just a few).

Africa is estimated to bear nearly one quarter of the world burden of disease, but only three percent of the biomedical health workforce.[11] Staffing shortages limit the capacity to deliver health services, partly due to the ongoing brain drain of trained medical personnel, which AIDS has worsened. A study of nine HIV/AIDS-affected countries estimated physician losses from 1990 had cost more than US$2.5 billion in public education expenditures, with Britain the greatest beneficiary and the United States second (Mills, Kanters, Hagopian, et al. 2011). In Tanzania, for instance, medical staffing levels in inefficient and poorly re-sourced health facilities plummeted from the wholly inadequate level in 1981 of 19,000 people per physician and 3,300 per nurse to 24,880 and 5,470, respectively, in 1991, and one doctor per 100,000 people in 2010. In 1991, only half the rural health centers had antimalarial drugs in stock (field notes 1991). Privatization did not improve access, as few new clinics were located in underserved areas (Benson 2001).

SAPs are not the only destroyer of health services; corruption, too, has taken a heavy toll (U4 2009). Mobutu's Zaire was notorious, a worst-case scenario in the 1970s and subsequent decades, in which endemic corruption absorbed much of the foreign funds supplied by complacent donors. Uganda exited colonialism with one of the best records in health services, which Idi Amin undermined. Since Museveni's 1986 victory, extraordinary largesse from the international do-nor community has been diverted to the President and his cronies. The effect on fund-starved public health services is disastrous, despite high praise for the government's response to AIDS.

> Uganda has some of the worst health statistics in the world despite having received billions of dollars in foreign aid for health services. . . . Today this system is a shambles. Bats, snakes, and other wildlife have taken up residence in once-functioning rural clinics. I have seen fecal material rain down from crumbling ceilings of operating theaters. Power cuts and water shortages kill thousands of patients each year, and emergency operations on pregnant women are sometimes carried out by the light of torches made from burning grass. . . . Only half of Uganda's health workers show up to work on any given day. (Epstein 2014, 40)

Epstein's grim depiction applies to many countries. In Uganda and else-where, many underpaid health workers who remain in the fund-starved pub-lic sector demand fees (or bribes) above the state-imposed user charges; others neglect their service to moonlight in the private sector. Nurses and others are often perceived as rude and quick to blame patients for poor outcomes. Some steal medications and supplies to sell. Some hospitals and birthing centers hold women and infants hostage until families come forth with payment. Apparently some folk practitioners also resort to this as patients grow poorer and reluctant to pay (Beckmann 2010; Whyte 2014).[12] In sum, in most countries, adequate biomedical care remains accessible only to government and business elites and their relatives, while the wealthiest go abroad for care. Many poor sick people and their relatives resort to home remedies and folk practitioners. Countries such as Mauritius and the Seychelles that refused to bow to Structural Adjustment have entirely different health statistics and health-seeking behavior (Schoepf, Andrianisata, Bedja, et al. 2006).

In 2001, economist Jeffrey Sachs estimated that it would take US$25 billion annually to support public health systems that can rid the world's poor of major diseases, including HIV/AIDS, tuberculosis, and malaria, and can render motherhood safe. Even doubling that amount today, it palls in comparison with military expenditures, on which the United States spends $1 trillion annually and the rest of the world, together, nearly as much. At the same time, billions are lost in illegal transfers of funds from Africa to foreign countries (Kar and Cartwright-Smith 2011; Africa Focus 2015).

Consequences in the Time of AIDS

Lack of access to quality affordable public biomedical health care and secondary education has created barriers to understanding biomedical concepts of disease causes and prevention. When AIDS came upon the scene, such credibility as biomedicine had enjoyed was undermined in the eyes of many by the lack of a cure, by rumors and conspiracy theories, and by the racist constructions placed upon HIV transmission by some early researchers and mass media. AIDS offers a broad cultural field for polysemic interpretation in competition with accumulating biomedical knowledge, and is particularly difficult for lay people, including political leaders without training in contemporary biological sciences, to understand. The multiple disease processes of the AIDS syndrome wax and wane over time, while unseen, the HIV continues to destroy the immune system. Folk practitioners may interpret the next sickness as a new attack or attribute it to failure to follow prescribed rituals. With variable periods between infection and the onset of disease symptoms, AIDS appears to strike arbitrarily, so that folk practitioners' claims might seem plausible to sufferers, at least for a time (Schoepf 1990). In addition, due to the stigma surrounding AIDS as a sexually transmitted disease associated with "immorality," many families prefer to ascribe the illness and death to witchcraft rather than AIDS (for example, Rodlach 2006). While antiretroviral treatment (ART) has begun to make inroads on the hopelessness of AIDS, the stigma is not yet eliminated (White 2014; Schoepf 2016).

Several diseases that result from immune system damage and are characteristic in people with HIV/AIDS are widespread in Africa, especially among the poor. Some diseases of the AIDS syndrome, including prolonged severe diarrhea and wasting, skin diseases, and dementia, are stigmatized in many cultures. With plumpness considered a sign of health and beauty, many attributed sufferers' weight loss to moral transgressions, a sign of spiritual affliction and supernatural sanction. Persistent cosmological beliefs related to constructions of sexuality, reproduction, health, and gender made biomedicine just one among several competing sources of authority, as in the time of Janzen's 1970s research. In DRC, this was particularly true of the rural and urban poor, those who along with pluralistic health-seeking practices, believed in witchcraft as an explanation for misfortune (reviewed in Schoepf 2014). The following example highlights an inventive bricolage formed by integrating African, European and biomedical ideas of health care, although perhaps not in the way that international health officials who urged collaboration envisaged.

Ebale Mbonge's Clinic

One of the most impressive health care enterprises in Kinshasa was that of Ebale Mbonge, a well-known healer, reputedly connected to high-level political men. I visited in September 1986, in the company of Dr. Lurhuma, at the time the recently named Director of the Institut de Recherche Scientifique (IRSS), who had been invited by the healer.[13] The establishment occupied a large compound with a two-story house at one corner, fronting on the street. On the ground floor, the rear parlor housed a "museum" containing objects deposited by patients. Guided by two of the *muganga*'s public relations staff, we were asked to remove our shoes to inspect the museum. They pointed to three types of objects. The first artifacts were fetishes, including statuettes and medicinal products, which we were told were produced by sorcerers with intent to harm. Objects in the second set were inscribed with occult signs including yin and yang designs and variations on the crucifix. The third group were animist objects which I could scarcely distinguish from the first set; these, however, were said to hold healing powers.

A series of open sheds lined the compound's rear wall, and between the shed and a wide central space stood tented cubicles resembling open market stalls, each equipped with a chair and table. These served as (semi-)private ambulatory treatment rooms. The central open space also served a waiting area for patients and their therapy managers, as well as a dancing ground for divination ceremonies. In another corner of the compound stood two small adobe shacks, designated as the in-patient hospital, where we were taken to see three women, said to be AIDS patients, lying on mats in complete darkness. The *muganga*, Ebale Mbonge [EbMb], explained how sicknesses are caused.

EbMb: Sorcerers [*baloi* or *baloji*] command "sorcery airplanes" fueled by
  human blood on which they ride in the night. These planes are large
  enough to carry 500 seated passengers, the spirits of the ensorcelled. The
  chief sorcerers can also drink the blood which they drain from people they

killed themselves, or could send *bestioles* like mosquitoes to kill for them.[14] Satanic powers, devils, and the spirits of people killed by sorcerers also could kill using other airplanes, and also by using slippers, wires, mirrors and television sets. [He mentions several names of famous and powerful people he claims to have cured.] I even cured K., a well-known sorcerer of the Bakongo. He killed by tying knots in grasses that people brought to him, along with palm wine, cigarettes and *makasu* [home-brewed alcohol]. His right foot was swollen. Inside were the spirits of all those he had killed to serve as spirit helpers against others. His foot swelled and throbbed and hurt badly. He went to Mama Yemo Hospital and stayed for two or three months, without result. The rot [*pourriture*] was still there. The doctors advised amputation below the knee, so he fled and came here. We cured him instead of amputating.

Many people consult the *feticheurs* [fetish priests, also called sorcerers in Congolese French] about problems in begetting children and marital problems, and for success in commerce. The devils who work for people who consult the *feticheurs* have to be paid. The *feticheurs* do not actually say this. They leave it up to the clients. So when they fail to pay, family members are attacked following the consultation.

[My field notes continue with a page of EbMb's interpretation of Rosicrucian and Franc Mason beliefs, and various types of "devils" folded into the discourse of sorcery, too lengthy to be included here.] He asks my university, nods, and continues his monologue:

EbMb: In medical anthropology it is important to know why these powders that come from Chicago in the United States are able to heal. Here we heal mainly by operating on the invisible. In 1986, we have received 4,749 patients already. For some people we perform cures through purification with holy water used in baths, in enemas and by mouth. That is the way to eliminate [*dégager*] the bad pus that lodges in the stomach.

The *muganga* then introduced us to the rest of his establishment: "The men in white lab coats are the *banganga nzambi* [spirit doctors]; the men in pink coats are . . . [I did not hear the term]. The *muganga* continued using biomedical analogies: "At the reception, when a sick person comes to us, we give them a "*radioscopie*" [there is no actual X-ray machine]. The sick person goes into a trance and the spirit makes the diagnosis. For the analysis, we call the *responsable* [a family member or therapy manager] who accompanies the patient and interrogate him, and perhaps other family members also can enter in trance. They form a circle around the *nganga nzambi*. The ceremony takes place here on the dancing ground."

Some two dozen people sit there motionless on mats. The women wear white headscarves, like members of a religious congregation. They appear to be stupefied, hypnotized or in trance. Male treatment personnel make yapping sounds and move their arms over them, apparently to enter into contact with spirits. While EbMb talks with us, a man begins to scream and shout.

EbMb: That is a crazy man [*fou*], whose people have brought him to get him quiet. [He continues describing the healing ritual]: The person or spirit responsible for the affliction reveals himself. Then we cure the patient by a semi-direct treatment. I verify [*controller*] each day to see if the spirit power is present. But not with this new disease. AIDS is due to a power we have not yet mastered.

[We have moved to the rear of the compound, where Ebole Mbonge introduces us to four biomedical physicians in his employ, as well as to ten other folk practitioners. We are taken to observe the physicians at work. In one tented cubicle, a woman sits with her breast uncovered, showing an open wound on which a white powder is being sprinkled by a white-coated woman healer.]

EbMb: This woman came to us directly [without being referred]. Her maternal aunt is a sorcerer. She sent a stone into the woman's breast and this stone caused a cancer. We did the analysis here.

BGS to the woman healer [WH]: What is the treatment?

WH: There is a hard mass in the breast. I have faith, but I worked a bit in a hospital, so I know how to do biomedicine and spiritual healing. With the [application of] medicine, the wound has softened and we removed the pus. You can see, it is clean and now almost no pus comes out.

Prof. Lurhuma: What certainty do you have that this is actually a cancer? It could be a simple abscess.

EbMb: Our doctors certified that is cancer of the breast. We interrogated the spirits who diagnosed the causes.

Prof. L: Is this the diagnostic procedure?

EbMb: Yes. The spirit also can communicate the prescription. We can call on the spirit to give us the name of the proper doctor and the prescription.

Prof. L.: What other maladies can you heal with this method?

EbMb: We can operate, for example on appendicitis. We can cure sterility in women and men for whom no solution can be found in hospital. We call the reproductive organs to speak to us and tell us what is wrong. Maybe it is because of something the women did that caused pollution. Or for example, a woman may have her fallopian tubes [*les trompes*] blocked by certain substances or tied by the sorcerers. For the uterus, it's the same thing. . . . That is the way we come to link spiritual healing and science.

[Belief in sexual pollution as a cause of reproductive and sexual health disorders, including infertility, is widespread in the popular quarters of Kinshasa and other cities in the Congo, where other forms of sent sickness are situated chiefly within the family. A man may seek "medicine" to "poison" the man who has sex with his wife, thereby causing an affliction. A woman who has not been purified following a miscarriage may afflict her next partner(s) with an STI.[15]]

EbMb: We also do birthing here. Children who are *revenants* [that is, believed to be reincarnations of the dead, usually deceased relatives], especially, prefer to be born here, out of the reach of sorcerers. This child here is a reincarnation of Saint Joshua. The birthing attendant here is a gynecologist trained by the revelations of Sainte Anastasie. We also cure many who come with psychosomatic complaints. Come see my hospital for AIDS patients.

[Our host led us to another corner of the compound where he pointed to the two dilapidated adobe shacks, which he called the inpatient hospital, where three women, whom he designated as AIDS patients, lay on mats in complete darkness. A physician in the establishment later told us the women had been brought and abandoned by their families who wanted no more to do with them.]

EbMb: AIDS is considered shameful and families are afraid of the stigma. Maybe they do not want the complications [conflict] that follows from witch-finding diagnosis. I diagnose AIDS clinically. There is one woman, age 35 years, whom I sent to Hôpital Mama Yemo on July 28. They found her seronegative. But two months later, on 2 September, she was tested at the INRB [government lab] and found strongly positive. [Actually, that lab did not test for HIV at the time.]

EbMb comes to the point of his invitation, which is to obtain an affiliation that would legitimize his treatment center. Apparently, Professor Gilles Bibeau had already visited his center in the company of two research assistants, Matumona and Nsiala. According to EbMb, they agreed in principle to the affiliation with INRSS, possibly prior to Dr. Luhruma's being named Director. Neither assistant has mentioned this to us.

Prof. L.: I am not going to enter into discussion about this now. I will read the documentation and reflect on the matter.

[On the way back to the office in his car, Dr. Lurhuma is rueful:]

Prof L: What a charlatan! The sore on that woman's breast is undoubtedly an abscess, nothing more. In addition, the man is a sorcerer! He must be making a great deal of money from the credulity of so many people. He has powerful political connections. We must be very careful not to allow him to create a false impression. I am afraid that, simply as a result of our visit, he will advertise that we are collaborating.

BGS: As might the government for political reasons of its own? I am amazed at the amount of biomedical half-knowledge he has been able to integrate into his discourse, and also with the syncretic religious bricolage he offers. No wonder desperate sick people believe him. And imagine how desperate the employment shortage is for physicians who graduate from the UNIKIN Medical School (Kinshasa University). Look at those working for him, when there are so many sick people who need biomedicine!

[Although most biomedically trained physicians we met rejected the folk practitioners' claims, some of those who worked in the establishment of Ebale Mbonge, and earned more than doctors in the public health system, claimed that his cures had merit. Others remained silent (field notes, visit to establishment of Muganga Ebale Mbonge, September 1986).]

Other Types of Collaboration?

Green (1999) argues that in southern Africa, folk practitioners' ideas of contagion are sufficiently similar to those of biomedicine to allow them to counsel HIV prevention by abstaining from sex. I disagree (see Symonds and Schoepf 2000). One way that folk practitioners in DRC and elsewhere may counsel patients to rid themselves of disease is to pass it on to others. The method is an old one. Patients are advised to rub the afflicted body part with something attractive (a Zaire note in the 1970s; today, a dollar bill), or to wash with the bill, and leave it at a crossroads to be picked up by a passerby who at the same time picks up the affliction (elsewhere, see Ngubane 1976; Prins 1979). Formerly, a sufferer might be sent to bathe in the river and told to return without looking back or speaking to anyone until the attractive object had been set out at the crossroads. Another widespread notion with respect to contagion is that disease can be transmitted to one who walks or urinates on the place where a sick person has urinated (in this case, too, crossroads are particularly dangerous). An idea that applies specifically to sexually transmitted infections (STIs) is particularly pernicious. In Kinshasa and elsewhere, folk practitioners have advised afflicted men to have sex with a young, vigorous woman who takes on their affliction and then will shed it with her menses (field notes, Kinshasa 1987).

This is also an old idea. In the time of AIDS, this advice has translated into sex with a virgin free of HIV and resulted in the rape of young girls and even babies in several countries, particularly South Africa.

Sending Sickness

The two principal questions sufferers and their families ask are *why* has this misfortune happened to X at this time? And *who* has caused this misfortune? These are not questions to which biomedicine can supply answers that most people find satisfactory. Instead, they may turn to folk practitioners to identify the source of misfortune. AIDS has provided a fertile field for folk practitioners and patients' imaginations. Old ideas about supernatural or interpersonal causes remain salient for many, especially for rural people and others without secondary education. This is particularly true for elders, and even for some among the university-educated elites. However, even if they do not know of the cosmology or place much credence in it, younger people may be guided in their choice of health care modalities by their elders. They may turn to diviners who search for causes in the realm of spirits, by ancestors angered by breaches of rules of respect (or taboos), or in the envy of relatives, neighbors and others with evil intent. Practitioners in Zaire during the 1970s and 1980s often supplied indirect answers (especially in light of anti-sorcery laws remaining from colonial times) and allowed clients or their therapy managing group to interpret hints as they would.

Without wishing to exoticize witchcraft, which has parallels in the United States as well as in Europe, both historically and at the present time (Geschire 2013), accusations are a sign of mistrust in kin relations that has become acute in the time of SAPs and AIDS (Beckmann 2010; Dilger 2010; Schoepf 1990). Rising inequality, deepening poverty, and mysterious afflictions are accompanied by a dramatic increase in accusations of evil-doing. Integral to old ideas of causation, witchcraft (used interchangeably with sorcery despite the RB distinction) is no small matter. People accused of witchcraft, today as in the past, may be ostracized, killed, or driven to suicide (Douglas 1997; Yomba 1997; Lawyui 1998; Schoepf 2002). Newspaper accounts from rural Africa in the 1990s related numerous deaths of elderly women, especially those without kin, suspected of witchcraft.[16] Niehaus, who examines ways that cosmologies have changed over time in rural South Africa, suggests witchcraft accusations are "a complex discourse on social inequality, deprivation and envy" in which privilege is justified by "defining the desires of those who have been deprived as illegitimate and evil" (Niehaus 2001, 111). In other words, in contrast to what earlier might have served as a leveling mechanism, witchcraft accusations made against the poor legitimate the conspicuous wealth of those who earlier would have been obligated to share their wealth with kin and community. In Nso', Cameroon, powerful elder men who formerly would have been accused now may get off scot free (Quaranta 2010).

Where formerly elders were the ones accused of sorcery against younger kin in Congo, now children and youth are accused of "occult practices" and "mystical harms" (Yengo 1998). Geschire (2013) and Dilger (2010) also find that the strains placed on intimate relations by new forms of accumulation and commoditization that do not lend themselves to redistribution are particularly powerful. Although Whyte and her colleagues (2014) find many instances of strong solidarity and caring that enable people to access ART, one cannot automatically assume the family is a benign therapy managing group with the best interests of sufferers upmost in their complex motivations. At the very least, "witchcraft accusations have significant potential to break down social capital networks and exacerbate community tensions and fear" (Thomas 2007, 289). Some Zaire/DRC examples follow:

Chiefs were routinely suspected of killing members of their families through magical means to ensure or consolidate their power. Those killed were supposed to have been sent to the spirit world to work on the chief's behalf. In 1987, a member of the CONNAISSIDA team sought election to Parliament from his home district of Bandundu. When his son died of malaria, people there whispered that he had killed his child to obtain political power. Similarly, in 1990, when another team member's infant daughter died, her paternal uncles, who sought to inherit her father's property despite his testament, claimed responsibility for the death in an effort to frighten her into ceding the house. They also threatened her, and when she died two years later of "a long and painful illness," as AIDS was known, they claimed responsibility for her death as well. Still, her mother and younger sister who lived in the house held out against eviction. Devout Catholics, they refused to countenance sorcery as an explanation (SM, letter in files of the author, 1994).

A chief whose people died in great numbers was considered a bad chief whose subjects were justified in rebelling without fear of supernatural reprisals. The *vox populi* might occasionally win out against authority. In 1998, six local chiefs in Bandundu were believed by their people and police to possess a mystical ability to transform themselves into crocodiles. Since 1995, they were said to have eaten a total of thirty-three people; one chief confessed to eating five. The accused shape-shifters were arrested, but I have no information on the outcome of their case, or even if they were brought to trial. Earlier that month, real crocodiles killed some twenty people when they overturned a canoe. Sorcerers were believed to have caused the upset (news dispatches, AP, AFP and VOA, January 28, 1998). "There are no accidents in Africa," as the saying goes.

Some AIDS sufferers and their families may seek to avoid the shame and stigma of sexual transgression by claiming bewitchment rather than admitting to AIDS (Rodlach 2006). In several mature epidemics, HIV/AIDS has shifted from its initial impact on wealthy, educated urban men and their partners to afflict mainly poor people with little or no formal schooling, little access to biomedical health care, and little accurate knowledge of HIV prevention. This absence of modernity leaves the field to self-interested charlatans as well as to well-meaning herbalists who attempt to cope with AIDS and other infectious diseases associated with HIV. Some cite witchcraft or vengeful spirits as the cause, and may claim to cure AIDS or something they believe to be caused by sexual pollution. But in eastern Uganda, when AIDS is diagnosed, bewitchment is no longer suspected, as people now forgo expensive consultations with folk practitioners and seek antiretroviral treatment to "bring them back from the dead" (Whyte 2014).

Witch-hunting resonates with older beliefs, but it is by no means reserved to traditional healers, nor should it be labeled "indigenous." In the city, many who might have consulted folk practitioners turn to Pentecostal preachers and other pastor-prophets who promise to heal the faithful. Some add fuel to the fire of mistrust in intimate relations. Despite their ostensible rejection of the "evil spirits" of traditional religion, these pastors, some of them supported by religious congregations in the US (Obbo 2014; Schoepf 2014), have recreated demons, witches and others believed to exercise satanic powers and to lead people astray. Impoverished and demoralized by decades of privation, violence and AIDS, many families cannot feed their own children or those entrusted to them by deceased relatives. Biaya (1997) linked the plight of Kinshasa's then-estimated 30,000 homeless children to the destitution that followed adoption of Structural Adjustment measures and political conflict that made Kinshasa a site of evangelist fervor. Kinshasa and other African cities have witnessed an epidemic of accusations against children by Pentecostal pastors, leading to harsh mistreatment, torture, and even murders of those accused without drawing judicial response (Biaya 1997; Tonda 2000). Witchcraft accusations allow families to slough off unruly, burdensome, deformed or otherwise abnormal" children and orphans (Schoepf 2002; Aiguilar Molina 2005). I concur with Biaya (1997) and Mate (2002), that these beliefs, like those promoted by diviners in seeking evil-doers, allow the true causes of misfortune, poverty, inequality and structural violence to escape popular critique.

Not all medical anthropologists wish to see these ideas promoted (see Schoepf 2001). "Studies of healers' practices should not be construed as indicating scientific validation, nor should anthropologists be lulled into putting their work at the service of the publicity machines used by healers to attract clients" (Dozon 1995,193, my translation). In my view, the human right to health is better served by anthropologists and others advocating for monetary contributions by national governments and international donors in aid of establishing and maintaining quality biomedical services in Africa, free and accessible to all. Some people may continue to consult folk practitioners, but they will have a choice.

Notes

1. Also referred to as local and folk healers, or practitioners, among other terms.
2. GCM was the successor to the Union Minière du Haut Katanga (UMHK), nationalized by Mobutu.
3. Kaptchuk, quoted, *Harvard Medicine News,* January 10, 2014.
4. L-dopa was discovered by Dr. Melvin Yahr, working with my father, who also devised a method to rule out placebo reactors in a double-blind test to assess the effectiveness of Excedrin compared with regular aspirin (Sherman, Fiasconara, and Grundfest 1963).
5. The *Journal of Ethnopharmacology* is devoted to this research, much of it from Africa.
6. Note the importance of the crossroads, common in central Africa (Prins 1979; Schoepf above).
7. In the United States, believers in herbal remedies and aids to health spend some $90 billion annually on substances, including $25 billion on dietary supplements, all uncontrolled by the Food and Drug Administration (PBS Newshour, 3 February 2015).
8. I have heard nothing further from this initiative.
9. Janzen's 1978 *Quest for Therapy* was influential in this respect, as was the work of Charles Leslie.
10. Fassin (2000, Chapter 6) offers a scathing critique of the supposed "integration" of therapeutic systems.
11. WHO (2010) gives data on exceptionally deficient health worker staffing levels across the continent.
12. Apparently some traditional healers also resort to this as patients grow poorer and reluctant to pay what they consider exorbitant fees for poor results (Beckmann 2010; Whyte 2014).
13. Dr. Lurhuma, co-inventor of the bogus AIDS remedy MM-1, named after the two heads of state of its originators, Mobutu and Mubarak, died in 1995.
14. See Luise White (2000) for Africans' stories involving white vampires in colonial East and Central Africa and Peter Geschire (1995) for contemporary versions of zombies in rural Cameroon.
15. Lemba in southeastern Katanga told us of this before the advent of AIDS (field notes 1976).
16. In Tanzania, women, especially the elderly, were often suspected due to their red eyes, a common consequence of smoky cookfires.

Bibliography

Africa Focus. 2015. "Africa/Global: Stopping capital losses," *Africa Focus Bulletin*, February 5.

Aguilar Molina, Javier. 2005. *The Invention of Child Witches in the Democratic Republic of Congo: 2003–2005.* Kinshasa: Save the Children.

Bailint, Michael. 1959. *The Doctor, His Patient and the Illness.* New York: International Universities.

Beckmann, Nadine 2010. "The commodification of misery: Markets for healing, markets for sickness." In *Markets of Well-being: Navigating Health and Healing in Africa*, edited by M. Decker and R. Van Dijk. Leiden: Brill.

Benson, John S. 2001. "The impact of privatization on access in Tanzania." *Social Science and Medicine* 52: 1903–15.

Bernstein, Lenny. 2015. "A More Expensive Placebo is Often More Effective than a Cheap One." *Washington Post*, January 28.

Biaya Tshikala K. 1997. "Kinshasa: Anomie, 'Ambiance' et Violence." In *Jeunes, Cultures de la Rue et Violences Urbaines en Afrique*, edited by Georges Hérault and Pius Adesanmi, 329–82. Abidjan: Institut Francais de la Recherche en Afrique (IFAN).

Bibeau, Giles. 1979. "The WHO in Encounter with African Traditional Medicine: Theoretical Conceptions and Practical Strategies." In *African Therapeutic Systems*, edited by Z. A. Ademuwagun, J. A. A. Ayoade, Ira E. Harrison, and Dennis M. Warren, 182–86. Waltham, MA: Crossroads.

Bjilmakers, Leon, Mary T. Bassett, and David Sanders. 1996. *Health and Structural Adjustment in Rural and Urban Zimbabwe*. Uppsala: Nordiska Afrikainstitutet.

Buakasa, Gérard. "Itinéraire d'un nganga: Simon Makaya Ndonzoau (1905–1987)," *Anthropologie at Sociétés* 22(1): 153–81.

Cassiers, Daniel. 1973. "Courbe de poids des enfants de 0 à 2 ans dans les regions ruralse entourant les villes di Haut-Shaba," *Problèmes Sociaux Zairois* (Lubumbashi) 102–103: 41–45.

Cimpric, Aleksandra. 2010. *Children Accused of Witchcraft in West Africa: An Anthropological Study of Contemporary Practices*. Dakar: UNICEF, West Africa Regional Office.

Colson, Elizabeth. 2010 (2006). "The social history of an epidemic: HIV/AIDS in the Gwembe Valley, Zambia, 1982–2004." In *Morality, Hope and Grief: Anthropology of AIDS in Africa*, edited by Hansjorg Dilger and Ute Luig, 127–48. Oxford: Berghahn.

Colvin, Christopher J., Helen J. Smith, and Alison Schwartz et al. 2013. "Understanding Careeseeking for Child Illness in sub-Saharan Africa: A Systematic Review and Conceptual Framework Based on Qualitative Research of Household Recognition and Response to Child Diarrhea, Pneumonia and Malaria," *Social Science and Medicine* 86: 66–78.

Corin, Ellen. 1979. "A Possession Psychotherapy in an Urban Setting: Zebola in Kinshasa," *Social Science and Medicine* 13B (4): 327–38.

De Boeck, Filip. 2001. "Le Deuxième Monde et les Enfants Sorciers en République Démocratique du Congo," *Politique Africaine* 80: 32–57.

Devisch, Renate. 1985. "Pollution and Healing among the Northern Yaka of Zaire." *Social Science and Medicine* 21: 693–700.

Dilger, Hansjorg. 2010. "'My Relatives Are Running away from Me!' Kinship and Care in the Wake of Structural Adjustment." In *Morality, Hope and Grief: Anthropologies of AIDS in Africa*, edited by Hansjorg Dilger and Ute Luig, 102–24. Oxford: Berghahn.

Disengomoka, Ina, Pierre Delaveau, and Kaba Sengele. 1983. "Medicinal Plants Used for Children's Respiratory Diseases in Zaire. Part II," *Journal of Ethnopharmacology* 8: 265–277.

Douglas, Mary. 1997. "Sorcery Accusations Unleashed: The Lele, Revisited, 1987," *Africa* 69: 177–93.

Dozon, Jean-Paul. 1995. "Médecine Traditionnelle et Sida: Les Modalités de sa Prise en Charge par un Tradipraticien Ivoirien." In *Les Sciences Sociales Face au Sida: Cas Africaines autour d'un Exemple Ivoirien*, edited by Jean-Paul Dozon and Laurent Vidal, 187–95. Paris: Editions ORSTOM.

Epstein, Helen. 2014. "Murder in Uganda," *New York Review of Books* 61(1) (April 3): 40–42.

Fassin, Didier. 2000. *Les Enjeux Politiques de la Santé: Études Sénégalaises, Équatoriennes et Francaises*. Paris: Karthala.

Feierman, Steven. 1979. "Change in African Therapeutic Systems," *Social Science and Medicine* 13B (4): 277–84.

Geshiere, Peter, with Cyprian Fisiy. 1995. *Sorcellerie et Politique en Afrique: La Viande des Autres*. Paris: Karthala.

Geshiere, Peter. 2013. *Witchcraft, Intimacy and Trust: Africa in Comparison*. Chicago: University of Chicago.

Green, Edward. 1999. *Indigenous Theories of Contagious Disease*. Walnut Creek, CA: Altamira and London: Sage.

Grundfest, Harry 1959. "Synaptic and Ephaptic Transmission." In *Handbook of Physiology: Neurophysiology I*, edited by J. Field, 147–97. Washington, DC: American Physiological Society.

Human Rights Watch. 2006. *What Future? Street Children in the Democratic Republic of Congo*. New York: HRW.

IRIN. October 18, 2006. "Lesotho: 'Expert' Patients Lighten Load for Clinic Staff," *PlusNews*, Maseru.

———. August 5, 2008. "Religion—a Double-edged Sword in HIV Fight," *PlusNews*, Mexico City.

Janzen, John. 1978. *The Quest for Therapy in Lower Zaire*. Los Angeles: University of California.

———. 1992. Ngoma: *Discourses of Healing in Central and Southern Africa*. Berkeley and Los Angeles: University of California.

Kam-Hansen, Slavenka, Moshe Jakubowski, John M. Kelley, et al. January 2014. "Altered Placebo and Drug Labeling Changes the Outcome of Episodic Migraine Attacks." In *Science Translational Medicine* 6: 218–ra5.

Kar, Dev, and Devon Cartwright-Smith. 2011. *Illicit Financial Flows from Africa: Hidden Resources for Development*. Washington, DC: Global Financial Integrity, Center for International Policy. www.gfip.org

Kopytoff, Igor. 1980. "Revitalization and the Genesis of Cults in Pragmatic Religion: The Kita Rite of Passage among the Suku." In *Explorations in African Systems of Thought*, edited by Ivan Karp and Charles S. Bird, 183–212. Bloomington: Indiana University.

Lawyui, O.B. 1998. "Acts of Persecution in the Name of Tradition in Contemporary South Africa." *Dialectical Anthropology* 23: 83–95.

Lee, L. S., A. S. A. Andrade, and C. Flexner. 2006. "Interactions between Natural Health Products and Antiretroviral Drugs: Pharmacokinetic and Pharmacodynamic Effects." *Clinical Infectious Diseases* 43: 1052–59.

Luhrman, Tanya. 2012. *When God Talks Back: Understanding the American Evangelical Relationship to God*. New York: Vintage Books.

Lurie, Peter, Percy Hinton, and Robert A. Lowe. 1995. "Socioeconomic Obstacles to HIV Prevention and Treatment in Developing Countries: The Roles of the IMF and the World Bank." *AIDS* 9(6): 539–46.

MacGaffey, Wyatt. 1980. "African Religions: Types and Generalizations." In *Explorations in African Systems of Thought*, edited by Ivan Karp and Charles S. Bird, 301–28. Bloomington: Indiana University.

Marsland, Rebecca. 2007. "The Modern Traditional Healer: Locating 'Hybridity' in Modern Traditional Medicine, Southern Tanzania." *Journal of Southern African Studies* 33 (4): 751.

Mate, Rekopantswe. 2002. "Wombs as God's Laboratories: Pentecostal Discourses on Femininity in Zimbabwe." *Africa* 72 (4): 549–68.

Mills, Edward J, Steve Kanters, Amy Hagopian, et al. November 4, 2011 "The Financial Cost of Doctors Emigrating from sub-Saharan Africa: Human Capital Analysis." *British Medical Journal* online.

Mudimbe, V. Y. 1981. "Signes Thérapeutiques et Prose de la Vie en Afrique Noire." *Social Science and Medicine* 15B (2): 195–211.

Ngubane, Harriet. 1976. *Mind and Body in Zulu Medicine: An Ethnography of Health*. New York: Academic.

Niehaus, Isak, with Eliazaar Mohala and Kally Shokane. 2001. *Witchcraft, Power and Politics: Exploring the Occult in the South African Lowveld.* London: Pluto Press.

Obbo, Christine. 2014. "Sponsored Sexuality: AIDS and Tough Choices." In *Strings Attached: AIDS, and the Rise of Transnational Connections in Africa,* edited by Nadine Beckmann, Alessandro Gusman, and Catrine Schroff, 31–41. Proceedings of the British Academy of Sciences. Oxford University Press for the British Academy of Sciences.

Offit, Paul A. 2013. *Do You Believe in Magic? The Sense and Nonsense of Alternative Medicine.* New York: Harper Collins Books.

Packard, Randall. 1980. "Social Change and the History of Misfortune among the Bashu in Eastern Zaire." In *Explorations in African Systems of Thought,* edited by Ivan Karp and Charles S. Bird, 237–67. Bloomington: Indiana University.

Parent, Michel. 1961. "La Courbe de Croissance des Enfants Katangais entre 1 an et 3 1/2 Ans." *CEPSI Bulletin Trimestriel* (Elisabethville) 50: 27–38.

Park, Robert. 2000. *Voodoo Science: The Road from Foolishness to Fraud.* Oxford: Oxford University.

———. 2008. *Superstition: Belief in the Age of Science.* Princeton, NJ: Princeton University.

Patterson, David, ed. 1983. *Culpepper's Color Herbal.* New York: Sterling.

Peters, Pauline E., Daimon Kambembwa, and Peter A. Walker. 2010. "Contestations over 'Tradition' and 'Culture' in a Time of AIDS." *Medical Anthropology* 29 (3): 278–302.

Popat, Alpa, Neil H. Shear, Izabella Malkiewicz, et al. 2001. "The Toxicity of *Callilepis laureola*, a South African Traditional Herbal Medicine." *Clinical Biochemistry* 34: 229–36.

Prins, Gwyn. 1979. "Disease at the Crossroads: Towards a History of Therapeutics in Bulozi since 1876." *Social Science and Medicine* 13B (4): 285–315.

Quaranta, Ivo. 2010. "Politics of Blame: Clashing Moralities and the AIDS Epidemic in Nso' (Northwest Province, Cameroon)." In *Morality, Hope and Grief: Anthropologies of AIDS in Africa,* edited by Hansjorg Dilger and Ute Luig, 173–91. Oxford: Berghahn.

Rwangabo, Pierre-Claver. 1993. *Plantes Medicinales du Rwanda: Analyses Pharmacologiques.* Butare, Rwanda. Institut National de Recherche.

Rodlach, Alexander. 2006. *Witches, Westerners and HIV: AIDS and Cultures of Blame in Africa.* Walnut Creek, CA: Left Coast.

Sachs, Jeffrey. 2001. *Macroeconomics and Health.* Commissioned Report. Geneva: World Health Organization (WHO).

Say, Lalye, and Rosalind Payne. 2007. "A Systematic Review of Inequalities in the Use of Maternal Health Care in Developing Countries." *Bulletin of the WHO* 85 (10): 812–19.

Schellenberg, Joanna A., Cesar G. Victoria, Adele Mushi, et al. 4 February 2003. "Inequalities among the Very Poor: Health Care for Children in Rural Southern Tanzania." *Lancet* online.

Schoepf, Brooke G. 1971. "Raging Hormones or Raging Females?" Paper presented at the symposium "Anthropologists Look at the Study of Women," American Anthropological Association 70th Annual Meeting, New York.

———. 1976a. *Recherches en Anthropologie Médicale: Théorie et Perspectives Méthodologiques.* *Bulletin d'Anthropologie Médicale* (Lubumbashi) 1(2) August: 20–36.

———. 1976b. Pre-publication review of Janzen's *Quest* for University of California (ms. in files of the author).

———. 1990. "AIDS in Eriaz." In "AIDS on the Planet: The Plural Voices of Anthropology," edited by Gilbert Herdt, 13–14. *Anthropology Today* 6 (3):10–15.

———. 2001. "International Anthropological Research on AIDS in Africa: A Critical Perspective on the Crisis." *Annual Review of Anthropology* 30: 335–61.

———. 2002. "Mobutu's Disease: A Social History of AIDS in Kinshasa." *Review of African Political Economy* 994: 561–73.

———. 2014. "Hands across the Sea: Gender and the Politics of AIDS in the US and Africa." In *Strings Attached: AIDS, and the Rise of Transnational Connections in Africa*, edited by Nadine Beckmann, Alessandro Gusman, and Catrine Schroff, 43–67. Proceedings of the British Academy of Sciences. Oxford University Press for the British Academy of Sciences.

———. 2016. *An Annotated Bibliography of AIDS in Africa*. New York: Oxford University.

Schoepf, Brooke G., Claude Schoepf, and Joyce V. Millen. 2000. "Theoretical Therapies, Remote Remedies: SAPS and the Political Ecology of Health in Africa." In *Dying for Growth: Structural Adjustment and the Health of the Poor*, edited by Jim Y. Kim, Joyce V. Millen, Alec Irwin, and John Gershman, 91–125; 377–96. Monroe, ME: Common Courage.

Schoepf, Brooke G., John E. Andrianaisata, Said Ahmed Beja, et al. 2006. *Comprendre le Comportement de l'Épidémie du VIH dans les Isles Africaines de l'Ouest de l'Océan Indién: Pour une Plannification de la Réponse*. Pretoria: UNDP.

Sherman, Harold, J. E. Fiasconara, and Harry Grundfest. 1963. "Laboratory Evaluation of Analgesic Effectiveness in Human Subjects." *Experimental Neurology* 7: 435–56.

Spangler, Sydney A. 2011. "'To open oneself is a poor woman's trouble': Embodied Inequality and Childbirth in Southwestern Tanzania." *Medical Anthropology Quarterly* 25 (4): 479–98.

Swantz, Lloyd. 1990 (1978). *The Medicine Man among the Zaramo of Dar-es-Salaam*. Udevalla, Sweden: Bohuslaningen.

Symonds, Patricia, and Brooke G. Schoepf. 2000. "HIV/AIDS: The Global Pandemic and Struggles for Control." *Reviews in Anthropology* 28: 189–209.

Thomas, Felicity, 2007. "'Our Families Are Killing Us': HIV/AIDS, Witchcraft and Social Tensions in the Caprivi Region, Namibia." *Anthropology and Medicine* 14 (3): 279–91.

Tonda, Joseph. 2000. "La Violence de l'Imaginaire des Enfants-sorciers. *Politique Africaine* 75: 48–65.

Turshen, Meredeth. 1999. *The Privatization of Health Care in Africa*. Trenton, NJ: Africa World.

U4, Anti-Corruption Resource Centre. 2009. "Overview of Corruption in Tanzania." www.U4.no /helpdesk/helpdesk/query.cfm?id:201

van Puyvelde, Luc, Imrich Geiser, Pierre-Claver Rwangabo, and Boniface Sebikali. 1983. "Rwandan Herbal Remedies Used against Gonorrhea." *Journal of Ethnopharmacology* 5: 1–71.

White, Luise. 2000. *Speaking With Vampires: Rumor and History in Colonial Africa*. Berkeley: University of California.

Whyte, Susan Reynolds, ed. 2014. *Second Chances: Surviving AIDS in Uganda*. Raleigh, NC: Duke University.

World Health Organization. 1978a. *Health Care for All by the Year 2000*. Report of the World Health Assembly. Geneva: WHO.

———. 1978b. The Promotion and Development of Traditional Medicine. Meeting Report. Geneva: WHO.

———. 2010. *World Health Statistics*. Geneva: WHO.

SYMPTOMS AND THERAPEUTIC PLURALITIES

6 Wishful Doing

Journeying in a Nigerian Medical Landscape

Ulrika Trovalla

In memory of Dr. Mohammed A. Labaran. Even if your tired feet are now resting, I will always remember our journeys and how you opened my eyes to the Jos landscape.

WHEN WE SETTLED down around a table in the Nigerian city of Jos at the beginning of 2004, it became apparent that Labaran's troubles were mounting. After years of repeated religious and ethnic urban violence, the Nigerian Union of Medical Herbal Practitioners, Plateau State Branch in Jos had become divided and scarred in the same way as the urban landscape. It was not just that an "illegal election," according to Labaran, had been conducted and that he was thereby no longer the unquestionably elected secretary of the union, but he had also come down with a very bad cold. He kept blowing his nose. At one point he was even forced to go out to buy more toilet paper since he had finished a whole roll. "Enough with this catarrh," he exclaimed after blowing his nose, remarking that his condition was caused by the cold wind. This turned out to be an illness that, like his struggle to regain his position as the only elected secretary, would stay with him for the rest of his life. It was a struggle grown out of a body, a union, and a landscape in ailment. The urban landscape, Labaran's body, and the union merged together in an illness story that is narrated here.

As he tirelessly searched for ways to heal his illness as well as regain his lost position within the union, Labaran moved through Jos's highly heterogeneous medical landscape, with its ever-present churches brandishing big healing posters, its pharmacies, diagnostic centers, clinics, and hospitals of Western medicine, and its different consulting places, stalls, shops, temples, and clinics of the highly varied traditional medicine.[1]

The common denominator was not that these practices were "traditional" in the sense of being composed of local practices rooted in the past, but that they were not viewed as Western medicine. Verses from the Koran, persons possessed by spirits, talismans made by the Wicca movement in the United States, incenses imported from India, perfumes for calling on spirits, dried herbs with added perfume, and concoctions that had been decanted into second-hand bottles with labels giving dosage instructions were all offered as medicine. Their indications ranged from weight reduction, virility, blindness, broken legs, asthma, malaria, cancer, and HIV, to unemployment, lack of love, conflicts within families, stolen objects, elections, court cases, witchcraft, poison, and relationships with spirits.

For Labaran, the different medical logics behind the manifold forms of medicine he encountered through his journeys did not stand in conflict to each other, nor were the rationalities behind them—how their efficacy came about—necessarily known or considered of importance (see Last 1992). He strove to find treatments—relief of symptoms—rather than answers to the question of how the illness and the potential cure correlated with any abstract system (Whyte 2002, 178–79). More than any system or systems, it was Labaran's movements—his search—that gave the medicine meaning. The search tied together and formed relationships between the diverse diagnoses, prescriptions, and remedies. His unceasing travels forged the world through which his ailments and treatments came into being and became known. They were highly mutable walks; with every new footstep, new realities emerged—new realities with novel dangers, causes, diagnoses, and medicines. For Labaran, the world was an unfolding affair (Mead 1932, 1).

Through his walks, Labaran developed his understanding of his illness in relation not only to a medical landscape but to a landscape of conflict. On September 7, 2001, a once familiar city was thrown into disarray and confusion when a cleansing from within began, as Muslims in mainly Christian areas and Christians in mainly Muslim areas became targets of violence. This outbreak, which came to be known as "the crisis," brought with it a continuing cycle of escalating violence that has gained its momentum from a fusion of ethnicity and religion in the concept of "indigeneity" (see Suberu 2001, 17).[2] On one side of the clashes are Christians belonging to ethnic groups perceiving themselves as indigenous to the area, and on the other are Muslims, viewed as settlers, and belonging to ethnic groups often clustered together as Hausa-Fulani. The crisis has left the inhabitants of Jos with a landscape redefined into Muslim- and Christian-controlled zones (Danfulani & Fwatshak 2002, 253). Previous rules have been thrown into confusion. What a place is and how to behave to gain entry to it, which gates are secure to pass, which roads are safe to walk down, or whom to trust, have all become highly unpredictable matters (Andersson Trovalla 2011, 11–28, 133–146).

Just as in the landscape of Jos, new divisions and borders emerged among the members of the Nigerian Union of Medical Herbal Practitioners. The topography of the union was transformed. In 2004, just as the new year began, Labaran was very upset. For him, as a Muslim indigene—crossing the stereotypical distinction between the indigene Christian and the Muslim settler—things had become far more complicated. He recounted that the day before, the "Hausa faction" had held what according to him was an illegal election, to which none of the "indigenes" had been invited. He took out a piece of paper with a list of people who had been elected. He had been moving around showing it to a lot of different people, and the paper was already ragged. He commented, "See, they are all Muslims." He explained:

> There are now an indigene traditional herbalists, Plateau State, and a Hausa traditional herbalists, Plateau State. There is only supposed to be one Nigerian Union of Medical Herbal Practitioners in the State that is nationally recognized. However, because of the internal conflicts the Hausas have now brought themselves out and organized an election. This election is not recognized by the indigene herbal practitioners, so we now have two factions in the Union.

Previous friends had made plans behind his back. Relations between people had become blurred. An election had taken place in the union without any notification or invitation to him—a person who had long been at the core of the union's politics. In addition, he was also no longer the only elected secretary of the union.

As the future is always not yet known, uncertainty is an intrinsic part of all life (Dewey 1930, 213), but in Jos at the time this was brought to the forefront in all clarity. Years of conflict and tension had made life increasingly hard to predict. Even for Labaran, himself a doctor—a practitioner of traditional medicine—it had become far more complicated to navigate the conflict-ridden medical urban landscape. As I accompanied him on his daily movements through the city, rather than making calculated choices based on "trust" in systems, he "hoped" for beneficial outcomes (Lindquist 2000, 317ff.). Instead of being absolute cures, medicines emerged as incantations for futures hoped for. Building on John Dewey's (1930) pragmatist ideas of life as *uncertain* and George Herbert Mead's (1932) views of life as a constant *becoming*, the illness story told here brings to the forefront how Labaran's relation to his surroundings was characterized rather by a tentative, explorative, and *wishful doing* than by well-informed and calculated actions. For him, his search, his movements through the medical landscape, was in essence a series of uncertain walks through a landscape of hope—potential ways forward in a quest for futures wished for.

Movements of Danger

One day in 2004 when Labaran and I met with Bayo, another of Jos's practitioners of traditional medicine, he told me that when the crisis started, Labaran had changed clothes in his home. When he entered the house he had been dressed like a Christian, and when, some hours later, he left Bayo's home in a mainly Muslim area in the center to try to reach the village outside Jos where he lived, he had been dressed like a Muslim. Today, however, Bayo observed, Labaran looked like a Christian, with his yellow corduroy pants, shirt, and jacket. When I met Labaran the following day, he had put on a white gown over his corduroys and wore a small flat hat; he was dressed more like a Muslim. It was a Friday, and later in the day he attended the Friday prayer at the main mosque in Jos.

As borders became sharper, Labaran had an ability to move between and feel comfortable in many of Jos's different areas in ways that were unthinkable for most people. Born into a Muslim indigene family in the 1940s, Labaran had acquired skills needed for moving past the religious borders of the city. At an early age, at the same time his father and grandfather started teaching him medicine, he had also gone to school and learned how to read and write. In a way similar to his skills in moving between different areas, he could move between his own local language, Hausa, and English, and between what was written and spoken. He continually moved back and forth, communicating written and oral messages between practitioners and different factions in the union.[3]

Being the union secretary and at the core of its politics since its establishment in the early 1980s, Labaran had been moving across the city, visiting different members, looking for allies and support, for a long time. But union politics was no longer what it once was; visits, movements, and meetings had gained new dimensions. When the union was founded, its members were given an office at the Pharmacology Department at the University of Jos, an office which became a meeting point for practitioners with different religious and ethnic backgrounds. With the crisis, things changed: what used to be a room filled with as many as thirty or forty members during the weekly Tuesday meetings became an empty room.

Isaac, one of Jos's practitioners, explained that if he went to a meeting and spoke his mind, he knew that people who got annoyed or angry would never tell him to his face but would secretly send medicines that would make him ill. On another occasion, Samuel, one of Jos's indigene practitioners, explained that there would always be people who were not happy that you had a position within the union, and they would test you. He added, "Even our secretary has been tried." Labaran filled in and stated that people in the union had tried to poison him. He went on to refer to problems with the "Hausa faction" and said that he had been warned, since he was standing in their way. If he was not careful, they were going to kill him. Samuel emphasized that they would not kill him themselves, "physically," but through "poison." They would "either send poisonous missiles or injections."

As new fears were infused into the landscape, Labaran's abilities increasingly turned into matters of danger. On his movements through Jos, he carried his plastic bag with copies of important documents that he was ready to show at any time; and in the way his father had taught him, he kept two leather amulets fastened in his pocket with a safety pin. One was for protection when he traveled, the other for meetings and attacks by enemies. Once, when he showed me the amulets, he emphasized that if you moved around a lot, it was not good to do so without protection. Nor did he ever attend meetings or travel without consulting his spirits. A few nights in advance, he would check with his spirits on whether he would benefit from the event and whether he would die or survive. As he said, he had enemies and needed to know who they were so he could know how to act. When he went to bed, he would contact the spirits by sniffing perfume and by bringing charcoal into the room. During the night the spirits would leave a message in his head, which he would write down half asleep, preferably with charcoal. When he woke up, he would reflect on the writing and use it as guidance. Labaran's preparations and precautions highlight the felt dangers that surrounded his movements, but more than that, his lack of success in retrieving his position in the union or finding a cure for his illness intermingled with and connected to his mobility. At one point, Labaran's own spirits even told him that he had to stop running around so much and start taking care of himself. His spirits' statement was echoed at the time in diagnoses made by other practitioners.

When we entered Houwa's room, it was already filled, mostly with expectant and patiently waiting women. Houwa, a Muslim Fulani woman in her fifties, was the queen of *bori*, a group of practitioners who obtained medicines through spirit possession. For one of the spirits, an old *mallam* (Koranic scholar) by the name of Mohammed, a blue cloth, a blue hat, a white rosary, kola nuts, and perfume were laid out. The excitement in the room increased, and Houwa sat down in the middle of the floor with her legs crossed. She closed her eyes and started to breathe deeper and deeper. After some time, one woman removed the white cloth that had been put over Houwa and greeted the spirit Mohammed. He was given his clothes, the kola nuts, the white rosary, and the perfume. He put on the clothes, poured the whole bottle of perfume in a semicircle in front of himself, then put a kola nut in his mouth, and, in very traditional Hausa, started speaking in a dull and, because of the nut, somewhat slurred voice.

After some women had approached the spirit for advice, the spirit called Labaran to come forward. Labaran very humbly went down on his knees in front of him. The spirit told him that he had once done a lot of good things and people had listened to him, but today nobody did. It did not matter how much he worked and moved around; nothing would work anyway. The illness he had was not going to kill him, but all these other problems might. However, there was a medicine that could help him, and the spirit told Labaran to take out a paper and a pen. The spirit listed five food items that Labaran should collect and then throw into running water. Labaran was totally silent the entire time, listening very respectfully and writing everything down. He ended by bowing very humbly and thanking the spirit.

Around the same time, while visiting David, one of Jos's practitioners, and browsing through his many photocopied books of talismans from all over the world, Labaran started to cough so badly that he almost could not breathe. David gave him some salt, and it helped a bit, but Labaran's cold was worse. Like the warning spirit, David declared that someone was causing the illness because Labaran was blocking the person's way. He directed our attention to a talisman for protection against evil. The talisman looked like a diagram of a chemical compound. He pointed to the lintel above the entrance in his home where he had attached two of those talismans and told us that nothing evil, neither illness, nor thieves, nor anything else, could enter when he had this medicine. He described how he had made the talisman into stickers that people could buy and put on their cars. With the sticker, nothing bad could happen with the car. Considering the dangers connected to Labaran's constant movement, David gave him a medicine for protection against anything evil. It was a leather capsule sewn together with white stitches and inside was the paper with the photocopied talisman that had been folded in a specific way. Labaran put the new protection in his pocket with his two amulets, showing us how he attached all three to the inside of his pocket with the safety pin.

Consumptions of Hope

As Labaran's movements in Jos became increasingly dangerous, there emerged an increasing need for protection. Around the time of his visits to Houwa and David, Labaran told me that he had taken Mummy's advice. Mummy was the wife in the family that I was staying with at the time. She had told him that he should take vitamin C for his catarrh. In pharmacies in Jos at that time one would find a great variety of vitamins and multivitamins that were both imported and Nigerian produced. Labaran had bought thirty vitamin C tablets and had managed to consume them all in one day. He described having sat with a watch and taken two tablets every five minutes. He felt much stronger, even though he still had his cold. As he kept taking thirty tablets a day, vitamins, like the amulets in his pocket, became Labaran's travel companions. By boosting his defense, they became a counter-medicine that was constantly fighting the poisons of the surrounding world from inside his body. They were protective amulets that, instead of keeping in his pocket, he consumed, like the water with dissolved ink from an Islamic verse prepared by a *mallam*. Through consuming them you made sure that the prayer was safely kept inside your body.

Time went by, and Labaran's cold persisted. His walks through Jos continued, and during our regular rests in Jos's many facilities for food and drink, Labaran started to drink juice, preferably products enhanced with different health-promoting additives. One of them was Five Alive, the most common juice drink seen in Jos at the time. The word *Alive* brought with it connotations of a healthy body and future, and on the tetra pack was written "citrus burst: five fruit juice: with added calcium + vitamin C." Another side carried the message "It's a **perfect** start to the day and has **calcium** for added **goodness**." Many people besides Labaran turned to medicinal food to try to boost their bodies and protect themselves against present and future ills. Jos was plastered with posters and large signboards advertising foods and drinks enhanced with various invigorating and health-promoting nutrients. Food containers were equally covered with long lists of vitamins and minerals.

Labaran's drinks continued to change as he tried to bring forth futures he wished for. There was a number game going on in Nigeria in 2004. The idea was to collect soft-drink bottle caps that had a specific text inside the cap. After collecting them, you were supposed to send them to the soft drink company along with your choice of numbers. Once a week, there was a nationally televised drawing of numbers, and you could win one million Naira. Labaran started collecting bottle caps intensively. Every time we stopped to rest, he ordered soft drinks. He explained that if he won the million he would invest it all in shares and live on the profit. He would not let everybody else beg from him, because then he would have nothing left.

In the nights, Labaran started asking his own spirits which numbers he should choose. He also found out later on that David had a talisman that could help him get the right numbers. He contacted David, who, after some convincing and after pointing out that he himself never would use this kind of medicine, gave him a photocopied talisman and instructions on how to prepare it. Labaran was supposed to take it with him when he went to bed. When he woke up in the morning, the numbers would be there in his head. When we left David, Labaran was very happy about the talisman, but he also went on to talk about Indian medicine being very strong. Mummy had been born in India, and he wanted me to ask her for numbers to the lottery. I told him that she did not know anything about medicine, but that did not matter; she was powerful because she was from India. After some convincing, Mummy gave him the numbers 12, 13, and 17. The collection of numbers and bottle caps was something that occupied Labaran for several months, but in the end none of these efforts paid off.

An idea that was brought to the forefront, as Labaran relentlessly searched for tools that potentially would bring forth wished-for futures in the form of health and success, was that in itself, uncertainty is nothing bad. Its openness holds the seeds for hope, luck, and miracles as well as for disasters (Dewey 1930, 213). No matter whether they came in the form of a folded talisman or a tablet bought from a pharmacy, as tools to produce certain consequences, the enhanced food products, the vitamins, the bottle caps, and the amulets in Labaran's pocket were all "intrinsically relational, anticipatory, predictive" (Dewey 1929, 185), directed towards futures wished for as well as feared. Functioning as incantations—portrayals of "a subjunctive world"—a world of possibilities rather than certainties (Good 2005, 153), they were tokens of hope (Whyte 2002, 178).

Elusive Conditions

Labaran's daily movements through Jos emphasized how with every new emergent present a new reality came into being, with its own unique past and future (Mead 1932, 1, 23, 29, 48). He continually and relentlessly reinterpreted the world—what it had been, what it was, and what it was going to be. What was held true yesterday was quickly discarded and replaced by today's truths, only to be rewritten with the truths of tomorrow. For Labaran, it was no easy task to find the causes or the cures for either of his conditions. Not only was the future uncertain, but so, too, were the present and the past. They were "hypothetical" possibilities, a "possibly real present, past, and future," that were altered as new presents emerged (Mead 1932, 12, 173). For Labaran, the cure to all his troubles was to be found in correctly deciphering the past. Rather than being a fact that imposed itself upon the present, the past offered itself up as matters of potentiality (Jackson 2005, 356ff.). By persistently trying to reveal the forces of the past that had created his predicaments, he tried to find medicines that would cure him and give him back his position as the unquestionably elected secretary of the union. As, with every new step, he reinterpreted the past, his predictions of the future were also revised accordingly.

With his steady intake of vitamin C, Labaran started to feel better, but some weeks later when we were on our way to the Ministry of Health for some union politics, he revealed that his catarrh had returned due to the cold weather we were experiencing. From his plastic bag he pulled out a package of Koflin, a medicine against colds that could be bought in any pharmacy in Jos. He had used it before and knew that it worked well. At the ministry we bumped into Cheto, a middle-aged "orthodox" doctor who worked as a general practitioner at the ministry. Labaran described for Cheto how he often got tired after eating and experienced shortness of breath when walking up stairs. Cheto responded by explaining that it could have something to do with his heart. We should come to his office so that he could listen to his heart and take his blood pressure. He declared that he would treat Labaran's high blood pressure with digitalis.

Two days later when we visited Cheto in his office, he immediately wrote a referral for Labaran to bring to the clinic downstairs, where his blood pressure would be taken. After a while Labaran returned with a nurse, who gave the test results to Cheto. Sitting in his revolving leather chair behind his desk, looking serious and facing Labaran, Cheto started talking about the symptoms, which indicated a weakened heart that was becoming enlarged. He looked at Labaran's feet and noted that they were not swollen, which indicated that the condition was at an early stage. Cheto wrote more referrals for new tests and sent Labaran off for blood and urine tests. Cheto continued writing referrals for an x-ray and for a heart specialist at the hospital. He wanted to see the size of Labaran's heart. After leaving Cheto, Labaran was very pleased about all the tests. Later, when Labaran finally brought all the results, Cheto explained that Labaran did not have a heart problem but pneumonia and prescribed antibiotics for him.

Even though Labaran's health problems temporally subsided during his intake of antibiotics, they soon returned with full force. Nothing seemed to help, and he believed that the spirit had been right. He recalled that the spirit Mohammed had said that the illness was not going to kill him, but all his other troubles might. Somebody was after him, and this was why nothing was helping. Another practitioner had also told him that someone was trying to poison him, and Labaran added that he believed it was someone in the union. He no longer thought it was his heart or pneumonia that was causing his problems. He stated that he had never been ill before, but now he could not get rid of the illness. This proved that someone was poisoning him.

Some weeks later, Labaran was feeling a bit better. For six days he had been taking a medicine that he had obtained from yet another practitioner of traditional medicine. He mixed the medicine with charcoal, set it on fire, and inhaled the smoke. The man who gave him the medicine had told him that it was the spirits that were causing his illness. Labaran explained that he no longer believed that someone was poisoning him, but it had been the spirits all along. Before we parted company that day, he related that on his way home he was going to pick up his suit at the dry cleaners. Moving around, visiting people and trying to convince them to attend, he had been planning and organizing for tomorrow's union meeting for several weeks.

At ten o'clock the following morning, when the meeting was supposed to start, I found myself waiting outside the office along with a few medicine practitioners. A bit before eleven Labaran arrived, not wearing the newly dry-cleaned suit but the dirty gown from yesterday. He looked very old; he was limping and held himself up with the help of his umbrella. He told us that he had woken at five in the morning and had not been able to breathe. He was coming directly from the emergency room at Jos University Teaching Hospital, where he had received immediate treatment; they had given him an adrenaline injection. Getting very excited, he announced several times, and with large gestures, that the injection had had a lot of force. He explained that he had suffered an asthma attack. After being treated by seven doctors and receiving the remarkably powerful adrenalin injection, he had dismissed the spirits as the cause of his illness. He was now convinced that he had asthma and needed asthma medicine. He had received two prescriptions for tablets and one for an inhaler.

In his patient book from the hospital was a note that he should go for a follow-up on the following Monday. After the checkup, Labaran recounted that the first person to see him had been doing his internship at the hospital. Noting that Labaran's illness had not disappeared, he had called in a doctor. The doctor in turn had called in around ten different interns to look at Labaran. The doctor had asked if they could tell him what was wrong with Labaran. They had all answered incorrectly. From his plastic bag, Labaran took out a paper from the hospital which stated that he had been given the diagnosis of bronchial asthma. While showing me the papers, he described the tests the doctor had wanted him to take, which included a new x-ray as well as blood, saliva, and urine tests.

Illness stories, Byron Good acknowledges, "are stories that change as events unfold. They point to the future with both hope and anxiety, and they often maintain several provisional readings of the past and the present" (2005, 144), alternatives which keep an openness to a world of possibilities and miracles (153). As Labaran reinterpreted the cause of his illness from cold weather, enemies, a heart problem, pneumonia, poison, and spirits, to asthma, it was not only his view of the past that changed, but also his choice of medication. As Mead wrote, "We determine what the world has been by the anxious search for the means of making it better" (1932, 90). He had tried a great number of different forms of medicine. Besides Cheto, the spirit Mohammed, David, Mummy, and the doctors at JUTH, he had also taken medicine recommended by ten other practitioners, including Samuel, Isaac, and himself. Among other things, he had used talismans, manpower medicine, powder that would make everybody like you, cold medicine, antibiotics, vitamins, medicinal food, and herbal and Western asthma medication as well as talking and sacrificing to the spirits.

Still, after all the medicines Labaran had tried, his problems did not disappear. Since he had to be sitting up to be able to breathe, he had trouble sleeping. He also had shortness of breath when he was eating. When he explained his trouble to one of the professors in the pharmacology department, the professor seemed convinced that it was asthma, and he recommended that Labaran try the orthodox medicine sodium cromoglycate. He should take one tablet a day, and he should also start exercising. Every day he should go jogging for ten minutes. It would be good for his lung capacity, and that in turn would help with his asthma.

On our way home from the professor, Labaran bought some honey, an ingredient in a new medicine that he was preparing from a recipe he had been given from yet another traditional medicine practitioner. The next day, Labaran told me that he had been running back and forth in one spot for ten minutes, and that after doing this for three days he would increase it by five minutes. He added that the people in the village had laughed while he was running. He had also checked out the medicine that the professor had recommended. It would cost 45 Naira per day and he thought it was too much, but he would nonetheless try it for ten days. A week later, on another visit with the professor, Labaran declared that the new asthma medicine had worked very well. Compared to previous medicines that had been based on incorrect diagnoses, the new medicine had a lot of strength. Labaran described how he was getting well and that he was jogging one and a half kilometers every morning.

Snuff: *Wishful Doing*

Towards the end of 2004, Labaran, after sneezing persistently, went to buy traditional snuff that he thought would help. He explained that he had never tried it before, but he had seen other people take it when they were sneezing. Labaran's constant search for new medicines was done in a tentative, exploratory, and speculative mode. As his readings were continually put to the test against the unfolding outcomes—only to be rewritten by them—his knowledge of possible problems and the medicines he collected was an experimental knowledge rather than an abstractly rational one (Dewey 1930, 100, 160–161). He inhaled some snuff and started to sneeze even worse; his asthma became severe and he experienced serious problems breathing. His inhaler was finished, and he kept taking tablets against asthma but got no relief. We decided to go and buy an inhaler. We soon found a pharmacy, but it had only tablets, so we continued on to another but received the same message. Since his breathing was getting worse and worse, Labaran waited there for me to come back. After trying several pharmacies, I finally found an inhaler and hurried back. As he inhaled, the asthma attack immediately subsided. Labaran blessed me and said I had saved his life. Completing the blessing by making the sign of the cross, he declared that he would not take snuff again.

Being able to move past the plenitude of seemingly impenetrable borders in the landscape, Labaran brought different forms of medicines together through his walks. It was through his own journeying—his searches—that this medical landscape, a topography of possible ways forward, came into being. Still, even for him, an unusually skilled navigator, his quests often turned out to be beyond any form of prediction. In his awareness of possible failures—potentially ineffective, incorrect, fake, or even poisonous medicines—Labaran, rather than being perfectly informed and in mastery over his own future, made his search for medicine in a subjunctive "mood of doubt, hope, will and potential" (Whyte 2005, 251). As much as it was an experimental doing, Labaran's pursuit was a *wishful doing*: actions made with an awareness of the uncertainty of outcomes and future perils but with a hope of bringing forth futures wished for.

Epilogue: *Like a Spirit*

Labaran possessed an exceptional ability to move in Jos. In a way, he was perceived to be everywhere and nowhere at the same time. Isaac explained that one could never find him; he was like a spirit. When I returned to Jos in 2012, I had been trying to get in touch with Labaran for over a year. Calls to his mobile phone were not getting through, and messages sent through other practitioners did not reach him. When I arrived I met up with Isaac, who in a bit of shock told me that he just had found out, from a member of the "Hausa faction," that Labaran was not journeying the streets of Jos anymore. He had left us four months ago. He described how Labaran's mobile phone had stopped working a long time ago and that he had been looking for him for so long. Since Isaac, like so many others, did not know where Labaran lived, he had tried to find him in places that he knew he often visited. When Isaac had arrived at one such place they had told him that Labaran had been there yesterday but had moved on to another place. Isaac would then quickly try to reach the other place, only to find out that Labaran had just left. Isaac had then left his telephone number in all these places, but he did not hear anything from Labaran. He then went back to the same places again, only to hear once again that Labaran had been there yesterday. Up to Labaran's death Isaac had still not heard anything from him: "I no take eye see him before he don passed."

Although Labaran's talents for maneuvering the anxious and nervous landscape of Jos, its medical topography, and the geography of the union exceeded those of most people, he never recovered his health or his position as the union's only elected secretary. Instead, his abilities came to be perceived as a contributing factor in his suffering. For Isaac, Labaran's death, like his illness, merged together with the conflict-ridden urban landscape and connected with his comings and goings. Isaac recalled how in 2010, Labaran's movements had caused him to get caught in a Christian roadblock. Labaran had been at Isaac's house in a Christian neighborhood in Jos when violence broke out across the city, and they had all thought it would be safer for Labaran to try to get to a Muslim neighborhood. However, on his way he had been stopped at a Christian roadblock. They had wanted to kill him since he was a Muslim, and Labaran had kept screaming that he was an indigene. Somehow he had been able to escape and found his way back to Isaac's home. Isaac explained that he had been wearing his "Hausa clothes," his gown, so they could all see that he was a Muslim. Isaac had given Labaran a shirt and trousers to put on. He then left Isaac's home again and safely managed to reach his friends in a Muslim neighborhood. Isaac concluded that although it was asthma that had killed Labaran, in reality it was the fact that he was moving around too much and too recklessly that had brought about his death. By constantly exposing himself to the perils of Jos, he had not, in Isaac's words, been taking care of himself.

Notes

1. For a more detailed illustration of the variety in how traditional medicine was practiced in Plateau State, see Amma Oppong (1989).
2. Today there is a long list of ethnic groups that are officially perceived as indigene to Plateau State. Among them are Berom, Nges, Tarok, Geomal, Youm, Montol, Rukuba, Challa, Jarawa, Atem, and others (FMIC, 2005).
3. In union contexts, discussions were often translated for different members, and as all union documents were written in English, it meant that letters, invitations, minutes, and membership certificates, etc. often had to be read and translated for members who did not understand English or could not read. Even if Hausa is a *lingua franca* of Jos—along with English and Pidgin, to certain degrees—not all people could communicate with each other directly.

Bibliography

Andersson Trovalla, Ulrika. 2011. *Medicine for Uncertain Futures: A Nigerian City in the Wake of a Crisis*. PhD Thesis, Uppsala University, Sweden.

Besmer, Fremont E. 1983. *Horses, Musicians, & Gods: The Hausa Cult of Possession-Trance*. South Hadley, MA: Bergin & Garvey.

Danfulani, Umar Habila Dadem, and Sati U. Fwatshak. 2002. "Briefing: The September 2001 Events in Jos, Nigeria." *African Affairs* 101 (403): 243–55.

Dewey, John. 1929. *Experience and Nature*. London: George Allen & Unwin, Ltd.

———. 1930. *The Quest for Certainty: A Study of the Relation of Knowledge and Action*. London: George Allen & Unwin, Ltd.

Federal Ministry of Information and Communications (FMIC). 2005. Plateau State. *Nigeria Direct: The Official Information Gateway of the Federal Republic of Nigeria*. www.nigeria.gov.ng /NR/exeres/78852F93-7328-480F-8627-D29475F788E2.htm (accessed 24 October 2008).

Good, Byron. 2005. *Medicine, Rationality, and Experience: An Anthropological Perspective*. Cambridge: Cambridge University.

Jackson, Michael. 2005. "Storytelling Events, Violence, and the Appearance of the Past." *Anthropological Quarterly* 78 (2): 355–75.

Mbembe, Achille. 1992. "The Banality of Power and the Aesthetics of Vulgarity in the Postcolony." *Public Culture* 4 (2): 1–30.

Mead, George Herbert. 1932. *The Philosophy of the Present*. London: Open Court.

Last, Murray. 1992. "The Importance of Knowing about Not Knowing: Observations from Hausaland." In *The Social Basis of Health and Healing in Africa*, edited by Steven Feierman & John M. Janzen, 393–406. Berkeley: University of California.

Lindquist, Galina. 2000. "In Search of the Magical Flow: Magic and Market in Contemporary Russia." *Urban Anthropology* 29 (4): 315–57.

Oppong, Amma C. K. 1989. "Healers in Transition." *Social Science and Medicine* 28 (6): 605–12.

Schmoll, Pamela Gail. 1991. *Searching for Health in a World of Dis-ease: Affliction Management among Rural Hausa of the Maradi Valley (Republic of Niger)*. PhD dissertation. Department of Anthropology, University of Chicago.

Suberu, Rotimi T. 1997. "Religion and Politics: A View from the South." In *Transition Without End: Nigerian Politics and Civil Society Under Babangida*, edited by Larry Diamond, Anthony Kirk-Greene & Oyeleye Oyediran, 401–25. Boulder, CO: Lynne Rienner.

Wall, L. Lewis. 1988. *Hausa Medicine: Illness and Well-Being in a West African Culture*. Durham, NC: Duke University.

Whyte, Susan Reynolds. 2002. "Subjectivity and Subjunctivity: Hoping for Health in Eastern Uganda." In *Postcolonial Subjectivities in Africa*, edited by Richard Werbner, 171–90. London: Zed.

———. 2005. "Uncertain Undertakings: Practicing Health Care in the Subjunctive Mood." In *Managing Uncertainty: Ethnographic Studies of Illness, Risk and the Struggle for Control*, edited by R. Jenkins, H. Jessen, and Steffen, 245–64. Copenhagen: Museum Tusculanum.

7 The Individualization of Illness

Bewitchment and the Mental in Postcolonial Tanzania

Koen Stroeken

IN THE MID-1990s when I began my ethnographic fieldwork in Tanzania just south of Lake Victoria, the HIV epidemic had taken its toll in the city of Mwanza and was spreading fast in the rural areas. At about the same time, the rumor spread of two types of HIV/AIDS, *ukimwi*. The plain type of HIV, *ya hospitali* (of the hospital) or *ya kizungu* (European), was incurable, everyone knew. But the second type, HIV caused by witchcraft (*ya bulogi*), could be treated. The healer needed to identify the witch and then develop a socially and symbolically significant counter-remedy, possibly in collaboration with the witch's colleagues. Quite soon, however, a few healers became famous across Mwanza Region for claiming they had found the miracle cure for HIV witchcraft, which meant they did not even need to identify the witch and personalize the remedy. That was news at the time. The concoctions worked regardless of symbolic significance. Without the latter dimension of "magic," which circumvented the positivist criteria of biomedicine, the new type of "medicine" (*bugota*) pretended to rival biomedicine for efficacy, like a sort of science.

In this plain ethnographic observation discussed further on, we note a convergence of medico-anthropological issues in postcolonial Africa: the globalization of epidemics, the transformation and renewal of traditional epistemologies, and the role of biomedical knowledge and hospitals in Africa, including their impact on the local ways of thinking about illness and remedy. Since the spread of colonial hospitals, healers were compelled to rethink their trade and specialize in domains wherein the newcomers were unsuccessful. One such domain was hope: hope of recovery when even hospitals seemed to fail. The healers also specialized in hope's counterpart: despair and ways of coping. Both fed the discourse of witchcraft, whose institutionalization has escalated since the mid-1990s in Tanzania (Green 2005) and whose violent consequences seem a more recent phenomenon, at least going by the observations of early ethnographers, such as Evans-Pritchard among the Azande (Siegel 2006, 9). Before detailing our account, we cast a wider net that brings us first to more familiar terrain at home.

Witchcraft, Hope and Individualization

What do we normally mean by the popular expression "it's all in your head"? We are reassuring our interlocutor by referring to "it" as a problem that can be solved, on the grounds that it is not a problem in the real world out there but "merely" in one's mind. Since "it" is not a virus or other organic pathology, the problem can be fixed even if there is no cure. It can vanish by itself. How? Through a change of perspective, a mental change. Pivotal in this Western take on the human—in this Western "anthropology"—is the split between mind and matter. Cartesian dualism opposes the individual, called a subject and potentially solipsistic, to the outside world. Only in the latter realm do people and things have objective relations and are they consequential. In the mind—our first port of call—the world is malleable.

To speak of "witchcraft" has a similar effect. It reassures the victim of bewitchment that something can be done about one's condition, illness or misfortune, however desperate she may feel. A palpable person can be identified, after which the right intervention follows in the invisible world, such as counter-magic or the appeasing of protective ancestral spirits. Illustrative of this process is the hope HIV patients in Mwanza Region drew from the healer's claim of HIV-inducing witchcraft. As in the case of the mental change, here too the feared alternative was not the world of invisible forces but the hard reality of matter, the world of virus and bacteria—but also of poverty and misfortune—where ritual, magic or subjective intention are powerless. The literature has extensively dealt with the widespread attempt at coping with the hard facts of global economy, inequality and modernity in Africa south of the Sahara through witchcraft discourse and magic (Comaroff 1999, Nyamnjoh 2001).

What interests us in this chapter is the implication that the concept of witchcraft in rural Tanzania has changed over time, almost unnoticeably. Dualism, with a domain of matter presented as objective or "unmindful," is a newcomer on the scene of healing. Magic or ritual normally mean impact on the (material) world through symbolic (mindful) means, where the real and the symbolic are in continuity (Lock and Scheper-Hughes 1989). In this continuity human intuition and projection of ideas on nature are not seen as a liability, as in the mechanistic idea of objectivity since the nineteenth century (Daston and Gallison 2007). To paraphrase the ontological turn applied to animistic cultures (Holbraad 2012): before the dualism of object and subject, of outside world and individual perspective, the healer's intervention was a matter of changing the world, not just one's perspective on it. In Tanzania today, the present study argues, the split of mind and matter manifests itself in a new concept of magic, where witchcraft belongs to the domain of mental health and for that reason raises hopes for intervention.

In the mid-1990s when I did fieldwork in the Mwanza region, I could still observe the cultural contrast between the nascent towns along the main road to Dar es Salaam and the villages further away where views on health and healing were anchored in the local cosmology. Of course these views were chequered by Christian and Islamic influences, yet they were also supported by the community's *ihane* initiation, internalized traditions and norms, regular ceremonies involving the clan's ancestral spirits, and by youth's leisure practices and everyday beliefs. The healer's practices had medical "effectiveness" in local terms, for they restored the cosmology's envisaged condition, namely its "coolness" (*mhola* in KiSukuma) or peace. That peace could sometimes be attained at the expense of the individual. Healing rituals developed in continuity with animist cosmologies, which tended to relate micro-events to the entire moral order: a cut holy tree or an act of incest could ruin the chiefdom; the birth of twins that had not been ritually purified could cause famine across the valley; the supposed bitterness or jealousy of one person preoccupied the whole village for destroying happiness in the community; and addressing this "witch" also meant solving a collective problem; and so on. The state- and church-led implementation of hospital infrastructure worldwide altered the focus of healers and their patients. The focus no longer was on peace in the community that united the living and the dead, nor on the ritual process engaging the community of kin, neighbors and ancestors in the transformation of matter, but on the witch as an individual, identifiable and causing harm to another individual who can retaliate. This individualization of illness goes together with a separation between the mental and the physical, whereby the former domain falls within the expertise of traditional healers, and the hospital's reign in the latter domain is accepted as a given. When the hospital fails, hope is raised in traditional medicine. Hope, like belief, is an individualist concept. Dreams, suspicions, and divinations, constituting the field of "subjunctivity," thrive among people living in uncertainty while modernizing their healing traditions (Reynolds-Whyte 1996). The concept of traditional medicine itself in fact marks a paradigm shift for treating health as a separate domain in the hands of experts. The specialization in mental illness is a corollary.

This chapter collects evidence to make sense of these various tangles in postcolonial Africa under the heading of one process we loosely label individualization. The process implies a disintegration of the collective, or at least a focus away from the community towards self and other, which may not only have been the effect but also the cause of the European colonizing obsession, triggering various responses by subaltern groups also in the West (Mignolo 2000). A remarkable convergence arose from colonization, as well as from its immediate predecessor, the slave trade, and from its successors, nationalization, state-led identity politics and the formation of a postcolonial ruling elite (cf. Bayart 1993). The accumulated effect was to stimulate within the local health systems the existing type of belief that was most in continuity with this colonial and postcolonial disintegration. In many places that turned out to be witchcraft—the individualization of evil. On this cultural reality, we argue, postcolonial society in Tanzania converged, on top of the better known social effect of greater inequality. The market of healing became autonomous and booming, capitalizing on hope and despair, on people's sense of relative deprivation and intrusion, their suspicions of invisible forces at work, their dependence on secret expertise, and incomprehension of a fellow's bad or good fortune.

Culture as Collective Medicine

Before substantiating our claim on the individualization of illness and witchcraft today with qualitative research into divinatory practices in central Tanzania at the foot of the Uluguru Mountains, this essay will offer a literature review that reveals the remarkable association between mental illness and traditional medicine in postcolonial Africa. First, though, let us briefly introduce the idea of culture and cosmology as collective medicine.

If a process of individualization takes place, it will occur at different levels. Socially, individualization means that problems such as illness and misfortune are handled as personal issues. The alternative source of help, besides self-medication and individual consultation, can only be the State, which is a distant other, equally disconnected from a community, hence socially and culturally uprooting. Culturally, individualization means that the subject does not presume dependence of life and health on the larger whole and its condition; there is no direct relation or umbilical tie with clan, community and ancestors. Cultural individualization thus refers to the end of what Strathern (1988) describes in Melanesian culture as the "dividual." Whereas individuals need cures to ingest as patients, "dividuals" get better from changes at the collective level, which are embodied by each member, like fractals at the microlevel, for instance via the ingestion of symbolic material.

This brief section contextualizes Bantu healing traditions to familiarize the reader with the idea of culture itself as medicine. Medicine presumes some form of effectiveness. The question of effectiveness in biomedicine concentrates on curative particles operating in the body. We alter the question: can ideas prevent illness and actually cure people? More radically, can they do so at a collective level, by forming a worldview and entailing a way of life? Can culture, in the form of a moral order or medical epistemology or cosmology, heal? This shift in question is necessary, we will argue here, to understand the practices known as traditional healing in their own terms. The shift adds an ideational layer to the matter of medicine, to make up for our Western Cartesian model of science keeping matter and idea separated.

Traditional healing, also referred to as traditional medicine, comprises a wide range of practices such as collective rituals, group and private therapies, behavioral and dietary regimes, and the use of plant recipes. Because the practices fitting under the rubric of traditional healing lack cultural uniformity and undergo little or no institutional regulation, it is pointless to discuss the effectiveness of traditional healing as such. Assessments can be made of particular practices. Still, effectiveness, defined as the success in producing desired results is a culturally gauged matter; depends on what results are desired in a group. For example, healing across Bantu-speaking Africa has been attained by therapy management groups that developed therapeutic rituals (Janzen 1978). The rituals mending the patient's relations with kin and with ancestral spirits are of no interest to biomedical doctors, who address the health of the individual body. Therapy management groups seek what Devisch (1993) calls the resonance of bodily, social and cosmological fields through metaphorically potent material culture. The effectiveness of such healing is situated at a collective level. Now, we should ask whether, besides offering a treatment whose gains may be mainly behavioral or social (Kleinman and Sung 1979), the practices, beliefs and social relations together do not form a cosmology, operating at the fundamental level of a way of life, that may be *preventive* for certain afflictions. Such benefit should interest clinicians as well. For instance, the cultural dissonance between ideal and actual life-standard which Dressler's (1999) studies have associated with depression and high blood pressure can arguably be diminished by beliefs in the role of ancestral spirits. If the outcome of one's decisions is culturally considered as codetermined by the whimsical interventions of ancestors, then this should mitigate the individual's feeling of responsibility for unmet expectations, most probably lowering the blood pressure. Thus a cultural belief can operate as collective medicine. Patients' feelings of isolation and powerlessness, not uncommon in globalized settings, can in turn be tackled by rituals showing collective support, the pinnacle of which is the protection by the clan's ancestral spirits, avowed in public through oracle.

In other words, a cultural practice can "heal." By this we do not suggest, in functionalist mode, that cultural practices or beliefs necessarily serve the well-being of the individual or the group. But they can. Only in the Cartesian model of science is culture a mental thing, wayward and groundless, spiraling out in arbitrarily fettered signifiers of the imaginary, instead of operating in the real world. However, exactly when serving some form of collective wellbeing, cultural practices have more probability of surviving the innovations and intercultural exchanges of successive generations, and more probability of being encountered in disparate locations across cultures, as in the example of Bantu therapy management groups.

Mental Health and Traditional Healing in Africa: A Review

The following literature review demonstrates the affinity between traditional healing and the treatment of mental illness. The latter term is commonly used in public health research to refer to clusters of symptoms that point to psychiatric disorders classified in Western university curricula, which comprise depression, schizophrenia, dissociative disorders and post-traumatic stress disorders among others, but which will locally be denoted with other terms and through different (as well as less or more differentiated) classifications. A dual picture emerges from the literature. The concept of mental illness ensured healers a sizable piece of the pie on the health market, which was dominated by Western-style hospital care focused on treatable infectious diseases. Yet the traditional healer's increasing focus on therapy of the mind—rather than of society or the group or the world—also meant further dilution of the ritual cosmology in that community. Rituals and counter-magic were initially not intended as purely "mental" interventions, for African cultures had no tradition of Cartesian dualism. However, in postcolonial Africa, the Western doctor's discomfort over complex mental symptoms did in practice mean that the socially defined domain of "mental health" became the healers' specialty, often (but certainly not always) despite themselves.

Treatment of mental illness is not merely one of the many specializations in the field of traditional healing. It has become the main one, justifying the persistence of that field all over medically pluralist Africa. This is the least one can conclude from a review of the public health literature. Over the last ten years, a lot of public health research has been conducted into traditional medicine in Africa. This section deliberately considers public health research (via the search engine Pubmed) because medical anthropologists have long overlooked or marginalized this discipline, while it is no secret that in number of publications, number of funded projects, and involvement of local researchers the scientific domain of public health has far overshadowed any other in Africa, including anthropology. Unlike anthropological collaborations, the public health teams typically consist of local academic researchers. By local we do not mean a homogenous cultural reality, though. African university-educated researchers feel little affinity with their uneducated compatriots engaging in medicine. But on the latter's expertise in "mental" affairs the researchers seem to agree, to the extent of an internalized episteme.

When searching on Pubmed (the main database for medical research in the broad sense) using the terms "Traditional medicine OR traditional healing OR traditional healers AND Africa AND mental" we obtained 205 articles in total. Forty-eight dated from 2000–2010. After exclusion on the basis of irrelevance (e.g., other afflictions such as stroke; "mental" as a kind of effect; pharmacological study; other region than Africa), we were left with 31 recent papers dealing with traditional medicine and mental health across Africa. All of these will be discussed next, because the force of our argument on the growing matter/mind dualism and "mentalness" of traditional healing rests on the remarkable yet previously unnoticed consonance in the literature.

First of all, traditional healers attract comparatively more cases of mental illness. In Tanzania's metropolis Dar es Salaam, 48 percent of the 176 clients in traditional health centers (an urban version of the village healer's compound) suffered from mental illness, while among clients of primary health care centers only half of that proportion (24 percent) did (Ngoma et al. 2003). Second, the first stop for African patients suffering from mental illness is generally the traditional healer. In Abidjan, most of the 27 teenagers received in a mental health unit had either consulted "tradithérapie" first or, to a lesser extent, churches/ prayer camps (Yao et al. 2008). Half of the 90 patients in a mental health center in Tunis had consulted a traditional healer; the majority of them did so before trying other means (Zaghdoudi 2008).

Third, the choice of traditional medicine is not out of necessity or due to lack of alternatives. Patients rate their satisfaction higher after traditional therapy, as confirmed by Shibre et al. (2008), who interviewed mental health patients of healers and of health centers. Ethiopians migrating to Toronto many years later retain this preference for traditional healers (Fenta et al. 2006). In a cross-sectional study by Mirza et al. (2006) involving 821 Tanzanians on Pemba Island, people were attitudinally positive about both primary health care and traditional healing of mental illness, but the practice significantly favored the latter. The association between mental and traditional healing is so deeply ingrained among local public health researchers that in the rare case when practice turned out differently in rural Africa, as in a large sample of Yoruba speakers in Nigeria (Gureje et al. 2006), the authors suspected flaws in the research methodology (in this case the socially desirable answers that lay interviewers might prompt). University education anywhere is a product of globalization, also culturally. So, if the local trend in globalized areas is towards equating the traditional with the mental, hence reproducing the West's Cartesian dualism, then more of the same can be expected from the researchers coming from these communities.

Medical pluralism in sub-Saharan Africa (Slikkerveer 1982) is taken as an established fact by now. Indeed, the preferences observed by the studies above are statistical, so a client's use of one sector does not exclude the use of another as well. The antagonism between the sectors varies between settings. The association between traditional and mental and between modern and physical seems characteristic of globalizing rural Africa, but does not hold for the most urbanized settings. Biomedicine rules in urban areas such as Kumasi, Ghana, where only 6 percent of 322 patients in a mental health unit first consulted a healer and 14 percent first saw a pastor (Appiah-Poku et al. 2004). Is urbanity the reason for this limited success of traditional healing in mental health, or does the specific local history of mental illness treatment account for it? Another example is South Africa, where 29 percent of 3651 respondents opted for Western and 20 percent for alternative practitioners, 11 percent for religious-spiritual advisors and 9 percent for traditional healers (Sorsdahl 2009). In Peltzer's (2000) study, 104 South African patients tended to rate the effectiveness of Western treatment of mental illness higher, even if many of them combined it with traditional healing. Peltzer (2009) later on established that the proportion of South Africans consulting traditional or faith healers had dramatically decreased over the past 13 years, from somewhere between 3.6 and 12.7 percent to only 0.1 percent today. It is in a domain such as traditional mental healing that one observes how different South Africa and many African cities are from the rural areas of the continent.

The concept of the mental, in opposition to the physical, also seems to drive the field's differentiation. In areas with much influence from Christian denominations or Islam, the preferred treatment of mental illness is not by medical doctors nor by traditional healers, but by a third category: spiritual advisors and faith healers. In a sample of 2078 Nigerian respondents (Adewuya and Makanjuola 2009), the 41 percent faith consultations are still closely followed by the other options: traditional healing (30 percent) and hospitals or biomedicine (29 percent). The authors note that preference for faith healers and traditional healers increases with female gender, "belief in supernatural causes of mental illness," and lower education, among other factors. Faith healers and spiritual advisors have become a third source of treatment, which in some (especially west African) communities with a long tradition of Islamic or Pentecostal worship is more culturally rooted than traditional medicine. In these contexts resurfaces a medical dualism where mental issues are believed to require spiritual guidance, while matters of the body are reserved for medics.

The general call in the literature for dialogue between the various sectors is based on the cultural challenges proper to mental health treatment (Nelms and Gorski 2006; see Makanjuola et al. 2000 for Nigeria; Mkize and Uys 2004 for KwaZulu-Natal; Kendall-Taylor et al. 2009 for Kenya). Psychiatric researchers stress the role that traditional healers can play in integrating mental health services in primary health care (Anders 2003; see Alem et al. 2008 for Ethiopia). Patients, however, rather appreciate the segregation of the hospital and the traditional healing compound. Local divination and healing no longer means involvement of the group. On the contrary, the healer's compound guarantees privacy for the individual patient, whereas the hospital is the new locus of public discourse, mostly state-sanctioned. Hence, patients prefer traditional healing in a separate location (Al-Krenawi et al. 2001) or, when they continue to use traditional herbs in the hospital, they do not mind doing so clandestinely (Langwick 2008). The patients' de facto medical pluralism contrasts with the integrative, less open-ended approach to this relation by medical doctors. Even when medical professionals, for example in South Africa, acknowledge the limits of Western psychiatry (Yen and Wilbraham 2003a) and for that purpose discuss the alternatives, they appear to have assumptions about African culture and "African madness" that prevent them from taking traditional healers seriously (Yen and Wilbraham 2003b). A more open, constructivist (versus substantivist or hierarchical) approach by psychiatrists is to accept another type of effectiveness than the biomedical, and seek the empirical basis for affinity between African healing rituals and psychoanalytical therapy (Berg 2003, Maiello 2008). Nevertheless, here too the locus of healing is the individual, not the community, as medical anthropologists reflecting on the psychoanalytical import of ritual have underlined (cf. Boddy 1989, Devisch 1993).

Patients in low-income countries are used to making autonomous decisions about their health, since the first phase commonly is self-medication after which they monitor outcome (Cocks and Dodt 2000). As Johnson (2009) demonstrated in a study of explanatory belief models regarding the causes and treatments of depression among 246 Ugandan patients, lay psychiatries overlapped as much with biomedical as with traditional healing epistemologies. Patients first look at the symptoms and subsequently define a range of afflictions that more or less correspond to a certain type of treatment, rather than the other way around. Those empirical, affliction-based rather than principled decisions could explain the popularity of traditional healers for mental illness, and the aforementioned element of patient satisfaction. An explanatory model that is culturally accessible for the patient (and that predicts the illness's outcome) may be especially reassuring in mental illness. But also the contents of beliefs subtending traditional medicine may have a therapeutic and even preventive effect on the (potentially) mentally ill. The final set of papers from our review should clarify this.

The etiology of traditional healers is remarkably similar across the continent, at least going by the medical studies in our review. From Morocco (Stein 2000) to Malawi (Crumlish et al. 2007) to rural South Africa (Janse van Rensburg 2009; Modiba et al. 2001, for rural South Africa) mental illness is considered the work of either witches or spirits. In rural Africa the cosmology of spiritual and magical forces permeates traditional medicine. Healers are people able to engage with those invisible forces, which makes them privileged experts for mental health patients coping with disabling, yet largely invisible symptoms. Belief, a mental process, is not a sufficient explanation. The mental and material sides of phenomena are reunited as the etiology of spiritual and magical forces refers to a certain class of experiences, something empirically based. In a study of Ugandan healers, the idiom of spirit possession turned out to express what the psychiatrist's DSM-IV classifies as dissociative disorder (Van Duijl et al. 2005). Niehaus et al. (2004) showed that more than half of Xhosa patients with schizophrenia had a history of spirit possession. A "spirit" working in oneself points to health impairment in Mozambique (Igreja 2003), where new spirits were invented to articulate the postwar situation and where almost one out of five respondents claims to have a spirit, with more spirits standing for more impairment (Igreja et al. 2010). In brief, traditional healing has found a way of integrating post-traumatic stress disorder in its etiology just as Western psychiatrists have, and maybe–as far as we can tell– independently from the West.

Much more could be said about these studies in public health. For our purpose they illustrate the long-term process that took place since colonization. The initiated medium ritually restoring the peace between community and ancestors, whose breach was indicated by illnesses, has ceded the way to the bifurcation between modern medicine treating physical symptoms in hospitals and the traditional healing of individual patients with psychiatric or mental symptoms. The medicinal crossover is taken care of by individuals (cf. Langwick 2007). It is clear, however, that the above literature on patients' decision-making in response to mental symptoms only scratches the surface of more complex distinctions made on at least two levels. First, clients both in village and town have assumptions about which particular afflictions, within the clinician's list of mental illnesses so to speak, will be better treated by healers. Indicative in this respect is the recent study by Abbo et al. (2009) of 387 patients of traditional healers in Uganda. Of those patients with a mental illness (totaling 60.2 percent) certain conditions such as psychosis (29.7 percent) were more prevalent. We cannot exclude that the bias of consultations towards traditional healers at the expense of hospital doctors corresponds to an actual bias of effectiveness in treating the particular illness (which given the ongoing struggle of biomedicine with psychosis is not farfetched). But the bias also stems from a belief that the most severe psychical conditions belong in the knowledgeable hands of the healers. This brings us to the second level of complex distinctions made by clients which the above literature has failed to tackle: local classifications that ignore the Cartesian division and have their own empirical basis, which Western psychiatry ignores (Stroeken 2012). On these local classifications lacking in public health research, anthropologists have focused because of their preference for ethnography as a primary method, to which we turn next.

Qualitative Data on the Individualization of Healing

Now that we have extensively underscored the association in contemporary Africa of traditional healing with mental health, and subsequently the local associations between mental illness and spirits or witchcraft, it is time to verify the claim of this chapter, namely that these associations are no longer articulated in collectively oriented practices, as proposed in the previous section on the collective wellbeing obtained in certain cultural beliefs and practices. Nowhere in the above studies were the healing practices depicted as community activities or public ritual enactments of the cosmology of the group. Granted though, the collective or social dimension in traditional medicine, beyond mental versus physical, was not the topic of their study. To know more about the explanatory frameworks in local mental health, such as the changed concepts of witches and spirits, we need qualitative data from fieldwork. In Northern Tanzania, Sukuma practitioners are valued for serving clients' personal desires independently from community norms and collective wellbeing (Stroeken 2010). The extent (and pace) of this process is hard to determine because of the lack of longitudinal data across the whole region. But based on participant observation and ethnography during two consecutive periods of each one year, followed in the next decade by regular return visits, we should conclude that the communal rituals of divination, which were practiced in the frame of *ihane* initiation, have become very rare in northwest Tanzania. The following data detail the same trend of individualization for oracles collected among six diviners working at the foot of the Uluguru Mountains in central Tanzania. Three vignettes illustrate five aspects of individualization: the written word and contract (versus tradition), the individual life-force (versus collective peace), the remedy's physical effectiveness (versus procedural correctness), public orthodoxy (versus pluralist praxis), and the mental (versus the nondual or the "dividual").

In the region of Morogoro, about 300 kilometers west of Dar es Salaam, there exist two types of healing, according to popular understanding. The first type is conducted by the Koran healer, *mganga wa korani*, the second by *mganga wa kibuyu*, healer of the calabash, who adopts local (i.e., Luguru) traditions of divination and treatment. Islamic faith healing has a long tradition here, fairly close to the Swahili-speaking coast with its Arabic influences. But to use the term faith healer for the first type is not entirely correct, since the words of God are only part of the remedy. Before reciting Koran verses as a possible treatment, the healers want to determine a person's life-force, *nyota*, and for this purpose they use divination techniques inspired on Luguru practices. Conversely, healers of the calabash often refer to the Islamic concept of *majini*, spirits, and to the related Swahili idea of *mapepo mabaya*, evil or bad winds. The addition of the adjective, implying there would be good winds too (*mazuri*), is indicative of the syncretism of traditional and Islamic healing, for in Islam natural or ancestral spirits cannot be good (unlike angels). Some healers situate themselves explicitly in the middle between Koran and calabash, claiming to have medicine that unites the powers of both types.

As healers are not registered, finding them is a matter of asking around in the village. This is not an obvious matter. More than in Mwanza region, where Sukuma-speaking farmers live, many people in this area relatively close to Dar es Salaam and the capital Dodoma will deny that they condone such traditions denounced by official religions, school and government. Although the government does not officially forbid them, divinations are private affairs. Some highly ranked politicians in the region who have successfully competed for office are said to consult diviners. But they do so clandestinely. A diviner's reputation is spread by word of mouth. In town they advertise their trade by sticking small posters with a list of illnesses and their phone number onto old telephone posts. For the researcher in rural areas it is a matter of asking the right people at the right time. Local pharmacy shops (*maduka ya dawa*) and their clients are often helpful. Male smallholder farmers are too.

The first thing to note is that healers and diviners nowhere have an official function, nor are they seen as fulfilling a community task. Secondly, all diviners concentrate on cases of bewitchment or spirit possession, with mental illness as a major symptom. A third trait, illustrated in the first vignette as well, is that consultation boils down to a commitment between two individuals (with one caretaker) and this possibly before the eyes of God, an impersonal entity replacing the collective and community of old.

In Mlali village, near Morogoro, people greeted me politely, as the elderly wife of a successful farmer and a lady owning a small business, but they denied the existence of healers in the neighborhood. Deeper into the village, an elder smallholder farmer and Muslim brought me discreetly to a man who lived up the hill towards the Uluguru mountain and immigrated there some twenty years ago. Assertive and talkative, he initiated conversation as soon as we approached his modest compound. He had worked on the island of Nansio as a specialist in Koran healing. For him, healing is praying to God in a mixture of Arab and Swahili while standing behind the seated client and blowing incense their way. His garment is black and his headscarf bright orange. Writing plays a central role in the prior diagnostic session. The words of prayer speak to the issue written down by the client on a piece of paper, along with the client's name and sometimes their address and phone, but always with the reason for the visit and the sum he or she is ready to pay to solve the issue. The writing constitutes a contract between healer and patient, obliging the client financially but at the same time initiating the treatment, as the diviner has a basis to start from. The Koran is a written source of healing, and so are the verses on paper folded into amulets, which faith healers sell. As a client, I said I needed protection from harm on the many trips ahead. The healer then requested I sit down on the mat while he would recite a protective prayer. In his prayer to God the healer remained as true as possible to the information he got from me. He mentioned that the names of parents and ancestors are not known and that the destination of the client's trip is not known. The elder accompanying me acted as caretaker, facing me and the healer. Sitting down and looking up to the standing healer, he seemed intimidated by the incantations summoning the mercy of God. On the way back to the main street he said he would understand if I needed to check on another specialist.

The second vignette demonstrates that neither village community nor clan or kin are seen (anymore) as necessary stakeholders in dealing with family problems and witchcraft. What cures is not the group, cosmic forces, or the will of the ancestors, but a powerful thing acquired and hidden in the forest.

In the village of Vikenge an inhabitant claimed to know of no healers in the area. But many, he added, can be found in neighboring Changarawe. The local bar owner directed me to a female healer, one of the calabash. Again the tiny fenced compound bore no external signs of healing practice. Only within, behind the house, the little grass hut for divination could be noticed. To my show of interest in healing, she replied that today was indeed Tuesday, the day she receives spirits. She invited me to come back after sunset, and so I did together with a female friend. We had to wait for her husband, who had just dropped off a mental health patient to receive a bag of rice in return for curing him. The husband had no qualms about referring me to his wife for questions regarding diagnosis and classification of illnesses. One of his children had already intervened after his hesitation and told me that his mother will know. The husband's role, as is often the case in such small healer settings, is that of managing the financial affairs and doing the manual work of collecting and processing the plants. He also acts as mediator, to translate her spirit's words to the client as she reaches a state of mediumistic trance. So we entered and sat down in the grass hut. I placed the requested 1200 Tsh (0.6 Eur) on a small plate covered by three big shells. The husband told the client to hold in his right hand a brown polished stick made from a branch to which the problem was to be stated aloud. The client expressed worries about two family members whose demeanor had suddenly changed. When the diviner said she felt the spirit coming, her husband took and handed the stick back to her. This natural mediator now held the problem and would convey it directly to the spirit. As she started breathing a bit heavily, a low voice came into her. It spoke in a mixture of Swahili and Luguru. After every meaningful answer, she prompted her husband back in her own voice to translate in clear answers in Kiswahili. The main message was that the client's family problems were caused by *mapepo mabaya*, "bad winds." They could be treated by removing an intruding agent, labeled in general terms as *dudu* (insect), which now inhabited the body of the victim. The victim, who lived in Europe, could come over to Tanzania or could be cured at a distance by writing his name on a tag which tied to a tree in her medicinal forest nearby would become the subject of treatment. The main curative act is to touch a thing called *nyota* ("star," figuratively life-force) in that forest. To our query what really caused the simultaneous change in the family, the diviner said that the victims were disturbed (*ku-vurugwa*) by a certain person. The suggestion was that of witchcraft. The price of the cure would be at least tenfold the amount paid for the oracle.

In the third vignette, we observe the mixing of healing methods, on the grounds that what counts is not compliance with tradition, but the individual's sense of being cured, the visible result. Interesting is the use of the Islamic concept *ushirika*, literally polytheism, for witchcraft. While orthodox religion denounces the belief in polytheism as evil, the local healers adopt the term to fight the evil, *in casu* the witches and other forces acknowledged by "polytheists." At the same time, the healers do not defy orthodoxy. They could not, as their isolated, individualized position in the community deprives them from authority. The local cosmology their creativity stems from has little authority because it lacks cultural reproduction and rooting. As initiations have stopped, cosmology becomes a matter of the state and the churches.

As I got a lift to Milela, somewhat further away from the main road I saw a pharmacy-shop owner talking to her client, a young farmer in his working outfit with two machetes, small and big. After some chatting, I asked as usual: "I am looking for an indigenous healer. There should be one living nearby, isn't it? Can you tell me in which direction to walk?" (*Natafuta mganga wa kienyeji. Lazima mmoja aishi karibu, siyo? Nielekee wapi?*) The young farmer showed me the way, directing me to go behind the Catholic church and close to where the agricultural fields begin. Usually healers live at the outskirts of the village, in the vicinity of uncultivated terrain and more forested parts where medicinal plants can be encountered. His wife was alone with the kids living in a tent, which was exceedingly hot. The adobe blocks were drying in the sun for a house to be, on their tiny plot. She spoke with much admiration about her husband who was down in the valley helping to cultivate someone's field. She had him called for. They were poor, still waiting for the village to grant them fields of their own. Even after he had managed to summon the rains last year after a period of ongoing drought, the village council ignored him, he would tell me later. Yes, knowledgeable he was, the healer, his wife reassured me: *anajua sana!* Just recently they had a patient with serious mental illness, running naked in the street; he tied him down and gave him medicine until he got better and went home again. The healer, a muscled young man in his thirties, finally arrived and sat down with his toes covered in red-brown mud and a broad shining smile. He gave me the four-legged low stool of the elder. His mother is from Mgeta, in the Uluguru Mountains, and his father from further away, Kisaki. His specialty is Kiluguru spirits that originate from the Kolelo cult, which has a shrine in the Uluguru Mountains. His wife had to write down the name Kolelo for me because, she said laughingly, "*hasomi*" ("he does not read"), he is illiterate. In his explanations, he appeared yet another example of a bright and creative mind dealing with the lack of school education by obtaining *elimu ya mzimu*, knowledge of the spirit. In the new Tanzania, the illiterate explore their skills of intuition and charisma. How did he become a healer? He chose an interesting verb: his *mzimu*, spirit, is *wa kuoteshwa*, "of being made to grow" (with the stem *–ota*, to grow). How it will grow is not in the individual's hands, but the growth can be made to happen. In 2003, he got ill, with much pain including seizures (*kifafa*). He realized the illness would last unless he accepted becoming a healer. The elder healer he stayed with helped him to dream the requests of his ancestor. On the night before he was declared cured, he had dreamed that his guiding spirit belonged to his father's side. This was confirmed by the healing vocation of his father's sister. Since that day he wears three types of bracelet on his right arm in honor of the paternal ancestors. By now he claims to possess 169 spirits.

The medicine he prepares mostly consists of powder of grounded roots, which depending on the illness can be boiled or mixed in cold porridge. The leaves can be dried for infusion. Strong medicine is kept in bottles of liquid made of water and plants. Most original to me was his divination technique, which illustrates why they are called healers of the calabash. The receptacle for medicine is used for oracles. He performs his oracles with a remarkable tool he named Adija. The letters are engraved on a shiny reddish dark-brown calabash connected with a palm-size mirror via two thin strings of tiny white and black pearls, each a mere foot long. The middle of the strings carries a pair of small medicinal bottles, one smaller than the other and each covered with the black hair tuft of a cowtail. Both halves of the strings are strengthened with two wooden amulets on each side. Inside the calabash is a transparent liquid with the power to "pull" (attract) the spirit (*kuvuta mzimu*). The healer emphasizes that the liquid combines the forces of both Koranic and calabash healing. To attract the spirit, the liquid is dipped on the forehead with the stick forming a lid, covered with a hair tuft on top and tied with a little red banner. The information on the life-force (*nyota*) of the client is transmitted, "like an x-ray" said the healer, through the two bead strings to appear in the mirror. There the healer can "measure" (*kupima*) the life force. The diagnosis will determine whether the illness is caused by the power of God, *ya Mwezimungu*, or by superstition, *ya ushirikina*, literally "polytheism," the Arabic notion of heresy and most common term for witchcraft in this region. In the latter case evil spirits, *majini*, may have been sent, "thrown" (*kutupiwa*) by a person enraged (*-chuki*). In most cases healers assume the cause of illness to be the evil of humans, "as God is not evil." By saying this, the healers who grew up under both Islamic and Christian influences indirectly raise the question of theodicy for the many lethal illnesses that according to the hospital would be natural, and not the result of people's evil acts. People's witchcraft vindicates God's providence in view of the existence of evil and the innocent suffering. Theodicy could not be an issue in the Bantu cosmologies of capricious spirits, with an impersonal creator-divinity lingering in the back.

Conclusions

This essay describes the changes taking place in traditional healing. We contend that the general trend in postcolonial Tanzania has been away from collective village-based or clan-based practices and towards individualization of treatment, via a healer's private ceremony and oracle. In most of Africa, the literature review indicates, the healer is expected to specialize in mental problems. The renewed success of Pentecostal churches can be seen as a parallel process: as the formation of new therapeutic collectives that aim at wellbeing, albeit for participants sharing an individualist cosmology anchored on personal prosperity.

Individualization went hand in hand with a cultural division of traditional medicine into a physical (or biological) part, dealing with plant medicine, and a mental (or spiritual) part, concentrating on ritual therapy. To comply with government expectations, traditional healers in Tanzania indeed attempt to professionalize into associations and thus integrate themselves into the health system by implementing this cultural division socio-structurally. Healers have been accused of acting as witch-doctors, that is of increasing suspicions in the community, of identifying innocent people as witches (leading allegedly to witch-killings—a major topic in Tanzanian media since the late 1990s), and of encouraging the use of medicinal ingredients from human victims (such as the so-called albino murders for *mwanga* magic, publicized worldwide since the mid-2000s). An equally vivid, ongoing stream of media reports has articulated the plea of traditional healers, united in national or regional associations, to consider them as experts of plant medicine in the first place and to downplay the significance of witchcraft discourse in traditional medicine, even to reject witchcraft references as the work of charlatans and their gullible clients. In this plea of healers, we witness the reinvention of traditional medicine made in the image of the Western doctor. According to that same image, the government approves of the market of healing being flooded by medicinal pills in sachets claiming anti-malarial and numerous other effects largely unproven. At the same time, healers have never been so busy accommodating the patients and their caretakers who expect full-fledged detections of witchcraft, on the grounds that if the cause of illness were not witchcraft-related, they should have gone to the hospital. Suffice to add to this paradox the discomfort of biomedicine with mental illness, the long absence of psychology in the media and the shortage of psychiatric care, and we may better grasp the accelerating bifurcation in traditional healing between deritualized plant medicines or "pharma-philia," on one side, and spirit- or witchcraft-related therapies for the individual(ized) mind, on the other.

Bibliography

Abbo, C., S. Ekblad, P. Waako, E. Okello, and S. Musisi. 2009. "The Prevalence and Severity of Mental Illnesses Handled by Traditional Healers in Two Districts in Uganda." *African Health Sciences* 9: S16–22.

Adewuya, A. and R. Makanjuola. 2009. "Preferred Treatment for Mental Illness among Southwestern Nigerians. *Psychiatric Services* 60 (1): 121–24.

Alem, Atlay, Lars. Jacobsson, and Charlotte Hanlon. 2008. "Community-based Mental Health Care in Africa: Mental Health Workers' Views." *World Psychiatry* 7 (1): 54–57.

Al-Krenawi, A., J. Graham, M. Ophir, and J. Kandah. 2001. "Ethnic and Gender Differences in Mental Health Utilization: The Case of Muslim Jordanian and Moroccan Jewish Israeli Out-patient Psychiatric Patients." *International Journal of Social Psychiatry* 47 (3): 42–54.

Anders, Sherry L. 2003. "Improving Community-Based Care for the Treatment of Schizophrenia: Lessons from Native Africa." *Psychiatric Rehabilitation Journal* 27 (1): 51–58.

Appiah-Poku, J., R. Laugharne, E. Mensah, Y. Osei, and T. Burns. 2004. "Previous Help Sought by Patients Presenting to Mental Health Services in Kumasi, Ghana." *Social Psychiatry and Psychiatric Epidemiology* 39 (3): 208–11.

Bayart, Jean-François. 1993. *The State in Africa: The Politics of the Belly*. London: Longman.

Berg, Astrid. 2003. Ancestor Reverence and Mental Health in South Africa. *Transcultural Psychiatry* 40 (2): 194–207.

Berry, Katherine, Christine Barrowclough, and Gillian Haddock. 2010. "The Role of Expressed Emotion in Relationships between Psychiatric Staff and People with a Diagnosis of Psychosis: A Review of the Literature." *Schizophrenia Bulletin*, doi:10/1093/schbul/sbp162.

Boddy, Janice. 1989. *Wombs and Alien Spirits: Women, Men and the Zar in Northern Sudan*. Madison: University of Wisconsin.

Bustillo, J., J. Lauriello, W. Horan, and S. Keith. 2001. "The Psychosocial Treatment of Schizophrenia: An Update." *American Journal of Psychiatry* 158: 163–75.

Cocks, M. and A. Dold. 2000. "The Role of 'African Chemists' in the Health Care System of the Eastern Cape Province of South Africa." *Social Sciences and Medicine* 51 (10): 1505–15.

Crumlish, N., P. Samalani, A. Sefasi, A. Kinsella, E. O'Callaghan, and H. Chilale. 2007. "Insight, Psychopathology and Global Functioning in Schizophrenia in Urban Malawi." *The British Journal of Psychiatry* 191: 262–63.

Devisch, René. 1993. *Weaving the Threads of Life: The Khita Gyn-Eco-Logical Healing Cult among the Yaka*. Chicago: Chicago University.

Dixon, Lisa B., Faith Dickerson, Alan S. Bellack, Melanie. Bennett, et al. 2010. "The 2009 Schizophrenia PORT Psychosocial Treatment Recommendations and Summary Statements." *Schizophrenia Bulletin* 36 (1): 48–70

Fenta, Haile, Ilene Hyman, and Samuel Noh. 2006. "Mental Health Service Utilization by Ethiopian Immigrants and Refugees in Toronto." *Journal of Nervous and Mental Diseases* 194 (12): 925–34.

Geertz, Clifford. 1973. *The Interpretation of Cultures*. London: Fontana.

Green, Maia. 2005. "Discourses on Inequality." *Anthropological Theory* 5: 247–66.

Gureje, Oye, Victor Lasebikan, Lola Kola, and Victor Makanjuola. 2006. "Lifetime and 12–month Prevalence of Mental Disorders in the Nigerian Survey of Mental Health and Well–Being." *British Journal of Psychiatry* 188: 465–71.

Igreja, Victor. 2003. "'Why Are There So Many Drums Playing until Dawn?' Exploring the Role of Gamba Spirits and Healers in the Post-war Recovery Period in Gorongosa, Central Mozambique." *Transcultural Psychiatry* 40 (4): 459–87.

Igreja, Victor, B. Dias-Lambranca, D. Hershey, L. Racin, A. Richters, and R. Reis. 2010. The Epidemiology of Spirit Possession in the Aftermath of Mass Political Violence in Mozambique. *Social Sciences and Medicine* 71 (3): 592–99.

Janse van Rensburg, Bernard. 2009. "A Changed Climate for Mental Health Care Delivery in South Africa." *African Journal of Psychiatry* 12 (2): 157–65.

Janzen, John M. 1992. *Ngoma: Discourses of Healing in Central and Southern Africa*. Berkeley: University of California.

Johnson, Laura, Med Mayanja, Paul Bangirana, and Simon Kizito. 2009. "Contrasting Concepts of Depression in Uganda: Implications for Service Delivery in a Multicultural Context." *American Journal of Orthopsychiatry* 79 (2): 275–89.

Kendall-Taylor, Nathaniel, Caroline Kathomi, Keneth Rimba, and Charles Newton. 2009. "Comparing Characteristics of Epilepsy Treatment Providers on the Kenyan Coast: Implications for Treatment-seeking and Intervention." *Rural and Remote Health* 9: 1253.

Kleinman, Arthur, and Lilias Sung. 1979. "Why Do Indigenous Practitioners Successfully Heal?" *Social Science & Medicine* 13 (1): 7–26.

Kuipers, Elizabeth, Juliana Onwumere, and Paul Bebbington. 2010. "Cognitive Model of Caregiving in Psychosis." *British Journal of Psychiatry* 196: 259–65.

Langwick, Stacey. 2008. "Articulate(d) Bodies: Traditional Medicine in a Tanzanian Hospital." *American Ethnologist* 35 (3): 428–39.

Maiello, S. 2008. "Encounter with a Traditional Healer: Western and African Therapeutic Approaches in Dialogue." *Journal of Analytical Psychology* 53 (2): 241–60.

Makanjuola, A., M. Adelekan, and O. Morakinyo. 2000. "Current Status of Traditional Mental Health Practice in Ilorin Emirate Council Area, Kwara State, Nigeria. *West African Journal of Medicine* 19 (1): 43–49.

Mignolo, Walter. 2000. *Local Histories, Global Designs: Coloniality, Subaltern Knowledge and Border Thinking*. Princeton: Princeton University.

Mirza, I., M. Okitapoy, and R. Jenkins. 2006. "Knowledge and Practice of Help-Seeking for Treatment of Mental Disorders in Pemba Island, Zanzibar." *Tropical Doctor* 36 (3): 140–44.

Mkize, L., and L. Uys. 2004. "Pathways to Mental Health Care in KwaZulu-Natal." *Curationis* 27 (3): 62–71.

Modiba, P., H. Schneider, K. Porteus, and V. Gunnarson. 2001. "Profile of Community Mental Health Service Needs in the Moretele District (North-West Province) in South Africa." Journal of Mental Health Policy and Economy 4 (4): 189–96.

Mshana, G., K. Hampshire, C. Panter-Brick, R. Walker, and the Tanzanian Stroke Incidence Project Team. 2008. "Urban–rural Contrasts in Explanatory Models and Treatment-seeking Behaviours for Stroke in Tanzania." *Journal of Biosocial Science* 40: 35–52.

Nelms, L., and J. Gorski. 2006. "The Role of the African Traditional Healer in Women's Health." *Journal of Transcultural Nursing* 17 (2): 184–89.

Ngoma, M., M. Prince, and A. Mann. 2003. "Common Mental Disorders among Those Attending Primary Health Clinics and Traditional Healers in Urban Tanzania." British Journal of Psychiatry 183: 349–55.

Niehaus, D., P. Oosthuizen, C. Lochner, R. Emsley, E. Jordaan, N. Mbanga, N. Keyter, C. Laurent, J. Deleuze, and D. Stein. 2004. "A Culture-Bound Syndrome 'Amafufunyana' and a Culture-Specific Event 'Ukuthwasa': Differentiated by a Family History of Schizophrenia and Other Psychiatric Disorders." *Psychopathology* 37 (2): 59–63.

Nyamnjoh, Francis. 2001. "Delusions of Development and the Enrichment of Witchcraft Discourses in Cameroon." In *Magical Interpretations, Material Realities*, edited by H. Moore and T. Sanders, 28–49. New York: Routledge.

Peltzer, Karl. 2000. "Perceived Treatment Efficacy of the Last Experienced Illness Episode in a Community Sample in the Northern Province, South Africa." *Curationis* 23 (1): 57–60.

———. 2009. "Utilization and Practice of Traditional/Complementary/Alternative Medicine (tm/cam) in South Africa." *African Journal of Traditional, Complementary and Alternative Medicine* 6 (2): 175–85.

Shibre, T., A. Spångéus, L. Henriksson, A. Negash, and L. Jacobsson. 2008. "Traditional Treatment of Mental Disorders in Rural Ethiopia." *Ethiopian Medical Journal* 46 (1): 87–91.

Sibitz, I., A. Unger, A. Woppmann, T. Zidek, and M. Amering. 2011. "Stigma Resistance in Patients with Schizophrenia." *Schizophrenia Bulletin* 37 (2): 316–23.

Slikkerveer, Leendert. 1982. "Rural Health Development in Ethiopia: Problems of Utilization of Traditional Healers." *Social Science & Medicine* 14 (21): 1859–72.

Sorsdahl, K., D. Stein, A. Grimsrud, S. Seedat, A. Flisher, D. Williams, and L. Myer. 2009. "Traditional Healers in the Treatment of Common Mental Disorders in South Africa." *Journal of Nervous and Mental Diseases* 197 (6): 434–41.

Stein, Debra. 2000. "Views of Mental Illness in Morocco: Western Medicine Meets the Traditional Symbolic." *Canadian Medical Association Journal* 163 (11): 1468–70.

Stroeken, Koen. 2010. *Moral Power: The Magic of Witchcraft*. New York: Berghahn.

———. 2012. "Health-care Decisions by Sukuma 'Peasant Intellectuals': A Case of Radical Empiricism?" *Anthropology & Medicine* 19 (1): 119–28.

Taylor, T., H. Killaspy, C. Wright, et al. 2009. "A Systematic Review of the International Published Literature Relating to Quality of Institutional Care for People with Longer Term Mental Health Problems." *BMC Psychiatry* 9: 55.

Van Duijl, M., E. Cardeña, and J. De Jong. 2005. "The Validity of DSM-IV Dissociative Disorders Categories in South-West Uganda." *Transcultural Psychiatry* 42 (2): 219–41.

Yao, Y., Y. Yeo-Tenena, E. Tetchi, C. Assi-Sedji, Y. Bombo, L. Kouame, S. Soro, and R. Delafosse. 2008. "First Therapeutic Recourse of the Teenagers Received to the Service of Mental Hygiene of the INSP of Abidjan." *Mali Médicine* 23 (3): 55–60.

Yen, J., and L. Wilbraham. 2003. "Discourses of Culture and Illness in South African Mental Health Care and Indigenous Healing, Part I: Western Psychiatric Power." *Transcultural Psychiatry* 40 (4): 542–61.

Yen, J., and L. Wilbraham. 2003. "Discourses of Culture and Illness in South African Mental Health Care and Indigenous Healing, Part II: African Mentality." *Transcultural Psychiatry* 40 (4): 562–84.

Zaghdoudi, L., L. Mnif, R. Rafrafi, R. Ghachem, and R. Labbane. 2008. "The Practice of Traditional Therapies in Psychiatric Environment: About 100 Cases. *Tunis Médicine* 86 (6): 560–63.

8 Ihahamuka—PTSD in Postgenocidal Rwanda

Culture, Continuity and Change in Rwandan Therapeutics

Christopher C. Taylor

In MUCH RECENT anthropological writing, the concept of culture—once the core concept of the discipline—either receives scant attention or is avoided altogether. The reasons for this are multiple. Many anthropologists criticize the culture concept for being overly totalizing. Not all members of a society, it is said, internalize their putative culture in the same way. Differences in age, gender, class, or ethnicity prevent this from occurring. Secondly, the culture concept has been criticized for being overly deterministic. Not everyone marches to the beat of a single drummer, so how much causal weight need we attribute to culture when we observe wide variations in individual behavior?

Globalization theorists such as Arjun Appadurai join in the anticulturalist chorus. According to them, commodities, ideas, music, sports, and people traverse the planet in a dizzying testament to the human ability to mix, match, and hybridize. It is conscious choice which dictates cultural forms and not the reverse.

> As group pasts become increasingly parts of museums, exhibits and collections, both in national and transnational spectacles, culture becomes less what Bourdieu would have called a habitus (a tacit realm of reproducible practices and dispositions) and more an arena for conscious choice, justification and representation, the latter often to multiple and spatially dislocated audiences. (Appadurai 1990, 18)

Indeed, it would appear that something of an international haute bourgeoisie has emerged in recent decades and that its members retain very little of the local cultures from their places of origin. Bereft, or perhaps free, of the cultural influences of their natal regions, they fashion themselves by their choices in consumption and self-presentation. But it is legitimate to ask how many people belong to this international haute bourgeoisie and how pervasive is its influence?

However, even as many contemporary anthropologists appear to be turning away from "culture," or at least that part of the concept understood as "a tacit realm of reproducible practices and dispositions," in favor of notions such as agency and conscious choice, many experimental psychologists are showing that we may not control our behavior as much as we would like to believe. One such psychologist is Jonathan ST B.T. Evans, who critically reviews the current psychological literature on "dual processing theory" (Evans 2008). Dual processing theory posits that two mental systems coexist within our minds, and that working in tandem, they guide our reasoning and social cognition. The first system, system one, operates implicitly and automatically, while system two operates explicitly and consciously. According to proponents of dual processing theory, system one acts quickly and without being encumbered by conscious reflection, but it serves a subordinate role to the slower workings of system two, where decision-making ultimately occurs. Evans disagrees.

> However, this happy state of affairs, which leaves "us" in control of our behavior, is contradicted by much psychological research. Many researchers have emphasized the fact that unconscious processes may control our behavior without us being aware of them doing so. (Evans 2008, 258)

Perhaps it is scholars who study the darker side of human behavior, as in violence, terrorism, and genocide, who have a greater appreciation of the less-than-conscious processes that motivate action in these domains. When violent actions are organized collectively by state or quasi-state actors, we readily apprehend the conscious side of things, as the state or quasi-state spares no effort in legitimizing its violence according to readily articulable political, economic, or moral goals. Often, the state appeals to cost/benefit considerations and promotes actions that seem reasonable or at least defensible in the context of a supposed threat to the prevailing socio-moral order. However, what the state asks its citizens to do during times of violence includes things that would be unreasonable or indefensible during times of peace. It asks its citizens to risk death, and it asks its citizens to kill. Frequently, during such times the amount of killing and the "techniques of cruelty" (Foucault) employed take on a dynamic of their own, which defy reason and transgress the boundaries of ordinary sociality. The contradiction here has to be suppressed, if not fully hidden. This is attempted by the state's unwitting appeal, not only to reason, which is on the surface, but also to subjacent cultural codes that are tacit and even unconscious in nature. This means that at one level the polity's organized violence is supported and institutionalized in the form of explicit ideologies which make destructive acts appear justified for the maintenance of collective well-being. But it also means that the motivations which compel actors to commit violence and to face death derive from sources that the perpetrators themselves are not fully aware of. Frequently, the media and public rituals such as executions serve as the means by which overt and conscious ideologies are validated and communicated to the mass of the polity's followers. But at another level, and more importantly for the purposes of this chapter, media and public rituals also convey less apprehensible messages reflecting the community's deep desires, fears, and sentiments. These latter are less accessible to conscious apperception, more archetypal in nature, and less likely to be construed by social actors as having obvious and clear-cut ideological content.

Following Aijmer's discussion of violence (2000), whose analytical scheme bears close resemblance to that used by Godelier (1996) in an apparently unrelated matter—the ambiguities left unresolved in Mauss's discussion of the gift—one could posit the existence of three dimensions to state violence and to the political rituals that enact or serve to justify it: the imaginary, the symbolic, and the real. At the least apprehensible level is what Godelier terms the imaginary. The imaginary consists of iconic symbols loosely organized into diffuse cultural codes. These constitute the base of the social imagination in its envisioning of possible worlds. This material is only intuitively cognized by social actors and consists of what Roy Wagner (1986) would call "symbols that stand for themselves," or in other words, symbols that are not readily translatable into a verbal or discursive idiom. These symbols and diffuse codes constitute the body of any community's tacit assumptions about itself and the world, while subtly and almost imperceptibly revealing its profoundest fears and desires. This level is the least accessible to the social actors themselves and to their exegesis. In those instances when an outsider indicates material from this level to the social actors who actually live it, their verbal responses are likely to be ad hoc rationalizations or secondary elaborations (Aijmer, op. cit.). Despite the relative inaccessibility of this iconic imaginary base to the persons who embody it, it precedes and conditions everything that is more conscious in nature. In this respect, Godelier explicitly marks his difference from both Lacan and Levi-Strauss, who see the symbolic (discursive) as logically prior to both the imaginary and the real (1996).

At the next level, which Aijmer terms the discursive and Godelier terms the symbolic, verbal elements come to the fore. It is here that volitional phenomena are manifest as social actors verbalize what their intentions are and act out these intentions in consonance with avowed pragmatic ends. This is the domain of language, discourse, and narrative. People will usually be able to identify and verbalize what the ideologies of their supporters and opponents are and explain the pragmatic ends that are served with any particular statement or action. It is here that strategization is most apparent, as social actors weigh the consequences of one course of action against others and then behave accordingly. This is also the level where disagreement, conflict, and struggle are most manifest.

The most visible level of state violence is that which Aijmer calls the ethological and which corresponds to what Godelier calls the real. Violence has very real biological and psychological effects upon the people against whom it is applied: suffering, pain, injury, and death. Yet even this level is dependent upon its interaction with the other two levels in order for violent acts to attain their full amplitude of social meaning. It may not be sufficient, for example, to kill one's opponent; it may be necessary to mutilate, to destroy, or to dispose of the body in such a way that the victim's spirit not return to wreak vengeance on the perpetrator of the violence. As Aijmer puts it, while physical death may be irrevocable and nonnegotiable, social death may not (2000).

Although both Godelier and Aijmer posit the primacy of the imaginary, certainly these three levels are not hermetically sealed off from one another. It is possible for people to become aware of the iconic symbols that constitute their imaginary. Certain members of a collectivity, as with individuals in psychoanalysis, may have a *prise de conscience* in which the deeper levels of their socially shared fears and desires become manifest. When this happens, the iconic enters the realm of the symbolic and becomes susceptible to verbalization. The prediscursive rises to the discursive. In like fashion, this process can go the other way. Discursive material that had once been verbalized in the form of ideological statements and narratives can become so habitual as to become virtually unconscious. What was once stated and debated becomes tacit and implicit, joining the ranks of other phenomena constituting the *habitus* or the "things that go without saying" (Bourdieu 1977). Finally, it is also possible that at the level of the real or the ethological, the performance of violence radically reconstitutes the social and cultural order. In such a case, the older ideologies and deeper cultural layers may lose their salience, being replaced by something new.

My contention in this essay is that the pathological results of violence upon the human psyche, such as those that I observed in Rwanda in the wake of the 1994 genocide, follow a similar logic. Phenomena such as posttraumatic stress disorder (PTSD) can be examined from the vantage point of the imaginary (what I would call the pre-discursive), the symbolic/discursive, or the ethological/real. At the discursive level, the level of speech and language, I would agree with those theorists who emphasize conscious choice. At this level, it is agency which predominates as people pursue their political, economic, religious, or health-seeking aims. At this level, people are able to articulate what their goals are and what they need to do to attain them. It is also at this level that we witness a great deal of plurality as people act pragmatically, attempting first one course of action, then another, then another, if necessary, to obtain the desired result. John Janzen's *The Quest for Therapy in Lower Zaire* provides many examples of this. Sufferers seek relief from their symptoms first and foremost, and they care much less about the theoretical and ontological underpinnings of the therapy that is able to provide it. Pragmatic concerns govern behavior.

However, not everything which concerns sickness and the quest to be rid of it operates at a discursive level; not everything is conscious. We may choose our therapies, but we don't choose our sicknesses. They "choose" us. Elsewhere I attempt to demonstrate this with regard to the violence which occurred during the Rwandan genocide (Taylor 1999). Victims were killed in patterned ways, but neither surviving victims nor perpetrators could verbalize, much less explain, what those patterns were. In this chapter, I contend that there is also pattern and logic to how Rwanda's genocidal violence has afflicted those who survived it, but that this is not fully accessible to analytical frameworks that emphasize conscious choice. In other words, the ethological or real level of trauma depends for its expression upon the imaginary. I will discuss a malady called *ihahamuka* that I encountered among survivors of Rwanda's 1994 genocide during field-work there in 2005 and 2009. *Ihahamuka* is characterized symptomatically by a sensation that one's breath has become locked in one's chest. Sufferers say that the heart feels as if it has moved upward in the chest. There are feelings of suf-focation in some instances, and feelings that the words that one wishes to utter have become blocked in one's body. Many of the people (mostly Tutsi) who com-plained of these symptoms could be characterized socioeconomically as middle or even upper class. Most were bilingual in French and Kinyarwanda, most were practicing Christians, relatively well-educated, and most possessed a skeptical view of Rwandan 'traditional' healing. One might call them "Westernized." De-spite this, in order to fully understand *ihahamuka* we must look not at the dis-cursive level, but at a pre-discursive level, the level of implicit, even unconscious, cultural models. We must look at Rwandan traditional notions of health and healing. It is at this level that we see Rwandans, seemingly the most estranged from their "traditional culture," actually embodying it in ways of which they are not aware.

Background, Rwanda, *gacaca*, *ihahamuka*

In the central African country of Rwanda, infamous for the 1994 genocide that cost the lives of close to one million people, I have studied ethnomedicine and have also worked as an applied medical anthropologist. I started my first fieldwork there in 1983, at which time I was mostly interested in local Rwandan medicine, *ubuvuzi bwa kinyarwanda*. I studied notions of the body, notions of sickness, and the local treatments. Ten years later, I worked in an applied capacity in HIV and STD prevention. Because of the onset of violence in April 1994, I and other members of the American community there had to be evacuated. I returned to Rwanda later to study *gacaca* and to work with Tutsi survivors of the genocide.

I first encountered *ihahamuka* during two periods of fieldwork in Rwanda in 2005 and 2009. My intention then was to study the local tribunals called *gacaca* which were set up to deal with the immense number of judicial cases that had followed in the wake of the 1994 genocide. By accident, I discovered that many of the people who attended *gacaca* meetings complained of a disorder that they called *ihahamuka*. According to these people, attending the locally organized *gacaca* meetings helped to relieve some of their symptoms.

Many of the latter participated in the *gacaca* tribunals, bearing witness to what they had experienced during the three months of genocide. Many other survivors did not participate in *gacaca* despite the fact that attendance was highly encouraged by the Rwandan government. According to these nonparticipants, *gacaca* attendance made them relive traumatic events that they preferred to forget. Others said that their testimony might alert "genocidaires,'" still at liberty, that they had knowledge that might inculpate them. They did not want to expose themselves to the reprisal violence of *Interahamwe* still residing in Rwanda. This fear was not unjustified. During my two stays in Rwanda, I heard several news reports on the Rwandan radio of *gacaca* witnesses who had been murdered.

Despite the reticence of some, many others, both Tutsi and Hutu, regularly came to *gacaca* meetings in their neighborhood or district. These were the people whom I interviewed most frequently for the purposes of this study. Often, these people were, in sociological terms, members of what one might call the Rwandan middle class. Many were relatively well educated. Many were Francophone and had well-paying jobs by local standards. Practically all of them had completed at least eight years of primary school, many of them had some secondary school background and a few had some university level education. All were Christian, either Catholic or Protestant. None of them admitted to having practiced traditional religious rituals such as *guterekera* (ancestor veneration), *kubandwa* (a traditional religion practiced in southern Rwanda), or *Nyabingi* (a traditional religion practiced in northern Rwanda). None of them claimed to have consulted a Rwandan traditional healer, and most indicated skepticism with regard to Rwandan traditional therapeutic practices.

At the same time, however, many of these people complained of an indigenous malady that they called *ihahamuka*. They described these symptoms as feelings of asphyxiation, breath that would get caught in the chest, and a sensation that the heart was pushing upward in the chest making it difficult to exhale. Others said that even their words were getting stuck in their throats. These symptoms were accompanied by feelings of anxiety, fear, and even panic at times. During my earlier periods of fieldwork in the 1980s, I had never heard Rwandan healers or their patients speak of *ihahamuka*. To me, this was a completely new disorder, even though it must have existed in the past as it is mentioned in I. Jacob's abridged version of the dictionary compiled by Rwanda's Institut National de

Recherche Scientifique. The noun *ihahamuka* is derived from the verb *guhaha-muka,* which means, "to be paralyzed by fear, to be unable to speak because of fear, or, to speak while trembling with fear" (Irénée Jacob 1984). *Ihahamuka* is not the ordinary term for fear in Kinyarwanda; the term *ubwoba* is. *Ihahamuka* is a special kind of fear and is not a synonym of *ubwoba.* When someone says *nahahamutse,* what is meant is: "I am paralyzed by fear, my breath and words are caught inside me."

Other researchers who have studied *gacaca* have also noted that Rwandan survivors often complain of *ihahamuka* (Burnet 2008). The term connotes obstruction, a notion which can be explicated by the cultural model which I hypothesize subtends much Rwandan thinking about illness (Taylor 1992). According to Western medical terminology, *ihahamuka* would probably be called a form of PTSD (posttraumatic stress disorder). Hagengimana and Hinton also discuss *ihahamuka* in their theoretical discussion of panic disorder, citing my earlier work on Rwandan medicine by way of explanation. While many Rwandan survivors definitely suffer from PTSD, that term does not address what is Rwandan about *ihahamuka.* Rwandans are somaticizing their distress after having lived through many days of extreme terror, but they are doing so in a specifically Rwandan way. Despite the many faults of *gacaca,* which have been amply described in the literature, attendance at the tribunals has succeeded in bringing some measure of relief to those suffering from *ihahamuka.* For better or for worse, *gacaca* has served as a kind of local remedy for some Rwandans to a local illness.

The Case of Daphrose

One person who sought relief from *ihahamuka* by participating at *gacaca* sessions was a woman named Daphrose. Daphrose was about forty-five when I met her in 2009, meaning that she had been about thirty when the genocide occurred. Daphrose was almost killed during the genocide, when Rwandan government soldiers came to her house in the Gikongoro section of Kigali on several occasions. Luckily, she was able to eventually save herself as she was aided in her escape from Rwanda by Hutu neighbors. After the genocide, she returned and reclaimed her house and property. According to Daphrose, *gacaca* attendance was almost a necessity in order to preserve her mental equilibrium. In this respect, she was unlike her sister Anne Marie who never participated in *gacaca.* Anne Marie explained to me that she wanted to forget everything about the genocide and did not want to stir up old and painful memories. It should also be noted that Anne-Marie was able to flee Rwanda well before Daphrose and had not suffered the same degree of trauma.

Daphrose accompanied me to two *gacaca* meetings. After our second meeting, she began to talk about the ordeal that she had endured during the genocide. On one occasion when Rwandan soldiers came to her house, one of them took her to her bedroom, commanded her to disrobe and told her that he was going to have sex with her. He told her to keep quiet so that she would not suffer worse. A clever woman, Daphrose quickly invented a story about her being HIV-positive and her not wanting to infect him. She said that when she died, she did not want to meet God with that sin on her soul. The soldier thought about this for a minute then let her alone. He told her that soon enough other soldiers would come and they would kill her. A few days later others did indeed come. Once again a soldier took her to her bedroom, ordered her to disrobe and to lie on her bed. He then inserted the barrel of his rifle partway into her vagina and told her that he was going to pull the trigger. In effect that bullet would have traversed her body from the vagina to her neck or head. [This method of killing resembles vagina to mouth impalement by spear, an atrocity that some Tutsi women did indeed endure during the genocide (Taylor 1999)]. Daphrose begged the soldier to kill her in some other way so as to leave her with a modicum of human dignity. Once again, the soldier thought about it and demurred. After these and other close calls, her escape, and later return, she suffered from *ihahamuka*. It was *gacaca*, she explained to me, that had cured her of this and that had permitted her to speak normally again.

Comment:
My hypothesis is that this technique of cruelty, shooting a bullet that traverses the body from vagina to mouth, and the disorder of *ihahamuka* share a common symbolic logic, but without conscious knowledge of this on the part of the actors. This observation comes close to what M. Taussig observes in his book *Shamanism, Colonialism, and the Wild Man*, in which he discusses the violence committed against the indigenous people of Putumayo (Colombia) and the work of the journalist Roger Casement who investigated the violence:

> From the accounts of Casement and Timerman it is also obvious that torture and terror are ritualized art forms and that, far from being spontaneous, sui generis, and an abandonment of what are often called the values of civilization, such rites of terror have a deep history deriving power and meaning from those very values. (1987, 133)

Let us examine Taussig's observation that torture and terror are "ritualized art forms." This implies that torture and terror have both form and content, and that the form the violence takes is perhaps equally as important as the content. There is an aesthetics of violence. The content of torture and terror is not difficult to understand. The torturer asserts domination over the victim. The torturer has the power to cause extreme pain or death. The victim is powerless and cannot look to his or her group for protection. However, torture and terror take specific forms, and it is here that one can talk about an "aesthetics of violence." Why beat people on the soles of their feet, for example? Why draw and quarter hanged criminals who are already dead? Why employ execution methods such as lethal injection rather than the guillotine, the garrote, or the electric chair? Form is clearly important, even though its analysis is usually neglected or ignored. Further on in Taussig's book, he does not pursue the insight about "ritualized art forms" very far. One expects, but does not get, an analysis of European ritual and aesthetics that might tell us something about a preoccupation with the demonic and the tendency to project fears about it on scapegoats be these internal to the society (e.g., sorcerers) or external (e.g., savages).

Closer to Rwanda, Liisa Malkii's book, *Purity and Exile*, discusses the techniques of cruelty inflicted upon Hutu in Burundi during the genocidal violence of 1972–1973. These techniques included: the impalement of men by spear from anus to mouth, the impalement of women from vagina to mouth, cutting fetuses from their mothers' wombs, forcing parents to ingest the flesh of their slaughtered children, and forcing parents to assume a sexual position with children by binding them together with ropes prior to killing them. She raises interesting questions concerning these forms of cruelty:

> It is relevant to ask how the accounts of atrocity come to assume thematic form, how they become formulaic. . . . The first thing to be examined is the extent to which the techniques of cruelty actually used were already meaningful, already mythico-historical. (Malkii 94)

> One need only inspect reports from Amnesty International and other organizations whose main purpose is to document human-rights violations to begin to see that the conventionalization of torture, killing, and other forms of violence occurs not only routinely but in patterned forms in the contemporary world. Torture, in particular, is a highly symbolized form of violence. At this level, it can be said that historical actors mete out death and perpetrate violence mythically. (94)

These are interesting observations, yet despite the statement that the violence in Burundi was mythico-historical and that it had pre-existing meaning, the analysis is not pursued far enough. She states that the violence that Tutsis inflicted upon Burundian Hutu was an attempt to dehumanize and humiliate them. While this is true with regard to its content, this does not address all that is ritualized, symbolic, or aesthetic in the techniques of cruelty. In genocidal Rwanda of 1994, similar forms of violence occurred: impalement, the evisceration of pregnant women, forced incest, forced cannibalism. There were also other forms of violence such as the severing of the Achilles tendon of humans and livestock, breast oblation, and the emasculation of men and boys.

In order to render these forms of violence comprehensible in terms of the local symbolism, one must first recall the lesson imparted by Pierre Clastres, that social systems inscribe their law onto the bodies of their subjects (1974). Male and female initiation practices come immediately to mind, but terror and torture do something very similar. Pursuing a related point, M. Foucault shows that even without resorting to torture, societies use measures of bodily discipline upon those who pass through its institutions such as school, army, asylum, and prison (1977). Clastres cites Kafka's book, *The Penal Colony* to support his idea that the body can act as a blank slate, a writing surface ready to receive the readable text of the law. Clastres pursues this insight by considering the cognitive role of the body in ritual. The body acts as a mediator in the ritual acquisition of social knowledge. This is inscribed upon the body through ordeal and pain and these prevent the subject from ever forgetting the lesson.

One can extrapolate from this lesson of Clastres and apply it to Rwanda and to its ethnomedicine. We see this in practices that aim to keep the body healthy or to cure it of its ills. As I have explained elsewhere (1992), a core metaphor subtends conceptualization of the body in traditional medicine. This is not the only core metaphor, but it is important and necessary to understand if we wish to understand the genocidal techniques of cruelty and the postgenocidal disorder, *ihahamuka*. This core metaphor consists of an opposition between orderly humoral flows and disorderly ones (blocked flows or excessive flows). Here, for the purposes of this paper, we will be concerned with flow/blockage oppositions. Analogies extend this metaphor to the unfolding of social life. In traditional medicine, healers attempt to correct imbalanced flows caused by human negligence and human malevolence (e.g., sorcery). Corporal fluids such as blood, sperm, maternal milk, menstrual blood, saliva, etc. figure prominently in symptomatology. Illness is characterized by excessive, inadequate and even completely obstructed flows.

Healers, however, never explain the disorders of their patients, nor the logic of their treatments in these terms. They merely say that they learned their treatments from their predecessors and continue to employ them because they are effective. This cultural model then, flow vs. blockage, does not appear to be a conscious one. This is in sharp contrast to similar "image schemata" (M. Johnson 1987) found elsewhere in the world. In India, for example, healers speak of the flow of kundalini, and in China, healers speak of the flow of qi. In both cases, interruptions in the flow of these substances provoke illness, and healers can explain illness in these terms. Despite the less than conscious quality of the flow/blockage metaphor in Rwanda, one finds it in other symbolic sources such as myth and ritual (cf. Taylor 1988).

One example where we can observe the operation of this metaphor in the social construction of the person involves birth. After parturition, the mother is supposed to be isolated for eight days (or fewer, in recent years). On the ninth day the child is brought out and presented to other members of the family and local community (*gusohora umwana*). This rite of passage can be performed only after the child's body has been examined and found to be free of anal malformations.

Those who are present at *gushora umwana* receive something to eat, especially the children present, who are given foods favored by children. The meal given to the children is called *kurya ubunyano* which means "to eat the excrement of the baby" for it is said that a tiny morsel of the baby's excrement is mixed into the food. This name refers to the fact that the baby's body has been examined and found to be an "open conduit," a vessel capable of receiving and passing on that which it has received, a body that has the ability to promote a flow process. The child's excrement is, in a sense, its first gift, and the other children are the first recipients of this gift. They in turn incorporate the new child into their social group by giving him or her a name that will remain a special name and, by symbolically integrating the baby into their bodies, a product of the baby's body.

The confirmation of the baby's body as an open conduit is a socially and morally salient image. If the body had been found to be "closed," it would be unable to pass on that which it had received. It would be a "blocked conduit," and, metaphorically speaking, incapable of reciprocity, or in Freudian terminology, an anal-retentive body. As such it would not be a "moral body." Reciprocity and generosity are essential components of the moral person in Rwanda, as is attested in the term for *man*, *umugabo*, which is derived from the verb *kugaba*, for which one meaning is "to give." The construction of the moral person is contingent upon the social attestation that the body physiologically embodies properties which evoke the capacity to reciprocate. These include the capacity to ingest and the capacity to egest, or in socio-moral terms, the capacity to receive and the capacity to give. Hence the importance of two bodily orifices, the mouth and the anus, and their functioning connection via the alimentary canal.

Now we are in a position to comprehend the deeper meaning of anus-to-mouth impalement and vagina-to-mouth impalement. Both turn the body into a "blocked conduit." In like fashion, when the soldier threatened Daphrose by telling her he was going to shoot his rifle through her vagina, he was threatening her with the punishment of turning her body into a "blocked conduit." He was impaling her, but with a bullet instead of a spear. In earlier days, cattle thieves were punished by anus-to-mouth impalement. When someone is punished in this way, a message is imparted that the body so destroyed is an immoral body, a body incapable of reciprocity, a body incapable of leading a proper social existence. When Tutsi men and women were killed during the genocide by impalement, their killers communicated the implicit message that they were destroying only bodies already known to be incapable of a moral life. These were bodies that might ingest and acquire, but would never pass on that which they had amassed.

With regard to illnesses related to sorcery that I encountered in earlier fieldwork on Rwandan traditional medicine, I found that the person who obstructs the proper flow of social life, who prevents women from being able to have proper menstrual flow and renders them sterile or who makes men impotent, thus also affecting their fertility, is considered the immoral person above all others. This person is called an *umurozi*, a poisoner or sorcerer. At the same time, many Rwandan traditional illnesses are characterized by disruptions in humoral flows. One finds women who have been prevented from having proper menstrual flow and in consequence are sterile, or women who have excessive menstrual flow and sterility. Among men, one finds impotence and consequently infertility, or sperm that are "too hot" and which endanger the fertility of their spouses. Other symptoms of disordered flows include dry mouth, invisible loss of blood due to sorcery, the vomiting of blood, blood in one's urine, and lack of urine. Now we can understand *ihahamuka*. It too is a flow/blockage disorder where breath, speech, or both become blocked in the body.

What is most surprising about *ihahamuka*, however, is that it has afflicted people whom I seldom encountered in my earlier studies on ethnomedicine in Rwanda. They were people who had been exposed to the influences of Western education, Christian religion, and notions of biomedicine. One encounters *ihahamuka* in the rural areas of Rwanda, of course, but in the *gacaca* hearings that I observed in the Rwandan cities of Kigali and Butare, the attendees were urban dwellers, relatively estranged from their traditions, bilingual people in many cases, and others who did not observe traditional ritual practices. They were people caught between two therapeutic worlds, not yet fully accepting of Western psychiatry but with little confidence in Rwandan traditional medicine. In like fashion, *ihahamuka* is not exactly the equivalent of PTSD. One might even ask whether Western psychiatry would be adept at treating it. *Ihahamuka* is an ethno-malady, specifically Rwandan, yet afflicting people who are Rwanda's most Westernized citizens, as well as others much less influenced by the West and by modernity. For sufferers of *ihahamuka*, this continues to be a dilemma. How to seek treatment for a specifically Rwandan illness, one not consciously chosen, when one rejects the efficacy of *ubuvuzi bwa Gihanga*? The answer in some cases was *gacaca*, the means by which they were able to surmount the paralysis of fear and to reassume the power of speech.

In recent decades, the discipline of anthropology has at times appeared to abandon cultural analysis in favor of approaches which emphasize conscious choice. This may have much to do with the fact that anthropology has turned in the direction of the political and the ideological. Politics and ideology are indeed realms that are discursive in Aijmer's terms or symbolic in Godelier's terms. Both are realms characterized by debate, contestation, and struggle, and these are governed by forms of statement and action that are largely conscious in nature. This paper does not deny that politics and ideology have their place in understanding our world and the peoples who live in it. However, not everything that human beings do is political, not everything is ideologically motivated. Not everything is determined by our conscious choices.

Recent work in cognitive psychology has shown that conscious choice may occupy less of a dominant position in our thought processes than we have assumed heretofore. This body of work has for the most part been ignored by sociocultural anthropologists, who have continued to make assumptions about the nature of human thought processes that are, at their worst, merely extrapolations from their own social and cultural experience. At the very least, these assumptions about human thought have not been tested or proven.

In the realm of African therapeutic practices, it is the contention of this chapter that analysis which places conscious choice at the forefront may be a bit myopic. There is more to the story, especially when one admits that sickness and disorder are rarely, if ever, the result of choice. Such a sickness is *ihahamuka*, which I encountered in postgenocidal Rwanda. People afflicted by *ihahamuka* did not choose it. Moreover, if we wish to understand it in any way that would transcend the usual Western labels, such as posttraumatic stress disorder, we need to look at the practices of Rwandan traditional medicine (*ubuvuzi bwa Gihanga*). When we do this, we see that *ihahamuka* bears many of the same characteristics of other Rwandan ethno-maladies. It is a flow/blockage disorder.

The point that culture still counts for something is a controversial one today, even though it was axiomatic just a few decades ago. The usual objection raised by many critics of the culture concept is that it has been reified, seen as a static thing and not as an ongoing process. There is, of course, evidence to support this. Most social groups studied by anthropologists today do not live under a bell jar. They are part of the world system of production, exchange, and consumption. They absorb the influences that come to them from the outside, choose some and reject others. Certainly at a superficial level, we observe them wearing Ray Ban sunglasses, Nike shoes, and T-shirts emblazoned with the emblems and slogans of North American sports teams. They speak to their friends on iPhones and may even have email accounts. But does this mean that at a deeper level, there are no longer any differences between them and every other consumer seated around the world commodity smorgasbord table? Have the forces of homogenization gone that far? I do not think so, and I also believe that it is in the domain of therapeutics that we can observe this. Ethno-maladies such as *ihahamuka* show us that we have to deal with heterogeneity as well as homogeneity, that there is continuity in African therapeutic systems as well as discontinuity, and that often this is manifest among people who we would least expect to show it.

Bibliography

Aijmer, Göran, and Jon Abbink. 2000. *Meanings of Violence: A Cross Cultural Perspective*. Oxford: Berg.

Appadurai, Arjun. 1990. "Disjuncture and Difference in the Global Cultural Economy," in *Public Culture* 2 (2): 1–24.

Bourdieu, Pierre. 1990. *The Logic of Practice*. Translated by Richard Nice. Stanford, California: Stanford University.

Burnet, J. 2008. "The (In)justice of Local Justice: Truth, Reconciliation and Revenge in Rwanda's Gacaca," in *Genocide Studies and Prevention*, 3: 173–93.

Clastres, Pierre. 1974. *La Societe contre l'etat*. Paris: Les editions de minuit.

Evans ST B.T., Jonathan, 2008. "Dual Processing Accounts of Reasoning, Judgment, and Social Cognition," in *Annual Review of Psychology* 59: 255–78.

Godelier, Maurice. 1996. *L'enigme du don*. Paris: Fayard.

Foucault, Michel. 1977. *Discipline and Punish: the Birth of the Prison*. New York. Vintage.

Hagengimana, A. and Hinton, Devin. 2014. "Ihahamuka, a Rwandan Syndrome of Response to the Genocide: Blocked Flow, Spirit Assault, and Shortness of Breath," Chapter 9 in *Culture and Panic Disorder*, edited by Devon Hinton and Byron Good.

Janzen, John M. 1978. *The Quest for Therapy in Lower Zaire*. Berkeley: University of California.

Jacob, Irénée. 1984, 1985, 1987. *Dictionnaire Rwandais-Francais: Extrait du dictionnaire de l'Institut National de Recherche Scientifique*, 3 volumes, Kigali (Rwanda): L'Imprimerie Scolaire.

Johnson, Mark. 1987. *The Body in the Mind: the Bodily Basis of Meaning, Imagination and Reason*. Chicago: University of Chicago.

Malkii, Liisa. 1995. *Purity and Exile*. Chicago: University of Chicago.

Taussig, Michael. 1991. *Shamanism, Colonialism, and the Wild Man: a Study in Terror and Healing*. Chicago: University of Chicago.

Taylor, Christopher C. 1988. "Milk, Honey and Money: Changing Concepts of Pathology in Rwandan Traditional Medicine." Ph.D. dissertation

———. 1992. *Milk, Honey, and Money: Changing Concepts of Illness in Rwandan Traditional Medicine*. Washington, DC: Smithsonian.

———. 1999. *Sacrifice as Terror: the Rwandan Genocide of 1994*. Oxford: Berg.

Wagner, Roy. 1986. *Symbols that Stand for Themselves*. Chicago: University of Chicago.

Hospital Ethnography

9 Ear Infections, Malnutrition, and Circuitous Health Care Treatments in Zaria, Nigeria

Elisha Renne

Child here, I don't want to hear you crying,
When you cry, my mind is upset, my heart is broken.

—Song, *Baba of Karo*

IN AUGUST 2007, when Salimatu took her son, Musa, who had a painful ear infection, to the recently opened tertiary care hospital, Ahmadu Bello University Teaching Hospital (ABUTH), at Shika, just north of Samaru and Zaria, in Kaduna State, Nigeria (Figure 1), she participated in a new system of health care in Zaria which linked primary health care with ever more specialized healthcare provision. This revised system has advantages—attendance by trained specialist doctors and better diagnostic facilities—and disadvantages—Salimatu made a total of three trips to healthcare facilities, with the costly trip to Shika to and from her house in Zaria City taking an hour each way. Whether she would have gone to Shika without financial and logistical backing, but rather would have resorted to her first avenue for treatment at a nearby pharmacy shop, is unclear.

Almost twelve years earlier, in January 1995, Hawa'u, the two-year-old daughter of another family who lived in the same house in Zaria City, was unable to walk. In order to diagnose the source of her problem, she was taken, first by her father and later by her mother, to Ahmadu Bello University Teaching Hospital, which was then located in the nearby neighborhood of Tudun Wada in the larger town of Zaria. After seven trips to the hospital, a doctor established that she was suffering from malnutrition and not TB; nutritious food and antibiotics were prescribed, the latter obtained from the hospital pharmacy. The expenses incurred as well as the costs of a high-protein diet would likely not have been possible without outside intervention. Despite improved biomedical diagnosis and tests, the constraints of poverty made following recommended treatments unlikely in both cases.

This chapter considers the complicated and circuitous pursuit of child health care in Zaria, a large university town in northern Nigeria. In the cases of both Hawa'u and Musa, their health problems—otitis media (an infection of the middle ear) and malnutrition—were conditions that were frequently seen by medical personnel at primary healthcare hospitals and clinics in Zaria City, a section of the larger town of Zaria. Despite major improvements made in ABU Teaching Hospital infrastructure and changes in protocol between the times of Hawa'u's and Musa's visits there, the difficulties faced and expenses incurred by their parents in seeking diagnosis and treatment of these relatively uncomplicated health problems suggest that the provision of simple tests and treatments for common childhood health problems might be better served by a range of local outlets—clinics, pharmacies, and community health centers. Rather than reducing parents' options to a referral scheme that would take them take them on an ever narrowing and lengthy pathway to health, expanding healthcare options more broadly based at the community level would facilitate children's health care in towns and cities in northern Nigeria.

Time and Place

This study took place during two different research periods, the first in the mid-1990s, when I had initially moved into a family house in Zaria City, and the second in 2007, on a return trip when two University of Michigan students accompanied me to conduct research on bednet use in one neighborhood in the city (Renne et al. 2008). During this interval, a large university-funded primary healthcare center, known as the Institute of Child Health-Ban Zazzau, had been built in the Ban Zazzau neighborhood of Zaria City in 2005. For families living in the area, the Ban Zazzau Clinic, as came to be called, provided a range of diagnostic and referral services from faculty and staff associated with Ahmadu Bello University, one of the oldest tertiary educational institutions in Northern Nigeria, and its well-established teaching hospital.

This study begins in Zaria City, the old walled section of the larger town of Zaria, and the former capital of the old Hausa Emirate of Zazzau. It consists of approximately forty neighborhoods (*anguwa*), of which Ban Zazzau is one. Elsewhere in the City, there is a large local government clinic (at Babban Dodo), the large state-funded Hajiya Gambo Sawaba General Hospital (at Kofan Gayan), as well as many small private clinics and pharmacies. In addition, many traditional healers serve City residents, and there are several markets where traditional medicines are sold. Where a mother takes her child for treatment reflects her assessment of the type and seriousness of the disease, the proximity of healthcare provision to her home, her perception of the expenses that treatment may entail, as well as any personal preference for traditional or biomedical treatment that she might have (Colvin et al 2013, Janzen 1978). Indeed, people availed themselves of different medical options—both biomedical and traditional—as seemed warranted (Kamat 2008). For families living in the house where I also resided in Anguwar Kwarbai, in the central part of Zaria City—not far from the Emir's palace, the main Friday mosque, and main local government offices, there were several healthcare options available.

Musa's Ear Infection and his Journey to Shika

Musa, Salimatu's eight-year-old son was miserable, crying and complaining of an earache that would not go away. Nothing seemed to help, so I suggested to Lila, a visiting University of Michigan student, that she go with Salimatu and Musa to the Ban Zazzau Clinic to see if doctors there could diagnose the problem. On August 6, 2007, as they were going, Salimatu crossed the street to the local pharmacy to see if they could get treatment for Musa there. While pharmacist recommended several things, Lila convinced Salimatu to go to hospital, to see a doctor first. (Indeed, Lila was puzzled about why Salimatu would go to the pharmacy before seeing a doctor, the reverse order of treatment to which she, an American, was accustomed.) When Salimatu and Lila got to the hospital, the clerk, Malam Ibrahim, helped them to get a registration card so that Musa could be seen by a doctor. Malam Ibrahim then took card to the office of the doctor who would see him—where they waited until the doctor had gone through the pile of cards until he came to Musa's card.

At ABUTH-Ban Zazzau, they do what is called Integrated Health Management, meaning that that staff examine a patient and diagnose the health problem on the basis of symptoms. Based on the doctor's diagnosis, Salimatu was given a list of medicines to purchase from the clinic pharmacy. These included Paracetamol, vitamin C (together coming to ₦10), a generic version of the antibiotic Augmentin (₦300),[1] and eardrops (₦300). However, the antibiotic that she was supposed to buy was not available in the Ban Zazzau pharmacy, so Salimatu had to get it at an outside pharmacy instead. The total cost for this first course of treatment was ₦610. When Salimatu returned from Ban Zazzau, she showed me the drugs she'd been given and also an order for tests. One test was for malaria, the other was for an ear swab to determine specifically the bacterial sources of Musa's ear infection. When I asked her when she wanted to go to Shika to have these tests done, she said that Musa needed to rest a bit before going, so perhaps in a few days.

Three days later, very early on the morning of August 9, 2007, Salimatu, Musa, and I left Zaria City by public transport to go to the ABU Teaching Hospital at Shika, about ten miles from our house. First we boarded a bus going to PZ, in the center of Zaria, then we boarded another bus going to Samaru, and finally a third bus to going to Shika. On getting to the main gate at the hospital, we had to walk down a long avenue leading to the main entrance. There we obtained directions to the lab, which was located some distance away, in a back building. After several wrong starts, we found it about two long city blocks from the front door of the hospital. One lab assistant then wrote the charge on the referral form and sent me to pay at the hemabiology cashier, which was around the corner. Salimatu and Musa sat down and waited for my return.

When I got to the cashier's office, I was told to that it would not open until 9:00 a.m. So I then went back to the main building to pay at the 24-hour cashier, waited in line, got my receipt, and then walked back to the lab where Salimatu and Musa were waiting. We entered the laboratory front office but were told that they did not have swabs. So I walked back to the main building again, where they had a pharmacy; I was told that they didn't have any swabs and that I should go to emergency stores. When I got to emergency stores, I was told that I needed to get a receipt for payment first, but I begged the attendants to let me pay for two swabs (₦20). I took the two swabs and walked back to the lab. There I was told to take Musa and the swabs to GP (General Practice) where a doctor was going to take the ear swab sample.

Musa, Salimatu, and I then trekked back to the main building where the General Practice patients were seen. We walked past a nurse and to the reception area; after waiting a bit, we were told to go to a nurse, who would swab the ear. She was helpful but wanted to know why I'd brought two swabs when they only needed one and said that I should have brought gloves for her to use. Once Musa saw the swabs, he began crying and wouldn't sit still. It was not easy getting a swab sample from his ear, but somehow the nurse managed to do so. When she was finished, we walked back to the main entrance, Musa crying the whole time. I left them to wait while I dropped the swab off at the lab, where I was told that the results would be ready a week later. I then rejoined Salimatu and Musa, and we walked back to the main road, where we caught a bus going back to Zaria, returning to the house in Zaria City about three and a half hours later.

When I returned to Shika on August 15, 2007, I was given the lab report based on Musa's ear swab sample. It stated that gram-positive cocci in pairs and in singles were present, as well as gram-negative bacilli and cells. In the culture that was taken, *Staphylococcus aureus* bacteria were also isolated. I was given a prescription for the antibiotic Ciprofloxacin,[2] for Musa to take, which he did. By the end of end of the month, he was feeling much better and his mother reported that Musa had no further problems with his ears (Figure 2). Clearly, the identification of the specific bacterial infection and the definite diagnosis of otitis media contributed to this good health outcome. However, the expense and difficulties of pursuing this therapy, particularly the referral for testing at the main hospital at Shika and the long distances that a mother and child would need to walk while there, raises the question of how many mothers would actually go there. Unless their child's condition was very serious, perhaps very few.

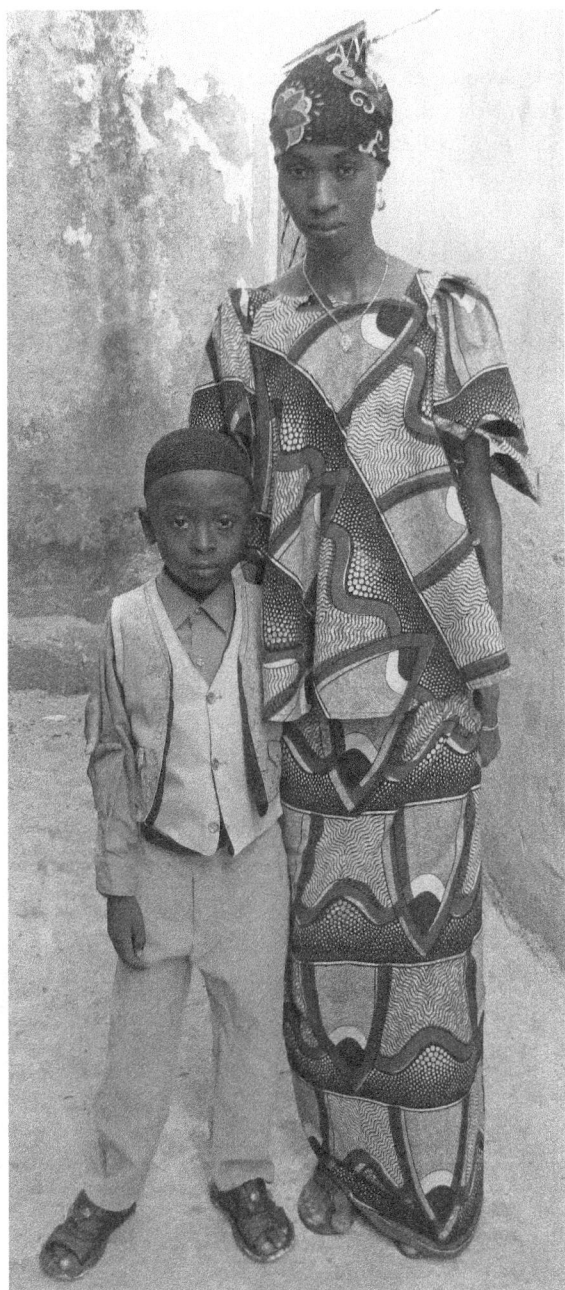

Musa & Salimatu, Zaria
City, 2009. Photo courtesy
of author.

Hawa'u Goes to the Hospital

Hawa'u, a two-year-old girl who could not walk, was living in the house in Zaria City where I rented two rooms in November 1994. She lived with her family, which included her father (whom we all called Mallam, literally "Islamic teacher"), her mother (Asma'u), and her older sister (Umma). Asma'u was pregnant, expecting to deliver her child in May the following year and Hawa'u had been weaned early, despite the fact that she was under two years of age at the time.[3] This early weaning contributed to what Asma'u said was Hawa'u's trouble, that "she had no blood in her body." As a result of this condition, she said Hawa'u was unable to walk. Rather, she moved about by crawling, although her spindly legs did little in the way of locomotion.

I traveled out of the city in late December, and when I returned in early January, Hawa'u was still not walking. I asked permission from her father, Mallam, for her to go to ABUTH in Tudun Wada for tests and treatment, if necessary. Mallam agreed, and on January 11, 1995 we went, together with Hawa'u, to Ahmadu Bello University Teaching Hospital. My comments concerning the six trips that we (Mallam, Aisha, Hawa'u, and/or I) took to ABUTH-Zaria may be seen in the following excerpts from my journal:

> [Trip 1, January 11, 1995], Zaria City: At first, going to the hospital with Hawa'u [and Mallam] who seemed to enjoy the outing until it came time for the stethoscope—the doctor was singularly unhelpful at first, desultory I'd describe his behavior, and I rather wonder about his course of X-rays and blood tests and talking to the nutrition specialist! Hawa'u wouldn't eat when she came home and would only drink water; also one eye was funny—although she was better and eating when I saw her. She gave me a very long and dirty look, though when I saw her later she sort of smiled. It's clear it's malnutrition but what, if anything else, we'll see.

The next day Mallam returned to the hospital alone [Trip 2] to make arrangements for tests; I later learned that he had to pay ₦50 to the hospital orderly who had helped him to obtain a registration card. A week later, Asma'u, Hawa'u, and I returned to the hospital for tests:

> [Trip 3, January 20, 1995] ZC: Left house around 8 am to get to hospital by 8:30 as we'd been told [in order to get the Montoux test/TB test]. The bus from house to hospital gate cost ₦10. The hospital was quite empty of people as we made our way toward the community health services part of the nursing school. But when we found the right room, there were already 7 women there waiting (women with 6 babies and 1 adult, to be given test). We sat around [waiting because] someone said that they needed 10 people before they could begin, something about the bottle of vaccine being opened. Then around 9:10 am the nurse come to say that the price of the medicine was now ₦62—so that

we'd have to add ₦22 to the ₦40 we'd already paid. Everyone stayed, even the woman who came with her three kids but only had money for one was allowed to stay (even though the nurse complained that she'd never come back to have her test read or pay back the money). She [the nurse] showed us the receipt for ₦620 [₦62 x10=₦620].

In the midst of the roll call and fee payments, one woman came in to have her baby immunized. She was told to come back on Thursday, but, in fact, the hospital had no DPT [diphtheria-pertussis-tetanus] vaccine at all; there was none in Kaduna State, and someone had gone to Kano and come back empty-handed. They'd also checked with the local government health people with no success. They were to go out with the EPI (early primary immunization) campaign but there is no material for inoculation.

After we'd all been accounted for, she [the nurse] began the test. She was quite good, joking with people, taking the little girl with the drip hanging from her arm out of order. There was the usual sense of a group of people helping each other, the man who offered the pen, etc. Just before giving the test, she [the nurse] gave a little speech in Hausa about not letting the child pick the scab, not getting the area wet. When she asked for questions, there was only one—from a man asking about the 72-hour waiting period which would have meant coming on Sunday. She said Monday was sufficiently good.

While we were at the hospital, I went to the pharmacy across the street to price the medication—Augmentin—written on the prescription that Mallam had been given for Hawa'u's treatment. My journal states that "Asma'u was suitably horrified when she learned the medicine prescribed was ₦500. We all agreed that this was ridiculous—for a 'broad-based' antibiotic."

The following Monday (January 23, 1995), Aisha went back to the hospital with Hawa'u for her TB reading, which was negative [Trip 4]. On Thursday (January 26, 1995), Aisha, Hawa'u, and I again took the bus to ABUTH for a final consultation with the doctor [Trip 5]:

We arrived at 8:30 am and there were already about 30 women with children waiting. So we got in line, got our prescription slip signed by the doctor, turned in our little registration card and then we were given our big [diagnosis] card. But by the time we had it, others, who'd received their [cards] first were in the attending room, filling theirs in so we had to wait until the next round. This was about 9:30 am. At about 9:50 am I decided to go back [to the house in Zaria City]. Aisha came back [to the house] at 1:15 pm; our doctor hadn't even come by the time I'd left. They asked why we hadn't filled the prescription for Augmentin they'd prescribed, so Asma'u said I'd priced it at ₦500. They said I should get it at the ABUTH pharmacy where it sells for ₦150. They diagnosed a minor infection causing her illness and the eye problem. She's to go back in 2 weeks for an eye checkup, then to attend Babban Dodo Clinic.

These trips to ABUTH-Tudun Wada were not all about the business of waiting, diagnosis, and treatment. There were some pleasantries as well, such as the courtesies shown during the TB test and one older man who was helping women at the Paediatrics Clinic. My journal shows that

> [There was a] funny man, everyone was calling him Baba Yaran [Father of the Children] who was helping women, telling them (not officiously, but jokingly) what to do about cards, etc. It's not clear to me if he is staff or some sort of volunteer.

On our return to the house that Thursday, Hawa'u finally was able to walk, although she did so with much reluctance (we encouraged her with sweets).

The next day (January 27, 1995), I went back to the ABUTH, to the pharmacy to get Hawa'u's Augmentin and eye medicine prescriptions filled [Trip 6]. After filling them, the staff gave me a receipt for payment, ₦121 (₦95 for the Augmentin and ₦26 for eye ointment), which seemed quite low compared with the local chemist prices of ₦400–500. In order to get the medicine itself, one had to wait in another line, so I decided to ask Mallam to pick up the medicine later that day [Trip 7]:

> He got the drugs but asked me if it mattered that the expiration date was past. So that's why they're selling at cut-rates. . . . I'd thought possibly it was subsidized. And the Augmentin is supposed to be refrigerated after mixing. (Journal entry)

With the improved diet that her mother had been advised to provide (with powdered milk, fruit, meat, and vegetables—which I helped to buy), Hawa'u was able to walk easily. "Asma'u just came by—Hawa'u is walking very well—it's amazing. It's been about 1 1/2 months, she wasn't walking at all" (Journal entry, March 2, 1995).

However, in early April, Hawa'u again became ill, and her mother took to the local pharmacy for an injection for fever and measles (a journal entry from April 7, 1995, says "The needle that Bashiri [the chemist] used to inject Hawa'u was huge—about 12-gauge. Plus all the other medicine she was given, no wonder she's coughing and vomiting. Poor kid, she's really sick."). Her condition seemed to get worse, and she became very thin, in part because she was only eating pap. Everyone said that it was *ba'kon dauro*, measles. When I suggested to Aisha that they take Hawa'u to ABUTH again to see if Hawa'u's illness wasn't something more serious, she declined:

> She doesn't want to go to ABUTH because she's afraid they will admit Hawa'u and she doesn't want to stay with her because of her pregnancy. Anyway, we'll see how she is tomorrow. (Journal entry, April 20, 1995)

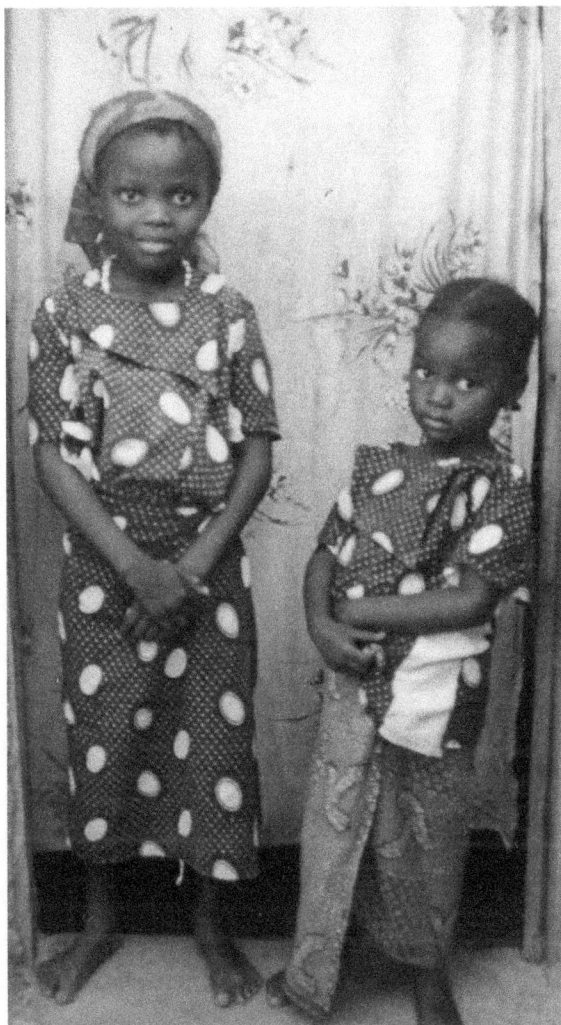

Umma & Hawa'u, Anchau, 1997. Photo courtesy of author.

The next day, Hawa'u seemed to be improving:

> Hawa'u is a bit better; she's crying more vigorously now. I will buy milk to-day and some oranges. She was so sick that Asma'u said that neither she nor Mallam slept. She's very emaciated but seemed to perk up yesterday when it got cooler. Wish I could remember the ORT salt/sugar formula but will also buy Lucozade today. Mallam also said that Hawa'u is better so we should wait on the hospital. He mentioned the money but Asma'u had said, "It's *wahala* ('trouble')" and she's right. (Journal entry, April 21, 1995)

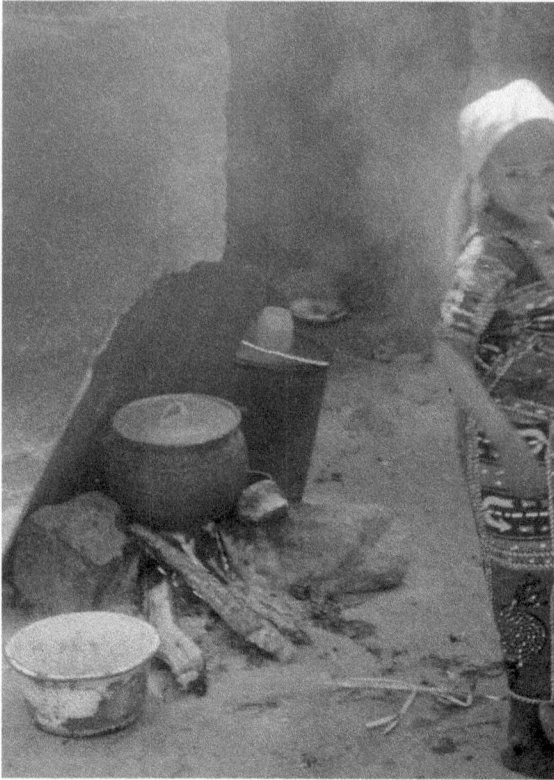

Cooking with wood in
house in Zaria City, 1995.
Photo courtesy of author.

A week later, Hawa'u had almost completely recovered; she was eating and putting on weight.

However, her mother, Aisha, who was eight months pregnant, looked hag-
gard, and she and her husband appeared to be having financial problems.[4]

One notable aspect about these excerpts that follow Hawa'u, through her
initial recovery from malnutrition in January to her recovery from measles in
April 1995, is the different decisions that her mother and father made about
where Hawa'u should be taken for diagnosis and treatment. The hospital sequence in January 1995 consisted of seven separate trips to the hospital for consultation with doctors, tests, and picking up medication. Since the bus from
Zaria City to the hospital gate cost ₦10 each way per adult, this sequence of diagnosis and treatment cost ₦120 simply for transportation. Additionally, there
were expenses for diagnosis, tests, and medicines, which brought the total sum
for the ABUTH-Tudun Wada diagnosis and treatment to around ₦650, a substantial sum in 1995.

Thus when Hawa'u became ill with measles in April 1995 and I suggested go-ing to the hospital again, her parents objected on the grounds of cost. However, there were other factors such as beliefs about contagion as well as simply having to go to so much trouble (*wahala*) to attend. This trouble consisted of making arrangements to go with Hawa'u, finding someone to care for Umma at home, dealing with the not always helpful hospital staff, and waiting for hours to be seen by a doctor. Furthermore, if Hawa'u had been admitted, Asma'u would have had to remain in the hospital with her, something which she did not want to do since she was pregnant. So Asma'u took Hawa'u to the pharmacy across the street from the house, where she was given an injection.

This particular form of health-seeking behavior, going to a local, private pharmacist for treatment, represents one of the consequences of the decline in public health care in Nigeria (Alubo 2001, 315):

> By far the most intricate network [of health care] is the business of running pharmacy/chemist shops. . . . By law only pharmacy shops can dispense pre-scription (ethical) drugs, while patent medicine dealers are restricted to com-mon remedies or over-the-counter medicines (OTCs). In practice, however, both sell prescription drugs; others even prescribe and effectively run clinics. (Igun 1994)

It was to one of these pharmacy shops *cum* clinic that Asma'u took Hawa'u. In-deed, several women in Zaria City reported taking their sick children to phar-macies within Anguwar Kwarbai for treatment—both getting injections and medicine—because they could not afford to or could not take time to go to the hospital. In one study conducted in Maiduguri, in northeastern Nigeria, in 1979, Igun (1987) notes five reasons for this preference of going to a pharmacy rather than hospital or local government clinic. The most frequently mentioned reasons for people's preference for treatment at a local retail pharmacy over hospital care were:

1. "treatment given without waste of time," i.e., no waiting" (31 percent)
2. "they are not crowded" (29 percent)
3. "there is no restriction on drugs that can be purchased" (26 percent)
4. "they give good treatments which are often better than hospital treatment" (21 percent)
5. "retail pharmacies hardly run out of stock of drugs" (13 percent)
6. (Igun 1987, 693).[5]

Igun (1987, 694) concludes that "access factors," namely "availability, accessibil-ity, accommodation, affordability, and acceptability," best explain his respon-dents' preference for pharmacies for health care. These factors also explain why Hawa'u's parents, Aisha and Mallam, preferred to take their daughter to a nearby pharmacy when she had measles, where treatment was easily available without a long wait, without the need to travel, and without great cost.

Lessons from Musa's and Hawa'u's Stories

> Poverty seems to be at the heart of the problem of childhood malnutrition in Nigeria. Unless and until the socioeconomic status of the vast majority of Nigerians improves significantly, malnutrition will continue to pose a serious threat to the growth and development of Nigerian children and to future national development.
>
> —Adelekan (2003, 181)

> Children in Maputo are exposed to [respirable suspended particulate matter] as wood and charcoal are the main source of energy for cooking in many homes. It may be argued that this is frequent in rural areas, but unfortunately it is also the case in the peripheral areas of the town, as well as in some houses within the town, as most people cannot afford to pay electricity or gas bills.
>
> —Da Costa et al (2004, 577)

A lack of nutritious food and excessive exposure to wood smoke contribute to two of the most common health problems—malnutrition and otitis media (infection of the middle ear)—for young children living in towns and villages in Nigeria (Adelekan 2003; Lasisi et al. 2007; Okafor 1984).[6] The study cited above examines the connection between otitis media and wood smoke from cooking in Maputo, Mozambique, although its findings have implications for children in Zaria City, where wood is commonly used for cooking. Indeed, food was cooked on wood fires in the main corridor that connected the inner and outer rooms of the house where Hawa'u and Musa resided (Figure 4). As the cheapest source of fuel for cooking, wood was also easily available in Zaria City as it was distributed on a regular basis by trucks whose presence in the early morning was signaled by their loud horns. While Da Costa et al. (2004, 576) cite other factors such as tobacco smoke, limited breastfeeding, and in some instances, living in overcrowded rooms, they found that wood smoke was a significant factor in middle-ear infections. Since no one in the house in Zaria City smoked, nor was Musa living in an overcrowded room (he shared two rooms with his mother), nor was breastfeeding an issue, it is likely that the wood smoke from cooking was the cause of his infection.

For Hawa'u, her inability to walk was diagnosed as a symptom of malnutrition, due in part to her early weaning but also due to a lack of protein-rich foods, particularly milk and meat. She was fed a starchy diet, consisting mainly of *tuwo* (a cornmeal porridge) with assorted vegetable-based soups, *miya kuka* (baobab leaf soup) being the most common one. The diagnosis of malnutrition was confirmed by Hawa'u's swift recovery upon being given a more balanced diet.

While these children's health problems might be attributed to their parents lack of education—about the dangers of wood smoke and the importance of good nutrition, both could also be attributed to poverty, as Adelekan has noted regarding malnutrition (see also Linnemayr et al. 2008). Yet the seemingly simple solutions to these two children's health problems—better diet, treatment with antibiotics and reduced exposure to wood smoke—are also related to the difficulties their parents faced when seeking health care in Zaria, Nigeria. Ideally, the parents of Hawa'u and Musa had several options for treating their children when sick. They could have attended the large state-sponsored general hospital at Kofan Gayan in Zaria City, the federally funded ABU Teaching Hospital (first at Tudun Wada and then at Shika) as well as the ABUTH Institute of Child Health at Ban Zazzau (after 2005), the local government health clinic at Babban Dodo, or one of the many privately run clinics and pharmacies in the City. They could have also decided to wait or to opt for self-treatment, based on the advice of local chemists, traditional herbalists, or trusted relatives and neighbors. In practice, their actions were constrained by a lack of cash, transport options, and sociocultural practices (e.g., seclusion), as well as by personal preferences, experience, and habit (Colvin et al. 2013).

Yet in the twelve years between the time when Hawa'u attended the ABUTH at Tudun Wada in 1995 and Musa attended the ABUTH at Shika in 2007, there were improvements for parents seeking health care for their children in Zaria City. The opening of the ABUTH Institute for Child Health-Ban Zazzau improved primary health care in the City, and it is well attended by mothers and children. However, the underlying problem of what Iyun (1987, 694) has referred to as "access factors"—specifically "availability, accessibility, accommodation, affordability, and acceptability"—persists. While diagnosis is provided free of charge at Ban Zazzau and medicines are sold at discounted prices at ABUTH, there are long waits to see doctors and nurses, prescribed drugs may not be in stock, and one needs to pay for transport to and from the clinic. The factors help to explain why Hawa'u's and Musa's parents continued to make use of the nearby pharmacy for their children's health care.

The disconnect between hospital care and the access factors mentioned above may clearly be seen in the stories of Musa, Hawa'u, and their parents and their many trips for diagnoses and treatment at Ahmadu Bello University Teaching Hospital. After Hawa'u's mother, Asma'u, first visited the hospital, the consulting doctor recommended that she attend the nutrition clinic. However, it was not a lack of knowledge about proper diet that was the problem but rather a lack of funds to purchase nutritious food that, along with early weaning, led to Hawa'u's condition. After the second visit, when Hawa'u developed an eye infection and the antibiotic Augmentin was prescribed, filling the government-subsidized prescription,[7] required three trips to the hospital pharmacy. Furthermore, not only had the use-by date on the bottle of Augmentin sold at the pharmacy expired but refrigerating the medicine once the bottle's seal was broken was out of the question. Not surprisingly, when Hawa'u developed a case of measles, her parents decided to take her to the nearby pharmacy for an injection, rather than going back to ABUTH or to a private or public hospital or clinic—which would have entailed considerable expense and trouble for all concerned. Three of the access factors—availability, accessibility, and affordability—contributed to their decision. One might also add another factor, appropriateness, to this list, for cases when, for example, drugs that must be refrigerated are prescribed to families living without electricity.[8] The growth in chemist shops as sites of healthcare services reflects their being seen as expeditious, efficacious, and less costly, and therefore more appropriate for the situation of many Nigerian families, in terms of time and money. Indeed, the deterioration of Hawa'u's parents' financial situation is suggested by the April 27, 1995, journal entry in which I note, "They must have sold the bedframe, only the 4-poster is there." Throughout this 1994–1995 period, Asma'u's material possessions (*kayan dakin*—literally, load of the room; what a wife brings with her when she moves to her husband's house) gradually disappeared as they were forced to sell or pawn her enamelware plates, bowls, and display cabinet. Salimatu, Musa's mother, also used her possessions as a backup bank account, and her four-poster bed was also sold; she used part of the proceeds to buy a sewing machine with which she hoped to improve her financial situation.

Yet one aspect of both Hawa'u's and Musa's stories that is striking is their resilience in the face of "numerous insults" to their well-being (Kunitz 1987, 400) that they have been subjected to in their lives. By focusing on how their respective "state[s] of good health" had been achieved, some effective health measures may more clearly be identified. First, a government program (perhaps assisted with NGO funds) could provide basic protein-rich foods at subsidized rates for women with children. For example, the Senegalese government introduced a World Bank–funded program, the Community Nutrition Project, in 1996, which provided monthly growth monitoring, educational sessions for mothers, and weekly food supplements in low-income urban areas (Gartner et al. 2007). This type of project or a type of conditional cash transfer program could help to address malnutrition in Nigeria. Second, since going to the local pharmacy was seen by many parents as a more practical solution in terms of cost, time, and treatment for their children, perhaps giving community chemist-shop owners additional basic child healthcare information, such as oral rehydration therapy (ORT, see Igun 1994) for diarrheal cases that they see, would be a useful goal. Yet these possible solutions to child health problems as well as this discussion of parents' micro-level choices and constraints concerning health care for their children are also related to macro-level structural problems, which reflect ongoing political and economic uncertainties in Nigeria.

The Political and Economic Context of Health Care in Nigeria, 1985–2007

> We found that most of the studies reviewed here were short-term qualitative studies comprised primarily of interviews and focus group discussions. Few involved multiple sources of data, long-term engagement in their field sites, or theory-driven study design. . . . Better understanding how care-givers and communities respond to childhood illnesses in the context of poverty, inequality, weak health systems, and continuing dramatic social change will require richer sources of evidence, including extended case studies and ethnography, that provide both sufficient depth—in order to understand specific contexts—as well as sufficient breadth—in order to understand the broader patterns common across contexts
>
> —Colvin et al. 2013, 75

By examining the health problems and care-seeking by the parents of two children living in the same house (but not simultaneously) in Zaria City over a period of twelve years, this study of the changes and continuities in parents' pursuit of health care in Zaria reflects the sort of "long-term engagement" that Christopher Colvin and his co-authors note is lacking in many studies of care-seeking for children's health in sub-Saharan Africa. Yet such long-term analyses would be incomplete without a discussion of "the context of poverty, inequality, weak health systems . . ."—in other words, the "structural violence" (Farmer 2004) under which Hawa'u, Musa, and their families have lived. Furthermore, the political economic contexts of healthcare provision in Nigeria needs to be included in this contextual analysis.

In the 1960s through the first half of the 1980s, drugs and services were provided free of charge in government healthcare centers throughout Nigeria. In Zaria, the Institute of Health of Ahmadu Bello University, consisting of a university teaching hospital with branches in Zaria and Kaduna, a secondary hospital at Malumfashi, two comprehensive health centers in Zaria City and Sabon Gari LGAs, and a campus health clinic, made health care available to approximately nine million people in the immediate and surrounding areas (Ejembi and Bandipo 1989, 6). This situation changed with the introduction in 1986 of an IMF-led Structural Adjustment Program, approved by the Nigerian head of state, General Ibrahim Babangida (although there was widespread public disapproval of his action). Under structural adjustment, user fees were introduced as a way of getting the health system to pay for itself. In addition, "patients were being asked to pay for most of the materials needed for their treatment. As a result most patients stayed at home and came to hospital only as a last resort if a serious complication developed" (Ekwempu et al. 1990, 57). Babangida sought to ameliorate this situation through the appointment of Professor Olikoye Ransome-Kuti as the Minister of Health in 1985, who was given the authority and wherewithal to establish primary healthcare (PHC) centers in Nigeria. As part of this program, immunization for six childhood diseases was begun in 1988 at PHC centers throughout the country. However, in 1990, the federal government shifted funding of these centers to local governments, which were unable (or unwilling) to support the provision of primary health care; routine immunization, in particular, deteriorated in the country. (Ransome-Kuti resigned his position in 1992.) The dismantling of the primary healthcare system in the early 1990s was matched by the many political changes that took place during the same period; from 1990 to 1993, Nigeria had a series of three heads of state. After a bloodless coup in November 1993, General Sani Abacha became head of state, a position which he held until June 1998.

It was during this time that Hawa'u went to ABUTH for diagnosis and treatment of her inability to walk. While Abacha's ascendancy to power led to a certain political stability, the economic situation was difficult for many. Hawa'u's father, Mallam, was unable to keep his Qur'anic students because their parents were unable to pay him, and he supported his family by working as motorcycle-taxi driver. Their financial problems persisted, and later in 1995, they moved to Mallam's home village of Anchau, where it was less costly to live and where Hawa'u lived for several years after.

For Musa, who was born in 1999, the same year when the election of President Olusegun Obasanjo reinstated democratic rule in Nigeria, the healthcare situation was somewhat improved, as some local government began to provide free primary healthcare services, particularly for antenatal care and immunization programs.[9] Yet for women and their children in Zaria City, these measures did not address other, infrastructural problems such as the provision of clean water and electricity, the lack of which impeded their ability to prevent illness and to maintain good health. Water has been a particular problem in Zaria, although in the house where Musa and his mother, Salimatu, stayed, the owner had built a deep well that provided water for those living there.[10] Musa also benefited from construction of the ABUTH Institute of Child Health-Ban Zazzau in 2005, although his mother continued to go to a nearby pharmacy until Lila accompanied them to Ban Zazzau in 2007. This preference for the use of local pharmacies reflects another aspect of child healthcare decision-making in Zaria City, namely the continuing devaluation of the naira (₦), which in 1986 was ₦4.6 to US$1 and in 2007 was ₦150 to US$1. Healthcare costs also increased as imported medicines and materials for diagnosis and treatment of illness became more expensive.

In March 2013, I visited the house in Zaria City and spoke with Salimatu and Musa, who is now attending secondary school. I asked Salimatu if Musa had had any further problems with his ears or with his hearing. "No," she replied, "he hasn't." The last time that I saw Hawa'u was in Anchau in 1997, although her mother, Asma'u said that she was doing well when I saw her two years later in Zaria.

The experiences of Salimatu and Asma'u reveal the ongoing constraints in ease of access to health care, which reflect continuing problems in government programs for child health—in part, the aftermath of earlier IMF-imposed requirements for reductions in government spending and, in part, a lack of political will, as evidenced by the fiscal mismanagement of government funds (Alubo 1990, Ityavyar 1988). Yet some federal health initiatives have helped mothers and their children in recent years. For example, the Subsidy Reinvestment Programme (SURE-P) was initiated in 2012 by the federal Ministry of Health with support from the World Bank and has provided conditional cash transfers to pregnant women to support their attendance at antenatal clinics (World Bank 2015). The federal government, also in 2012, began the "Saving One Million Lives" program, which includes several maternal/child health initiatives such as improving routine immunization, child nutrition, and malaria control through bednet use; the program organizers' goal was to save one million lives by 2015 (World Health Organization 2012). These shifts, from public funding of primary health care to user fees and back to federal support for primary health care raises broader questions about how to best go about addressing problems of child health care. In the late 1980s and early 1990s, the World Bank and the IMF emphasized individual accountability for health care and user fees, although as Alubo (2001) has noted, expectations that individuals acting alone can lower morbidity and mortality while living in impoverished conditions are unrealistic. In Nigeria, there has been some recognition of this argument; World Bank officials provided support for the SURE-P conditional cash transfer program in 2012. Yet despite recent Ministry of Health efforts to introduce programs such as the Saving One Million Lives initiative and the SURE-P cash transfer payments to mothers to improve maternal/child health,[11] the transitory history of such schemes underscores the likelihood that parents will continue to assess the "efficacy of treatment" in their pursuit of health care for their children. Through an examination of experiences of parents such as Salimatu, Asma'u, and Mallam as they pursued health care at ABU Teaching Hospital, their assessment of the efficacy of local retail pharmacies would seem to make sense. Indeed, expanding health care at the community level, particularly by providing simple tests and treatments for common childhood health illnesses such as otitis media and malaria, would improve children's health care in Zaria.

Acknowledgments

This study reflects the longstanding support for my research in Zaria, first conducted during my stay in the Department of Sociology, Ahmadu Bello University, Zaria, Nigeria, as a visiting Fulbright lecturer in 1994. Since then, I have worked, as a researcher from Princeton University and the University of Michigan, with ABU faculty on a range of research studies, and I would like to thank the current

Vice Chancellor, Ahmadu Bello University, Professor Abdullahi Mustapha as well as Dr. Salihu Maiwada, Dr. Ya'u Tanimu, and Dr. Dakyes Usman. Dr. Dapo Shittu and Dr. Mairo Mandara (the Gates Foundation's Nigeria representative), who have also been consistently supportive over the years. I would also like to thank Hajiya Hassana Hajiya, Malama Umma Yahaya, and Mrs. Zaineb DanLadi for research assistance and advice. Special thanks go to the women of Zaria City, who gave me the nickname Tambaya (Question).

Notes

1. According to the label, "Augmentin is bactericidal to a wide range of gram-positive and gram-negative bacteria including many B-lactamase producing penicillin resistant organisms" (see Foster 1991). Augmentin was also prescribed for Musa in 2007.

2. Ciprofloxacin, a second-generation fluoroquinolone, is a widely prescribed antibiotic used to treat a range of bacterial infections (Brownlee et al. 1992).

3. The cultural preference is to nurse for two years. *Baba of Karo* describes a couple who refused the customary interval of abstinence. When the wife became pregnant and the infant was born only one year after its elder sibling, special treatments were given to the older son to strengthen him in the face of early weaning (Smith 1954, 149).

4. Their financial problems persisted, and later that year, they moved to Mallam's home village of Anchau, where it was less costly to live.

5. Eighteen percent of Igun's 418 respondents said that drugs sold at retail pharmacies "are not adulterated," which is surprising as fake drugs are a continuing problem for Nigerian consumers. It may be that some respondents have noted hospital provision of drugs past their expiration dates, as was the case with Mallam, Hawa'u's father.

6. Both Lasisi et al. (2008) and Okafor (1984) discuss socioeconomic status as a significant factor in children presenting with otitis media, although they do not specifically mention wood smoke.

7. Monies from the Petroleum Trust Fund was used by officials to subsidize drug provided in government hospitals and clinics after General Buhari was appointed to head the fund.

8. The irregular provision of electricity and tap water is a longstanding problem in Zaria City (Liman 2001).

9. Nonetheless, immunization levels remained low in Zaria City; an outbreak of measles in November and December 2007 left fifty children dead (Aodu 2007).

10. Additionally, in 2007, the state government sponsored the building of solar-powered water pumps in various parts of Zaria City.

11. For example, the SURE-P program is scheduled to end in late 2015 (Okafor 2015).

Bibliography

Adelekan, Delana. 2003. "Childhood Nutrition and Malnutrition in Nigeria." *Nutrition* 19: 179–181.
Alubo, S.O. 1990. "Debt Crisis, Health and Health Services in Africa." *Social Science & Medicine* 31: 639–48.

———. 2001. "The Promise and Limits of Private Medicine: Health Policy Dilemmas in Nigeria." *Health Policy and Planning* 16 (3): 313–21.

Aodu, AbdulRaheem. 2007. "Measles Outbreak Kills 50 in Zaria." *Daily Trust* (December 5).

Brownlee, Richard E., Gregory Hulka, Jiri Prazma, and Harold Pillsbury III. 1992. "Ciprofloxacin: Use as a Topical Otic Preparation." *Archives of Otolaryngology, Head & Neck Surgery* 118 (4): 392–96.

Colvin, Christopher, Helen Smith, Alison Swartz, Jill Ahs, Jodie de Heer, Newton Opiyo, Julia C. Kim, Toni Marraccini, and Asha George. 2013. "Understanding Careseeking for Child Illness in Sub-Saharan Africa: A Systematic Review and Conceptual Framework Based on Qualitative Research of Household Recognition and Response to Child Diarrhoea, Pneumonia and Malaria." *Social Science & Medicine* 86: 66–78.

Da Costa, Joao Leopoldo, Albert Navarro, José Branco Neves, and Miguel Martin. 2004 "Household Wood and Charcoal Smoke Increases Risk of Otitis Media in Childhood in Maputo." *International Journal of Epidemiology* 33: 573–78.

Ejembi, C. L., and A. Bandipo. 1989. "The Impact of Nigeria's Structural Adjustment Programme (SAP) on the Health Care Delivery System." Paper presented at conference, SAP and the Future of Nigeria, CSER, Ahmadu Bello University, Zaria.

Ekwempu, C. C., D. Maine, M. Olorukoba, M. S. Essien, and M. N. Kisseka. 1990. "Structural Adjustment and Health in Africa." *Lancet* 336: 56–57.

Farmer, Paul. 2004. "An Anthropology of Structural Violence." *Current Anthropology* 45 (3): 305–25.

Foster, S. 1991. "Supply and Use of Essential Drugs in Sub-Saharan Africa: Some Issues and Possible Solutions." *Social Science & Medicine* 32: 1201–18.

Gartner, A., Y. Kameli, P. Traissac, A. Dhur, F. Delpeuch, and B. Maire. 2007. "Has the First Implementation Phase of the Community Nutrition Project in Urban Senegal Had an Impact?" *Nutrition* 23: 219–28.

Igun, U. 1987. "Why We Seek Treatment Here: Retail Pharmacy and Clinical Treatment in Maiduguri, Nigeria." *Social Science & Medicine* 24 (8): 689–95.

———. 1994. "Reported and Active Prescription of ORT for Childhood Diarrhoea by Retail Pharmacists in Nigeria." *Social Science & Medicine* 39: 797–806.

Ityavyar, D. 1988. "Health Services Inequalities in Nigeria." *Social Science & Medicine* 27: 1223–35.

Janzen, John. 1978. "The Quest for Therapy: Medical Pluralism in Lower Zaire." Berkeley: University of California.

Kamat, Vinay. 2008. "Dying under the Bird's Shadow: Narrative Representations of *Degedege* and Child Survival among the Zaramo of Tanzania." *Medical Anthropology Quarterly* 22 (1): 67–93.

Kunitz, Stephen. 1987. "Explanations and Ideologies of Mortality Patterns." *Population and Development Review* 13 (3): 379–408.

Lasisi, A., O. Sulaiman, and O. Afolabi. 2007. "Socio-Economic Status and Hearing Loss in Chronic Suppurative Otitis Media in Nigeria." *Annals of Tropical Paediatrics and Child Health* 27 (4): 291–96.

Liman, I. 2001. "Protest in Zaria over Power, Water Shortage." *Daily Trust* (March 1).

Linnemayr, Sebastian, Harold Alderman, and Abdoulaye Ka. 2008. "Determinants of Malnutrition in Senegal: Individual, Household, Community Variables, and Their Interaction." *Economics and Human Biology* 6: 252–63.

Okafor, B. C. 1984. "The Chronic Discharging Ear in Nigeria." *Journal of Laryngology & Otology* 98 (2): 113–20.

Okafor, Judd-Leonard. 2015. "SURE-P, CCT Sustainability Comes under Question amid Falling Oil Price." *Daily Trust* (January 6), www.dailytrust.com, accessed January 6, 2015.

Renne, Elisha, Kelly Kirby, and Roopa Akkineni. 2008. "Bednet Use and Malaria Knowledge in Zaria City, Nigeria." *Journal of the International Institute* 15 (2): 5.

Smith, Mary F. 1954. *Baba of Karo*. New Haven: Yale University.

World Health Organization. 2012. Nigeria Launches 'Saving One Million Lives' by 2015 Initiative. World Health Organization Workforce Alliance. www.who.int/workforcealliance/media/news/2012/1mlives/en/

———. 2015. Nigeria Subsidy Reinvestment and Empowerment Programme (SURE-P): Maternal and Child Health Initiative. Washington DC: World Bank, 09_ch9_fn.docxwww.worldbank.org/en/programs/sief-trust-fund/brief/nigeria-subsidy-reinvestment-and-empowerment-programme-sure-p, accessed January 19, 2015.

10 Therapeutic Eclecticism and Cancer Care in a Kenyan Hospital Ward

Benson A. Mulemi

Ms. souda, a 39-year-old single mother of two teenage daughters and two teenage sons, was in treatment for stage-3 cervical cancer. By the time she was diagnosed, it was already in stage 2. She lived in a one-bedroom flat with her children, about 16 kilometers from Kenyatta National Hospital, where she was undergoing chemotherapy treatment courses. However, at her advanced stage of cancer, admissions to the cancer ward were proving futile, especially in light of the hospital's lack of appropriate treatment technology. The brachytherapy machine had broken down. She had completed the scheduled radiotherapy and was waiting for one more course of chemotherapy, then another radiotherapy session. After these therapies, she would be looking forward to traveling to Uganda, her next destination, for brachytherapy sessions, if she had enough money for transport fare and other costs of seeking treatment in the neighboring country. I visited her at home. Here, with minor revisions, are my notes:

> As we chat, a middle-aged woman comes in her house to talk to Ms. Souda. The woman seems uneasy about the presence of "the visitors" in the house. After Ms. Souda introduces me as a "visitor from the hospital" the woman stays on for a little while and excuses herself. Later on Ms. Souda says that the woman sells soya milk to cancer patients and that she had also wanted her to begin on herbal treatment. Ms. Souda says that the lady has been encouraging her to begin taking herbal medicines since she had been in so much pain. Ms. Souda says that the lady is a member of the Seventh-Day Adventist Church and that her pastor deals in herbal medicine for cancer. Souda says that they know of "another woman with cervical cancer who is gradually getting well after using the herbal medicine." The woman who had visited promises to come back after I have left. Ms. Souda seems to be in dilemma on whether to start on the herbal treatment, because it would conflict with her hospital treatment and her faith as a member of the Jehovah Witness Christian movement. (Field notes, November 25, 2005)

Cancer patients undergoing treatment cycles in the Kenyan hospital oscil-lated between biomedical and alternative therapies, both at home and while in the hospital. Ms. Souda recounted the following:

> We even shared with my friend here (a fellow patient) so much yesterday. It was like we were taking a stand. . . . So we were saying if it is chemo (chemo-therapy), we go for chemo. If it is *mitishamba* (herbal medicine) we go for it with clean heart (clear conscience). So my friend was giving an experience. . . . There was a lady, I think they are both on the fourth course (of chemother-apy). . . she was lying next to another patient who had a breast cancer. . . . she was getting the chemo and at night she would take some things and rub on her breast . . . saying; 'my mother told me to rub this on the breast' . . . she has not gone for radiotherapy—before she goes for radiotherapy, she was told to go for *mitishamba* (herbal medicine) first then she comes back to hospital for further treatment. (Ms. Souda, cervical cancer patient, October 3, 2005)

The experience of hospital cancer care and treatment in Kenya represents a criti-cal juncture in the prolonged paths of health-seeking efforts of patients and their family members. This also paints the grim picture of cancer care in a resource-poor African health system with insufficient responsiveness to the patients' needs, a situation exacerbated by the double burden of infectious and chronic noncommunicable diseases. The adversity that cancer engenders transforms the hospital into an institutional space for therapeutic improvisations as all actors in cancer care, including the affected patients, draw on all available resources and knowledge in attempts to cope with the disease, relieve suffering, and restore health and a quality of life.

However, cancer care innovations in times of perceived despair and hope-lessness during hospital treatment are either official or unofficial; either accept-able as part of the hospital care enterprise or not. This may explain the tendency among many people undergoing hospital treatment to resort to discreet use of complementary and alternative medicine. Biomedical practitioners in the public domain often express disapproval of alternative therapies, which they may per-ceive as negating biomedical veracity and approved cancer-care protocols. While patients may wish to have other therapies perceived as complementary to bio-medical treatment of cancer in the hospital, the fear of reproach accounts for the clandestine use of alternative therapies simultaneously with hospital treatment. Biomedical practitioners are often concerned about the possibility of desperate cancer patients deserting potentially curative or palliative conventional thera-pies in favor of unproven treatment methods (Cassileth et al. 1991). While this apprehension may be genuine, some patients prefer to move eclectically among available therapies according to their perceived needs, rather than disavow hos-pital biomedical treatment and care completely (Cassileth et al. 1984, Thomas et al. 1991, Dein 2006). Hospital treatment interludes offer ample opportunities for sequential rather than simultaneous patterns of resort (Young 1983) among available medical systems with less anxiety about reproach from the authoritative agents of hospital biomedical care.

This essay draws on hospital ethnography in Kenya to explore the nature of medical pluralism in cancer care as enacted in the space intended for exclusive biomedical practice. The concepts of therapeutic eclecticism and community of care are used as heuristic devices to show how a hospital ward in Kenya serves as an arena of converging medical sectors, their agents, and consumers who either wittingly or unwittingly reenact medical pluralism that exist in the wider society. Cancer patients and their caregivers struggle to cope with the burden of cancer care by flexibly drawing on all the therapeutic sectors and knowledge available to them. The chapter also sets out to describe and analyze the enactment of medical pluralism within the hospital, which embodies the accuracy of biomedicine. The central premise of the analysis is that simultaneous or sequential patterns of resort to biomedical cancer management and other sources of care during hospital treatment cycles typify the quest to enhance hope in and synergy of available resources. It demonstrates how the pursuits of well-being shape therapeutic eclecticism and choices between hospital treatment and other forms of therapy. Therapeutic eclecticism inside and outside the hospital in Kenya is consistent with the imperatives of holistic cancer care. This practice underscores the need for policy guidelines regarding incorporation of complementary and alternative cancer therapies into programs aimed at improving the quality of life and well-being of patients and their families.

The Cancer Crisis and Medical Care Pluralism

The emerging global cancer epidemic and other life-threatening chronic diseases challenge the capacity of biomedicine to restore health and sustain affected people's well-being. In Kenya and other sub-Sahara African countries, the experience with cancer reflects limitations of existing therapeutic systems in providing definite etiological, diagnostic, treatment, and prognostic paradigms for effective care. This results from the inadequacy of the health system in providing essential cancer care expertise and technology that would facilitate early detection and referral for appropriate, timely treatment. Therefore, there are some patterns of delay in cancer treatment that are typical to affected people and shape their health-seeking behaviour in Kenya and other African countries. Significant delays occur between the development of symptoms, medical diagnosis, and the quest for treatment from different available sources. Typically, the first kind of delay happens between the recognition of the symptoms by either the affected person or his or her therapy management group (Janzen 1978) and medical consultation. The second delay occurs between the time of consultation and the final cancer diagnosis. The third delay takes place between the time of diagnosis and the initiation of proper treatment (Dein 2006, 95).

Self-medication and eclectic recourse to the popular folk and professional sectors of health care (Kleinman 1980) characterize all the stages of delayed professional biomedical treatment of cancer in the modern African hospital. These aspects have significant implications for the ultimate outcomes expected from hospital treatment. The interval between identification of cancer symptoms and seeking medical care is relatively shorter in developed countries. Such treatment postponement may last, for instance, between two to three months in about 20–30 percent of the female breast cancer patients in the developed world's multicultural health systems (Coates et al. 1992, Lauver and Ho 1993). Conversely, the intervals between cancer sign and symptom recognition and proper biomedical hospital treatment in sub-Saharan Africa and other regions of the developing world may be longer, stretching even to one year. Numerous phases of treatment deferrals typify the health-seeking behavior of patients experiencing chronic conditions in African countries. The analysis of maternal mortality by Haiti Barnes-Josiah et al. (1998) provides a framework for understanding treatment delays, a framework that is also relevant in explaining cancer care–seeking behavior that contributes to poor prognoses in Kenya today. The framework encompasses delays in deciding to seek appropriate medical help, reaching appropriate medical facilities, and receiving adequate care at the correct facility. Further, arrival at the appropriate facilities does not always guarantee timely, appropriate treatment in the Kenyan health system. Inadequate medical and institutional care, shortages, inappropriate care, and unresponsive healthcare services frequently worsen the often bleak prospects of cancer patients (Maseko et al. 2015).

African and other low- and middle-income countries lack the capacity to adequately address the growing cancer burden and other life-threatening public health challenges. These countries experience very low cancer survival rates because the treatment technology and oncology expertise available in developed countries have not materialized in the developing countries (Stewart and Kleihues 2003). In the developed countries, most cancers are preventable and curable; only about one third are incurable. On the contrary, in developing countries, only 10–15 percent of cancers are curable with appropriate treatment, less than 5 percent are preventable, and 80–90 percent are incurable at presentation (Musibi 2010). While there is a looming cancer epidemic in Africa, cancer care is widely neglected in the health system. Cancer has not been a priority for health ministries; nutritional, parasitic, and infectious diseases have presented a greater and more immediate challenge (Parkin et al. 2003, 2.) The struggle with cancer care in African homes and hospitals therefore reflects the low priority that has been given to malignant disease in the past and at present.

The rapid increase of the incidence of cancer in Kenya portends an epidemic, with cancer now the third cause of death after infectious and cardiovascular diseases. Increasing environmental pollution, cancers associated with viral and bacterial infection, changing lifestyles, and rising life expectancy also account for the significant place of cancer within the double burden of infectious and chronic noncommunicable ailments in Kenya and the rest of sub-Saharan Africa today (Okobia 2003, 90; Livingston 2012; Strother et al., 2014). Failure to diagnose cancer and its late detection contribute to the poor treatment and care outcome prospects. Patients often follow long therapeutic paths, in which facilities at all levels in the Kenyan health system lack the requisite cancer care expertise and technology. The patients and the practitioners who represent the available professional sectors—both Western and non-Western—fail to recognize the symptoms of cancers and may treat the wrong disease(s). Narratives in the Kenyan hospital ethnography of the predicament of misdiagnosis and waste of time for proper cancer treatment abound. Cancer progression goes unabated as health practitioners search for illness etiologies in vain.

Prolonged treatment proves futile when cancer illness is mistaken for diseases that are more commonly diagnosed in the health system. The symptom or sign confusion couples with the shortage of proper diagnostic technology and pathologists in the health system to account for the futility of much cancer treatment. Cancer patients and their caregivers often talk of experiences in which their chronic illness manifested signs and symptoms associated with HIV/AIDS, fever, typhoid, or amoebic dysentery, or conditions associated with folk etiologies and indigenous therapeutic systems. Referrals for appropriate diagnosis and treatment often occur at very late cancer stages, followed by often arduous yet futile hospital treatment efforts.

Thus cancer treatment in Kenya and many other developing countries may involve progressive physical and emotional deterioration and catastrophic livelihood vulnerability. Poor prognosis, relapses and metastases, debilitating treatment side effects contribute to increased suffering, desperation, and diminishing prospects of a quality of life, which encourage eclectic therapeutic behavior in spite of hospital treatment cycles. At this juncture negative experiences with the healthcare system and perceptions of treatment efficacy encourage the simultaneous and/or sequential resort to complementary and alternative medicine and biomedical regimes in the search for comprehensive relief from cancer (Dein 2006, 108).

Hospital Ethnography of Cancer Care in Kenya

The analysis in this chapter draws on twelve months of ethnography in Kenyatta National Hospital (KNH) in Nairobi, Kenya. KNH is the largest teaching and public national referral hospital in Nairobi, followed by the Moi Teaching and Referral Hospital in Western Kenya, less equipped than the former. The hospital receives patients referred from both private and public hospitals all over the country. The joint KNH and University of Nairobi Ethics and Research Clearance Committee approved the study proposal and fieldwork in the clearance for application number P155/12/2004. The ethnography was conducted between July 2005 and August 2006. I had return visits in 2007 and follow-up key informant interviews in 2010. The main ethnography site was the adult cancer ward, which admits both male and female patients. I moved flexibly between the ward and the Cancer Treatment Centre clinic and the radiotherapy department in the process of data collection.

All actors participating in cancer care, including the patients, and all the daily hospital activities in the clinical settings and their environs were integral parts of the ethnography. Forty-two patients (28 male and 14 female), 11 nurses, 3 doctors, and 11 family members were the main informants who were purposively selected and included in in-depth conversations and interviews on multiple occasions. All the participants granted informed consent either orally or by signing a consent form and retaining copies. I kept in mind the essence of commitment to the ethical standards of anthropological research and engaged in continuous negotiations for access to clinical and patients' spaces as an outsider social scientist (Mulemi 2010a, 2010b; Aagaard-Hansen and Johansen 2008). Focused informal conversations on multiple occasions with purposively selected patients, their relatives, and hospital staff constituted the main qualitative data-collection technique. Conversations centered on the use of complementary and alternative medicine, including African traditional medicine, during the hospital cancer treatment cycles in the ward and at home. Most informants indicated that relatives sometimes brought alternative medicine to the inpatients during hospital visiting hours.

Direct nonparticipant observation of hospital cancer care procedures, ward rounds, and clinic reviews and therapeutic relationships elicited more data. I was an obtrusive ethnographer in the hospital, and my participation was limited to ordinary social interactions. All the conversations and interviews were in either English or Kiswahili languages. I recorded observations and responses by taking notes and using a voice recorder and transcribed the data in English. Pseudonyms are used in this ethnography, and I have avoided descriptions that identify particular incidents in order to safeguard the privacy and anonymity of the study participants.

The second part of the ethnography entailed follow-up visits to ten purposively selected patients out of the hospital and at home to explore how they coped with cancer after or in-between hospital treatment sessions. Conversations outside the hospital elicited information on perceptions and attitudes about the hospital biomedical cancer treatment regimens and different forms of alternative therapies. Observations of the patients' surroundings outside the hospital and at home gave clues about the actual resort to alternative therapies. Most of the informants with assorted cancer care resources in their houses and around them felt less anxious about reproach regarding 'medicine mixing' if they described their extra resources as registered or improvised food supplements and alternative therapy products. In the Kenyan cancer care situation at home and in the hospital, many chronically ill patients and their caregivers regard patented food supplements and alternative medicines as either substitutes or complements to hospital treatment regimes. Misgivings about complementary and alternative medicine (CAM) among clinical personnel derive from awareness about the former attitude, which they associate with non-adherence to hospital treatment and uncertainties about biomedical treatment outcomes. Content analysis of current media reports on the cancer care crisis in Kenya supplements the interpretation of data in this chapter.

This chapter combines thematic analysis of transcribed conversations, in-depth interviews, and observation notes. I conducted the ethnography and transcriptions personally, and this facilitated familiarity with the data for thematic analysis of transcription texts (Miles & Huberman 1994). The analysis draws on the grounded theory approach to qualitative research (Glaser & Strauss 1967, Glaser 1978) to analyze and discuss the emerging themes on cancer care in Kenya. Resort to therapeutic eclecticism in cancer care in Kenya results from the desperation and state of hopelessness patients feel while in treatment for cancers in the advanced stages in a resource-poor health system. Patients and their caregivers—both formal and informal—wittingly or unwittingly engage in therapeutic eclecticism to increase the chances of positive treatment outcomes and relieving cancer suffering.

For the cancer patients and their family members, a tendency towards care pluralism in the medical settings and at home is part of their quests to maximize therapeutic synergy as well as expand and sustain a community of care for comprehensive support in the face of cancer-caused adversity. Thirty-two of the main respondents in my ethnography were either married or had been married (2 divorced, 3 bereaved), while ten of them were single. All the patients were subsistence farmers, although a few engaged in small-scale cash crop production. A few of the patients were also formally employed in low-wage work such as primary school teaching, clerical work, and low-grade technician jobs. Most of the cancer patients were not covered by the National Health Insurance Fund or any other health insurance.

Cancer Care Desperation and Medical Eclecticism

Variations in approaches to cancer treatment in the Kenyan health system are observed at the national referral hospital. This often begins with trial-and-error oscillations among therapies before diagnosis is definite. The search for primary causes of some cancers continues up to the national referral stage. In addition, weak policy guidelines on standardization of regimens as well as lack of drugs to sustain recommended protocols define the individual initiatives that character-ize attempts to help patients by 'doing something for them'. In this sense, differ-ent levels of hospital cancer treatment and care tend not to adhere to consistent approaches and procedures. There are variations in cancer treatment regimens, depending on the combinations of drugs in each. However, Dr. Subira, who pro-vided advice on pharmaceutical issues for the cancer ward at KNH, indicated that the whims of individual consultants and considerations of patients' ability to buy the drugs during shortages in the hospital influenced further discrepan-cies in chemotherapy preparations. Similarly, variations in the training of doc-tors prescribing cancer treatments contributed to the variations in therapy for the same type of cancer in different hospital units or at different times in a pa-tient's treatment. According to Dr. Subira, this unregulated flexibility of the bio-medical approach to cancer treatment negated aspirations for care optimization. Dr. Subira noted:

> We should ideally have a cancer treatment centre . . . where all the patients are seen by all the consultants, involving all the specialities; the surgical, the haemato-oncologists, the medical oncologists, the radio-oncologists. . . . If they were seen in one unit, by all those key players, and the doctors discuss the issues of the patients together . . . the patients would get the treatment that is optimal for them. But now it depends on where the consultation lands first. You might see two patients with same exact diagnosis, but one was probably referred to the oncologist in the haematology clinic and the other was referred to the oncologist in the radiotherapy clinic. . . . But you see there are a lot of other cancer patients in the other units where consultants apply their varied knowledge which none of us here knows about in their specialisations. . . . So every one of us tries to manage cancer in the way we believe we were trained to manage. You see those differences are there, and yet no one will put them down and ask them so you bring your papers let's see . . . you bring your pa-pers let's see. So everyone continues to manage depending on who is referred to whom. . . . But I have a lot of issues especially with prescriptions from units that are not well organized, or the units that are admitting oncology patients but do not have a resident oncology consultant. . . . There will be some mishaps in regimes and dosing. (Subira, July 4, 2006)

Therapy variations that may affect the optimization of cancer care in KNH result from various factors. In the excerpt above, inadequate harmonization of cancer treatment decisions stands out. Second, there are issues related to either inade-quate oncology expertise or variations in paradigms and assumptions about can-cer treatment among the qualified experts. This brings to the fore what Dr. Subira regards as "professional politics" and medical hierarchy, which define perceived authority about medical decisions and their implementation. This is also an issue that has consequences for organization as an important dimension of cancer care work (James 1992) in the contemporary institution of the hospital. However, as Dr. Peters points out, flexibility in cancer treatment decision-making, albeit not necessarily to optimize care outcome, may be clinical personnel's personal initiative to help suffering patients in spite of the prevailing scarcity of medical resources, such as the prescribed regimens. This constitutes therapeutic improvisations as part of the moral obligation "to do something" for suffering patients. Dr. Peters, for instance, noted:

> We admit them for three courses of chemotherapy and then radio (radiotherapy). Since they could not afford to buy the (drugs for) chemo (chemotherapy), we decided to admit, give radio, followed by weekly chemo, which is available most of the time in the hospital. We will assess after a few patients and see how they have responded. (Peters, June 10, 2006)

Helping to meet desperate cancer patients' care needs in the Kenyan hospital occasionally entails improvisation of medicine, which Livingston (2012) similarly observed in Botswana. As Dr. Peters pointed out, "radio-chemotherapy" improvisation was a desperate experimental ("trial") treatment protocol for patients with chronic illness and pain. It was also an innovative way of "doing something" for poor patients who could not afford drugs when the hospital experienced shortages that interrupted recommended therapy courses. With regard to Dr. Peters' observation in the excerpt above, a doctor in the cancer ward or treatment center in the Kenyan hospital would, for instance, adaptably interrupt chemotherapy, even in the first cycle, and recommend radiotherapy when a patient's condition was rapidly deteriorating rather than responding to the chemotherapy dosage. This unilateral decision to deviate from a conventional pattern of therapy cycles by virtue of the authority of medical hierarchy often entailed an "unpopular decision," which other clinical staff had qualms about. The manner in which radio-chemotherapy regimens were implemented for critically ill patients would also raise professional tensions. Dr. Peters and some nurses had reservations about some of the radio-chemotherapy sequences and preparations, which they thought did not conform to standard procedures for the combined therapy. This regimen is expected in specified time frameworks for patients with advanced esophageal, neck, and nasopharyngeal cancers at aggressive, inoperable stages. Some patients had to be treated by chemotherapy and radiotherapy on alternating weekly dosages determined by an oncology consultant.

The oncology consultants' and cancer ward personnel's initiatives to do something for the patients in the face of cancer drug scarcity constitute attempts at taking cancer care beyond mere physical needs. As James (1992) noted, comprehensive care includes deliberate attempts to address both the physical and emotional aspects of therapy. This calls for inventiveness and eclecticism that complement the medical approach to care and transform it into comprehensive biopsychosocial care. This is the essence of therapy eclecticism or pluralism aiming at holistic care in contemporary clinical psychology, psychotherapy, counselling, and alternative systems of medicine (Hollanders and McLeod 1999; Micozzi 2007, 284; Waldegrave 1984). Improvisation of medicine in the Kenyan cancer ward is a response to shortage of drugs, the challenges of addressing treatment needs of patients with cancer in advanced stages, and the global reality that some cancers are still untreatable.

All providers in hospital cancer care in Kenya therefore engage in therapeutic eclecticism, which is a process through which they draw on medical resources, paradigms, assumptions, and theories available to them in order to meet the needs of the affected people comprehensively. This further entails the agency of all care providers in hospital cancer management in the continuous processes of redefining cancer therapy (Mulemi 2014). However, the hospital staff guard against care eclecticism that deviates from the biomedical treatment protocols. This accounts for the discreet agency of inpatients and staff in the lower levels of the socio-medical hierarchy in redefining therapy drawing on licenced complementary and alternative medicine and unpatented African traditional medicine (ATM). Therapeutic eclecticism among the clinical personnel suggests they view the hospital as an arena of professional adaptability for effective care and moral space for sustaining patients' hope. Conversely, patients, informal caregivers, and nurses may regard the hospital as the space for compassionate therapeutic relationships. The hospital provides the space for creation and expansion of the community of care. Available medical systems converge in the clinical setting either covertly or overtly to provide the much desired therapeutic synergy in cancer management. This characterises African oncology practice in spite of the challenges that cancer poses to the perceived power and efficacy of biomedicine.

Complementary and Alternative Medicine (CAM) in Cancer Care

The responsibility of a pharmacist associated with the cancer ward was to ensure the availability of drugs to the patients. The pharmacist is to be consulted on the required treatment and pharmaceutical combinations and advises the hospital what to buy. Dr. Subira indicated that:

> it was the responsibility of the doctors to make patients understand the medication, cost implications, and the price variations depending on available protocol combination options. If the pharmacist and the ward physician failed to find cheaper alternative regimens, they would try to find out on how

to assist the patient, because it is not good to leave out the patient just because they cannot afford. (Subira, July 4, 2006)

The initiative in the excerpt above is an important basis for medical eclecticism that would be sensitive to patients' livelihood vulnerabilities that affect hospital treatment continuity in spite of persistent shortage of subsidized cancer drugs. The cost of cancer drugs and treatment uncertainties may affect patients' adherence to hospital therapies. The clinical staff on the cancer ward therefore work hard to ensure that the patients adhere to the treatment, taking into consideration all the factors that affect adherence to biomedical cancer therapies. During my ethnography, the clinical staff on the cancer ward vigorously discouraged patients from using traditional medicine while on hospital treatment due to "unfavourable drug interactions and confusing symptoms," side effects, and effects on treatment outcomes. Such opinions against sequential or concurrent resort to CAM and patented food supplements during hospital cancer treatment cycles do not deter patients and other caregivers seeking synergistic therapies. Conversely, the clinical staff may attribute failure of hospital cancer treatment to either the use of alternative medicine or the treatment cycle interruptions and delays they engender. Dr. Latiff, for instance, noted: "The only problem is that sometimes patients concentrate on those things and then they abscond from our clinic. . . . Most of the times they come back when they are worse off and we really need to restrategize the whole treatment plan radically" (June 10, 2006).

The challenges to enhancing responsiveness of the Kenyan health system to cancer care needs presents a public hospital as a microcosm for medical pluralism. During my ethnography, the cancer ward at KNH embodied the potential market space for the convergence of medical sectors available in the wider society. Different agents of the medical sectors converge in the hospital and various clinical spaces and wards at different times. Hospital staff in the lower social and medical hierarchies as well as patients and their social networks link the biomedical space to the activities of other medical and healing systems. Sellers of herbal medicine and other forms of CAM therefore become part of the cancer patients' care community within the hospital and beyond. Transactions in the CAM were rife, initially targeting some of the hospital staff who would extend their networks to patients with whom they had friendly care relations. The CAM transactions in the cancer ward and other hospital units therefore address a wide spectrum of healthcare needs that affect both the patients and the hospital staff.

Complementary African Traditional Medicine

Both the hospital staff and patients involved in the CAM and especially African Traditional Medicine (ATM) transactions are often concerned about incurring reproach, so they always strive to be inconspicuous. A patient support staff member on the cancer ward observed, for instance:

> Because these people are so desperate, they say why can't we try other medicines? . . . they bring those herbs and they administer in the ward, without even the knowledge of the medical staff! The patient is admitted, and then this "outside knowledge" is used in the ward, without the knowledge of the medical staff. Then you end up seeing a patient's condition changing abruptly. Then you might also blame yourself of mismanaging the patient but the patient was mismanaged from outside by the relatives and others. . . . there was a man diagnosed with breast cancer and had a post-operation wound. We came across people performing some strange things on him at the bedside. So we had to intervene, but it was too late because this had been going on for almost five days! Then finally the patient died. We ended up blaming ourselves for not being so keen to notice strange activities happening to our patients in the ward. (Mr. Kulal, ward assistant, July 11, 2006)

Transactions in CAM on the cancer ward as illustrated above reflect the practice of "healer shopping" (Kroeger 1983, 147) in the wider society of a resource-poor health system. This aspect of health-seeking behaviour entails resort to therapeutic intervention of another healer or caregiver for a single illness episode without referral from the first. Due to informal social interactions among hospital caregivers, patients and their family members may decide, without the knowledge of hospital staff, to engage in this form of therapeutic eclecticism, which is often blamed for unsuccessful biomedical care. However, many people who face situations of hopelessness in hospital management of chronic illnesses in Africa (Green 1992, Nkwi 1994) are bound to engage in healer- or care-shopping, which may shape current hospital care outcomes.

Extension of the Cancer Care Community

Hospital cancer care in Africa begins from a traditional, less institutionalized therapy management group (Janzen 1978) framework. While hospital care may promise to provide exclusive and efficient biomedical care, disappointments in oncology and lack of resources soon negate the hope of suffering patients and their caregivers. Therefore, the hospital, like the larger society, is an arena for the expansion of the cancer care community through interactions among people sharing the experience of coping with the disease and available therapies. Transactions in CAM on the Kenyan cancer ward in this sense are a microcosm of the proliferation of alternative remedies for cancer management in spite of the hopelessness the patients and caregivers experience during treatment cycles in the hospital and at home. The proliferation of alternative remedies for cancer management is a free-market phenomenon in which people choose the remedies that they perceive as efficacious or as contributing to therapeutic synergy within the rapidly growing medial pluralism in Kenya (Mulemi 2014, 179). However, owing to the uncertainty of treatment outcomes for cancer, being in the hospital tends to constrain the desire for eclectic choice among the available cancer care resources for those that would be more efficacious in restoring health and well-being and sustaining a better quality of life. Arguably, cancer is among the key noncommunicable diseases that require a wider care community beyond the confines of biomedical therapeutic models. Patients and their caregivers seek to expand the care community through healer-shopping in the prevailing therapeutic market place (Whyte 2014, 200–201).

The often discreet transactions in CAM on the cancer ward, as in many other units in Kenya public hospitals, point to the challenge of the double burden of disease on the healthcare system. However, the low priority given to cancer care promotes the proliferation of a unique kind of marketplace around the disease, as is the case with other neglected noncommunicable chronic diseases, such as diabetes. Care for chronic conditions other than HIV/AIDS receives low budgetary allocation in public health funding and still attracts very little donor support in Kenya and other developing countries (Whyte 2014).

In a case of a patient admitted on the Kenyan cancer ward during my ethnography, a doctor leading the ward round on September 9, 2005, suspected that he was using alternative medicines. The doctor complained that the patient's file showed an irregularity that he could not explain; he suspected that it resulted from using ATM. The doctor was about to scold the patient, but a nurse informed him that the patient was diabetic and was using other medicines apart from cancer chemotherapy. A pharmacist clarified that they always noticed when other "medicines, including traditional medicine, were being used beside the main chemotherapy" as this would be reflected in the blood test results. However the pharmacist noted that "the effect of alternative medicine may not necessarily be negative in cancer treatment, but the actual effect was not easy to determine" (Dr. Subira, July 21, 2006).

While cancer care should benefit from subsidized public health services in Kenya, persistent shortages of cancer drugs and treatment technology in public hospitals often renders both the caregivers and patients helpless. The challenge of treating cancer in advanced stages and the fact that available technology and expertise are ineffective often worsen the hopeless hospital care situation. Nurses often easily relate to the patients' experience and recommend to them sources of CAM and therapeutic food supplements. Several patients could recall instances when nurses promoted famous licensed practitioners in ATM and other CAM. This shaped the patients' help-seeking behaviour during and after the prescribed hospital treatment sessions. Mr. Beneas noted: "some begin here, then they resort to traditional medicine when they feel that the modern medicine would not cure them. . . . Some will stop the treatment in the hospital especially when the processes becomes too expensive and painful to sustain" (Beneas, Nurse, October 28, 2005).

Therapeutic eclecticism during and after the hospital treatment cycles therefore constitutes attempts at expanding care resources and increasing the chances of positive treatment outcomes. This includes access to additional socio-psychological support networks during hospital care. Similarly, the patients and their family members resort to both biomedicine and CAM to enhance two important aspects of responsiveness of a health system. First, patients aspire for autonomy, especially in seeking help during prolonged chronic illness. They want the opportunity to exercise self-directing freedom to enhance well-being, drawing on available resources and the care community. An important dimension to this is the right of the patients to information on his or her disease and alternative treatment options. However, members of the care community should have the capacity to facilitate informed choice rather than inhibit it through medical paternalism. This tendency is reflected in the fact that some cancer patients and caregivers in Kenya who wish to try CAM during hospital treatment cycles are restrained and clandestine. Similarly, patients' resort to CAM during my ethnography was often a response to perceived extremely negative side effects of available cancer treatment regimes. As indicated below, some patients and caregivers considered chemotherapy and radiotherapy both toxic and lethal, owing to the perceived rapid morbidity and mortality that coincide with cancer treatment. With this in mind, interactions with the agents of CAM offer a larger community of care where patients exercise their autonomy in other different ways. Arguably, the community of care within the CAM sector enhances the cancer patients' right to be consulted about therapy and choice of therapeutic options.

During my ethnography, patients, nurses, patient support staff, and members of patients' informal network of support constituted the community of care directly involved in the therapeutic marketplace on the cancer ward. Their tendency to seek more information on cancer therapy characterized their agency in redefining hospital treatment, albeit in a constrained environment. Nurses' portion in the care of patients suffering from the chronic condition and debilitating treatment side effects exposes them to the daily cancer care burden. They therefore have the opportunity to relate to the experience of suffering and limited efficacy of available therapies. In this regard the nurses and other patient support staff served as patients' link to simultaneous or sequential resort to CAM from the community of care inside and outside the hospital. Elsewhere, in United Kingdom and Australia, Tovey et al. (2007) found out that cancer patient support networks outside hospitals tend to coalesce around practices of eclectic appropriation of CAM in the wider society. Similarly, such practices would not preclude resort to hospital care and review when necessary after the final exit from regular biomedical cancer treatment courses in the Kenyan context. On exiting the hospital in Kenya, nurses take the responsibility to recommend patients to CAM clinics where they can establish continuity in encountering a regular community of care and support. On occasion, patients introduced each other to "doctors" and dealers in CAM. Thus, the hospital offers the space for convergence of therapeutic strategies that cancer patients can choose from in order to boost their quality of life. Similarly, it extends the community of care as patients seek information about therapy and care beyond the hospital.

Confidence in the potential of the hospital to restore cancer patients' health wanes with prolonged treatment. This prompts increasing interest in other therapies advertised in local media and described on the internet. Perception about the failure of "trial medicine" and the adverse negative effects of chemotherapy and radiotherapy contribute to increasing uncertainty. Observations and lived experiences of increasing debility and mortality in spite of the medical care available in the hospital decrease hopes for achieving the desired quality of life. During my ethnography, nurses tended to share the patients' hospital care misgivings more than the clinical and other technical staff did. On occasion, there was tension between physicians and patients about medicines that were harming patients, yet they could not be changed. In a study on the treatment of prostate cancer in Canada, Boon et al. (2003) similarly found out that patients tended to turn to the use of CAM because of their negative experiences with the healthcare system. Nurses in the Kenya ethnography seemed to concur with the patients, albeit unobtrusively, about perceived toxicity of chemotherapy regimens, as they were "just chemicals," as opposed to patented food supplements and CAM available on the local therapeutic market. Since nurses deal with cancer care work daily, they can relate to the associated emotional and physical labor (James 1992) more than other hospital staff. As Langwick (2008) reported about Tanzanian nurses, the nurses in the Kenyan cancer ward also helped patients to access traditional and other forms of CAM. They perceived their moral obligation in facilitating the patients' quest for therapeutic synergy and complementary community of care.

Dietary Supplements and Complementary Chinese Traditional Medicine

Several patients returned to the cancer ward in worse condition, and the doctors and nurses would scold them for having substituted their hospital treatment with ATM. Nurses, however, emphasized to them that the use of ATM and dietary supplements were not complete substitutes for the arduous chemotherapy and radiotherapy. For them, resort to ATM and other CAM would facilitate a quality of life either during or after hospital treatment, provided that the patients made "wise choices at the right time." This would "add life to their days, rather than days to their lives", and also motivate the nurses to continue taking care of the patients in spite of poor prognosis.

The nurses encourage the patients to take advantage of the dietary supplements that are abundant in the Kenyan therapeutic market today. Both patients and hospital staff often participate in the sale of dietary supplements from different international companies, and many people believe that the supplements alleviate an array of chronic conditions (Whyte 2014, 201). However, cancer patients are careful not to be blamed for their deteriorating conditions because of the use of the nutritional supplements. The most common companies that marketed the dietary supplements and were well known to cancer patients during my ethnography were *Golden Neo-Life Diamite* (South African, popularly abbreviated as GNLD); *Swissgarde* (South African), and *Tianshi* (Chinese). In a clinic review at the cancer treatment center in the Kenyan study hospital, a woman wondered whether she should continue buying and using "GNLD medicines" now that she had been admitted to the ward. The consulting doctor clarified that "the GNLD products are not medicines." He observed:

> Some people stop chemotherapy and resort to GNLD, but these are not substitutes for chemotherapy. So they should buy GNLD knowing that these are just supplements but they must continue with chemotherapy. (Peters, clinic consultation, March 27, 2006)

The increase of traditional Chinese medicine (TCM) in the management of chronic conditions in Kenya today accompanies the promotion of the *Tianshi* nutritional supplements in the prevailing local therapeutic market. During my ethnography, several cancer patients used Chinese medicine as an important alternative during hospital treatment or at the end, when doctors could not help them anymore. When the decision to "send patients home to rest" was impending, a negligible number of them contemplated palliative care through the hospice, but most of them planned to try Chinese medicine. TCM has gained popularity in the emerging medical pluralism in Kenya, particularly in urban areas. The claim of many people that TCM is relatively cheap in managing cancer and other chronic diseases belies the fact that prolonged cancer care drains personal assets. The rising cost of this CAM also derives from the fact that it is concentrated in Nairobi and other main cities in Kenya. Most of the poor patients lack the necessary support to sustain their consultations and cost of the array of therapeutic prescriptions recommended for them in a single treatment cycle. However, most of the people who use TCM praise it for effective management of multiple illnesses and alleviation of chronic suffering with negligible side effects compared to biomedical prescriptions. Similarly, Hsu (2002) found that the popularity of TCM in Dar es salaam, Tanzania, resulted from similar benefits relative to biomedicine and the perception that TCM was a superior form of traditional medicine compared to ATM. Processing and packaging traditional medicines as practiced in the TCM market increases the consumers' confidence and trust. Licenced practitioners of ATM tend to emulate this with an emphasis on marketing the products as scientifically tested for safety, efficacy, and quality. In order to appeal further to consumers, the herbalists advertise their products widely, emphasizing their rapid and effective synergistic qualities in relieving multiple ailments like those associated with cancer comorbidities.

Medical Pluralism and Holistic Cancer Care

Cancer contributes significantly to the double burden of infectious and non-infectious diseases in Africa. However governments of African countries, including Kenya, still prioritize infectious diseases and virtually neglect cancer care. The rising cancer epidemic occurs in the context of poor health system infrastructure and an array of livelihood vulnerabilities that hinder timely detection and treatment. Therefore, the burden of cancer and the morbidity it entails occur against the background of inadequate preparation to deal with its impacts on health, livelihood, and the well-being of affected people. The global challenge of cancer to the efficacy of biomedicine further complicates the hopeless situation of hospital management of the disease. Therapeutic eclecticism therefore characterizes people's recourse to both biomedical and complementary and alternative therapies in desperation. The eclecticism in the Kenyan hospital care of cancer involves the agency of all the providers of biomedically oriented health, patients, and the agents of other sectors available in the therapeutic market today. Owing to scarcity of cancer drugs, expertise, and other medical resources, the agents of biomedicine are involved in therapeutic eclecticism through improvisation of medicine (Livingston 2012). This entails inventiveness in which established treatment protocols may be altered in frantic attempts to assist patients amid limited biomedical cancer treatment options. Patients have little flexibility in exercising their rights to be consulted about treatment and grant informed consent regarding testing improvised regimens and regular arduous therapies. Consequently, patients have to endure the treatment offered by the doctors, in spite of their negative side effects and perceived inefficacy. Agents of biomedicine may therefore infringe on patients' autonomy and other provisions of a responsive health system. Treatment uncertainty, adverse negative side effects, and the perceived inefficacy in alleviating suffering underpin patients' own therapeutic eclecticism.

Cancer care burden and associated treatment adversities result in patients' preference for different therapies in a complementary fashion, rather than in isolation (Hök et al. 2007). Conversely, clinical personnel and other technical staff in the Kenyan hospital often stigmatize patients' therapeutic eclecticism, which they scapegoat for poor and fatal cancer treatment outcomes. However, therapeutic eclecticism among patients, their informal social support groups, and hospital staff in the lower medical hierarchy, such as nurses, is a coping strategy in the face of the perceived futility of hospital treatment and care. Eclecticism in this regard entails either simultaneous or sequential resort to available care resources in the therapeutic market. It allows members of the cancer care community, including the patients, to exercise adaptability in coping with cancer and its treatment challenges. Members of the care community are able to choose among a variety of available resources, techniques, and methods that are perceived to offer relief in times of hopelessness and critical chronic illness. Therapeutic eclecticism in cancer care therefore involves all the personal and collective initiatives in finding and improvising alternative modes of care to optimize care outcomes.

The medical pluralism enacted in the Kenyan cancer ward accentuates the need for personalized therapy and care that can meet the needs of each cancer patient in a resource-poor health system. Not all the needs of chronic disease sufferers are amenable to the medicalization approach, so therapeutic eclecticism may help address care needs more holistically. Second, therapeutic eclecticism in Kenyan cancer care points to the need for increased knowledge about CAM among all cancer caregivers. This would ensure regulation of available cancer treatment resources in order to enhance their safety, efficacy, accessibility, and affordability in holistic cancer management (Hassan et al. 2014, WHO 2001).

In addition, the analysis above indicates an important dimension to nurses' participation in patients' quests for alternative therapies. The agency as part of the care community within a clinical setting underscores the potential for fruitful communication about complementary alternative therapies between agents of biomedically oriented health care and other stakeholders in patient care. This can enhance holistic cancer care through appropriate therapeutic and care complementarity in the emerging medical pluralism, which the demands for adherence to the biomedical model of care tend to stifle in Africa. Increased collaboration among the stakeholders in cancer care is imperative for the promotion of integrative care, which is possible through respectful dialogue about complementary and alternative therapies with the representatives of the biomedical sector (Hök et al. 2007, 1650). Similarly, the experience of therapeutic eclecticism in the Kenyan hospital ward points to the need for more attention to formulation of policy to improve preventive, curative, and palliative care. In order to sustain these dimensions of care, more effort is required to build a more responsive health system that can cope better with the escalating double burden of infectious and noncommunicable diseases in Kenya.

Bibliography

Aagaard-Hansen, Jens, and Maria Vang Johansen. 2008. "Research Ethics across Disciplines." *Anthropology Today* 24 (3): 15–19.

Image text at top

Boon, H., J. Bell-Brown, A. Gavin, and K. Westlake 2003. "Men with Prostate Cancer: Making Decisions about Complementary Alternative Medicine." *Medical Decision Making* 23 (6): 471–79.

Cassileth, B., E. Lusk, and D. Guerry. 1991. "Survival and Quality of Life among Patients Receiving Unproven as Compared with Unconventional Cancer Therapy." *New England Journal of Medicine* 324: 1180–85

Cassileth, B., E. Lusk, and T. Strouse. 1984. "Contemporary Unorthodox Treatment in Cancer Medicine: A Study of Patients' Treatment and Practitioners." *Annals of Internal Medicine* 101: 105–12.

Coates, R. J., D. D. Bransfield, M. Wellesley, et al. 1992. "Differences Between Black and White Women with Breast Cancer in Time from Symptom Recognition to Medical Consultation. Black/White Cancer Survival Study Group." *Journal of the National Cancer Institute* 84: 938–50.

Dein, S. 2006. *Culture and Cancer Care: Anthropological Insights in Oncology*, London: Open University.

Glaser, Barney G. 1978. *Theoretical Sensitivity*. San Francisco: Sociology Press.

Glaser, Barney G., and A. L. Strauss. 1967. *The Discovery of Grounded Theory*. Chicago: Aldine.

Green, E. C. 1992. "Sexually Transmitted Disease, Ethnomedicine and Health Policy in Africa." *Social Science and Medicine* 35 (2): 121–130.

Hassan, A. A., A. Allam, S. Al. Kindi, G. A. Zeinah, S. Eziada, and A. Bashir. 2014. "Knowledge, Attitudes and Practices of Oncology Nursing Towards Complementary and Alternative Medicine in Qatar." *Palliative Medicine and Nursing* 1 (1): 1–15, accessed at http://dx.doi .org/10.14437/PMNOA-1-1-1 on February 2, 2015.

Hök. J., C. Wachler, C. Falkenberg, and C. Tishelman. 2007. "Using Narrative Analysis to Understand the Combined Use of Complementary Therapies and Biomedically Oriented Health Care." *Social Science and Medicine* 65: 1642–53.

Hollanders, H., and J. McLeod. 1999. "Theoretical Orientation and Reported Practice: A Survey of Eclecticism among Counsellors in Britain." *British Journal of Guidance and Counselling* 27 (3): 405–14.

Hsu, E. 2002. "'The Medicine from China Has Rapid Effects': Chinese Medicine Patients in Tanzania," *Anthropology and Medicine* (3): 291–313.

James, N. 1992. "Care = Organisation + Physical Labour + Emotional Labour." *Sociology of Health and Illness* 14 (4): 488–509.

Janzen, J. M. 1978. *The Quest for Therapy: Medical Pluralism in Lower Zaire*, Berkeley: University of California.

Kleinman, Arthur. 1980. *Patients and Healers in the Context of Culture: An Exploration of the Borderland Between Anthropology, Medicine and Psychiatry*, Berkeley: University of California.

Kroger, A. 1983. "Anthropological and Socio-medical Health Care Research in Developing Countries" *Social Science and Medicine* 17 (3): 147–61.

Langwick, S. 2008. "Articulate(d) bodies: Traditional Medicine in a Tanzanian Hospital." *American Ethnologist* 35 (3): 428–39.

Lauver, D., and C. H. Ho. 1993. "Explaining Delay in Care Seeking for Breast Cancer Symptoms." *Journal of Applied Social Psychology* 23: 1806–25.

Livingston, J. 2012. *Improvising Medicine: An African Oncology Ward in an Emerging Cancer Epidemic*. Durham: Duke University.

Maseko, F. C., M. L. Chirwa, and A. S. Muula. 2015. *Health Systems Challenges in Cervical Cancer Prevention Program in Malawi. Global Health Action* [S.l.] 8, Jan. 2015. ISSN 1654–9880. Accessed at: http://www.globalhealthaction.net/index.php/gha/article/view/26282 on Jan. 30, 2015. doi:http://dx.doi.org/10.3402/gha.v8.26282.

Micozzi, M. S., ed. 2007. *Complementary and Integrative Medicine in Cancer Care and Prevention: Foundations and Evidence-Based Interventions,* New York: Springer.

Miles, M. B., and A. M. Huberman. 1994. *Qualitative Data Analysis: An Expanded Source Book.* Thousand Oaks, CA: Sage.

Mulemi, Benson A., 2010a. *Coping with Cancer and Adversity: Hospital Ethnography in Kenya.* Leiden: African Studies Centre.

———. 2010b. "On Being 'Native' and 'Outsider' in Hospital Ethnography." *Viennese Ethnomedicine* XII (2–3): 6–14.

———. 2014. "Technologies of Hope: Managing Cancer in a Kenyan Hospital." In *Making and Unmaking Public Health in Africa: Ethnographic and Historical Perspectives,* edited by Ruth Prince and Rebecca Marsland, 162–83. Athens, OH: Ohio University.

Musibi, A. 2010. *Cancer in Kenya today.* Accessed at http://healthpromotionkenya.org/LIBRARY%20OF%20DATA/Cancer/Project%20Reports/CANCER%20IN%20KENYA%20TODAY.pdf on January 30, 2015.

Nkwi, P. N. 1994. "Perceptions and Treatment of Diarrhoeal Diseases in Cameroon." *Journal of Diarrhoeal Disease Research* 12: 35–41.

Okobia, M. N. 2003. "Cancer Care in Sub-Saharan Africa: Urgent Need for Population-Based Cancer Registries." *Ethiopian Journal for Health Development* 17 (2): 89–98.

Parkin, D. M., J. Ferlay, M. Hamdi-Cherif, F. Sitas, J. Thomas, H. Wabinga, and S. L. Whelan, eds. 2003. *Cancer in Africa: Epidemiology and Prevention.* Lyon: IARC.

Stewart, B. W., and P. Kleihues, eds. 2003. *World Cancer Report,* Lyon: IARC.

Strother, R. M., F. C. Asirwa, N. B. Busakhala, E. Njiru, F. Orang'o, F. Njuguna, J. Skiles, J. Mega A. Carter, G. J. L. Kaspers, B. Rosen, M. K. Krzyzanowska, S. Washington, A. Griest, A. Rosmarin, and P. J. Loehrer. 2014. "The Evolution of Comprehensive Cancer Care in Western Kenya." *Journal of Cancer Policy* 1: e25–e30. at doi.org/10.1016/j.jcpo.2013.04.001.

Thomas, K. J., J. Carr, L. Westlake, and B. T. Williams. 1991. "Use of Unorthodox and Conventional Health Care in Great Britain." *British Medical Journal* 302: 207–10.

Tovey, P., J. Chatwin, and A. Broon. 2007. *Traditional, Complementary and Alternative Medicine and Cancer Care: An International Analysis of Grassroots Integration.* New York: Routledge.

Waldegrave, C. 1987. "The Butchers: An Eclectic Approach to Family Therapy." *Journal of Family Therapy* 6: 247–63.

WHO 2001. *Traditional medicine strategy 2002–2005,* Geneva: World Health Organization, accessed online at http://www.who.int/medicines/library/trm/trm_strat_eng.pdf

Whyte, S. R. 2014. The publics of the new public health in Uganda, *In Making and unmaking public health in Africa: Ethnographic and historical perspectives,* edited by Ruth Prince and Rebecca Marsland, 187–207, Athens, Ohio: Ohio University Press.

Young, A. 1983. The relevance of traditional medical culture to modern Primary Health Care, *Social Science and Medicine,* 17(16): 1205–1211.

11 Elusive Paths, Fluid Care

Seeking Healing and Protection in the Republic of Benin

Carolyn Sargent and James Leslie Kennell

THE AVENUES OF TREATMENT and therapy for sickness that are available to the people of the Republic of Benin are many and varied, and therapeutic modalities are combined and overlap. Our ethnographic research, and that of others (Chary and Rohloff 2015, Janzen 2014, Rhine et al. 2014, Wendland 2014, Langwick 2015) suggests that patients, often with the advice of kin and friends, consult diverse practitioners as diagnoses evolve over time, as efficacy of treatments waxes and wanes, as symptoms are interpreted and reinterpreted, and as new counsel is offered by respected others. Consulting an herbalist, a ritual specialist, an evangelical preacher, and a physician for the same illness episode may seem incompatible, if not contradictory, acts. Yet from the patient's perspective, these may be initiatives drawn from a field of possibilities, not necessarily in epistemological competition, but rather, appropriate at a given moment in an illness trajectory.

In societies with multiple healing epistemologies, systems that are sometimes in competition may not be perceived as such at the level of individual experience. As Janzen suggests (2014, 23) it is important to examine not only healing modalities but also how individuals and their supporters negotiate approaches, practices, and knowledge—both therapeutic modalities and the existential experience of suffering and healing. Drawing on case material from northern and southern Benin, we find support for Rhine (20104, 3) who argues that we will benefit from attending to the dynamic capacity of local healing systems to grow and transform, especially in relation to biomedicine. Accordingly, binaries (traditional healing vs. biomedicine, for example) can obscure connectedness among modes of healing (Wendland 2014, 45; Janzen 2014, 23; Chary and Rohloff 2015, xx). We propose to give more credence to fluid, elastic domains of medical knowledge as we analyze how patients pursue elusive paths to alleviate suffering.

Therapeutic Options in Benin

Along with the National Health System (a biomedical-based system under the direction of the Ministry of Health), types of health care in Benin range from religious (both local and missionary) to foreign aid (NGOs and other donor initiatives) to black-market pharmaceuticals and various combinations of medical knowledge and materials. Among non-biomedical alternatives, we find herbalists, diviners, bonesetters, evangelical healers, midwives, and other specialists. Increasingly, quasi-biomedical practitioners, who combine herbalism with biomedical packaging, injections, and clinical paraphernalia (such as stethoscopes) are visible presences.

In 1998 the Republic of Benin began a process of governmental decentralization which, among many tasks, divided the existing provinces in half (renaming them *departements*) and restructured the National Health System. The process also divided the departements into communes and communes into *arrondissements*. The government's decentralization plan reorganized medical services into a hierarchical system following the new territorial organization and began construction of new medical facilities throughout the country. Each departement, depending on size, is divided into zones, each with its *hôpital de zone*, which is responsible for administering medical services for multiple communes and also provides surgical services for the entire zone. The capital, or county seat, of each commune has a central hospital, under the direction of the *hôpital de zone*, and each arrondissement has a branch clinic with pharmacy and maternity care, staffed with a head nurse, midwife, a few assistants, and an accountant/secretary. As of 2012, 30 of 34 health zones were fully functional, with 77 percent of the population living within 3 miles of a facility, but with only 45 percent utilizing the services provided (Cuellar et al. 2013).

Seeking a Cure along a Fluid Path: An Aja Case in Southern Benin

During two years of fieldwork among the Aja peoples of southwest Benin, I learned the significance of *zohwiʒi*, a classification for disease affecting the skin, which crosses multiple biomedical classifications regardless of their pathology: smallpox, measles, chicken pox, and some rashes, for example.[1] The disease is also intimately associated with Sakpata, the *vodun* (deity) of the earth. The Aja often directly translate *zohwiʒi* to the French term *la variole* (smallpox), and say that Sakpata is uniquely responsible for both sending and curing *zohwiʒi*. Seen as both blessing (being selected by the deity) and curse (suffering and possible death), the reaction to the sickness when it comes upon an individual, especially a child, varies and sometimes seems contradictory. For example, many devotees of Sakpata, who are said to be immune to *zohwiʒi*, long for the day their children may be either initiated into the possession group to receive immunity or be given the sickness by the deity, a true sign of the child's destiny.

Many Aja healers' explanation of general disease pathology is that disease is situated inside a person's body, usually the abdomen, and when agitated or coaxed, begins to work its way out of the body. A headache, fever, or pain in the abdominal region is often the first sign of a disease beginning this process but is not adequate symptomology alone to make a diagnosis. Thus, initial therapy is directed more toward coaxing or hastening the sickness out of the body in order to identify it and then determine curative therapy. The various processes and physical manifestations by which the sickness works its way out allow for direct diagnosis and further treatment of the sickness. During the dry season (November to March), *zohwiʒi* is often the sickness first suspected, especially in children, and when a child has a headache, fever, or abdominal pain, the first therapy often relates to the hastening of *zohwiʒi*.

Zohwiʒi is diagnosed by the way it breaks through the skin as it leaves a person's body: individual fluid-producing pustules of any size, which may be localized or cover the entire body. The nature of Aja disease classification—skin diseases particularly—and their relationship to Sakpata have significant medical, historical, and political ramifications in southwest Benin (Kennell 2011). In my research and work among the Aja in the Couffo region, *zohwiʒi* has always been an important aspect of Aja life and experience, from public health initiatives to religion (local and other) to politics as well as understanding Aja sensory illness experience (Kennell 2014). The following narrative describes the experience of one Aja family, their son, Jacques, and their efforts to navigate the varieties of available medical therapies, the place *zohwiʒi* holds in Aja experience, and the ways in which medical knowledge is understood and used in the search for healing.

When I first met with Jacques and his father near their home in the village of Kpomachihoue, Jacques, who was 8 years old, had a rash over much of his torso, arms, and legs. The dry, slightly-raised, grayish rash did not itch, Jacques affirmed, but his squirmy demeanor betrayed his discomfort. This initial meeting had been arranged by a friend of mine, a relative of the father who lived in another quarter of the Arrondissement de Hondjin, and who had been assisting me with a morbidity survey of the Hondjin community. Both Jacques and the father were well dressed for this special meeting, the father in an Oxford-style dress shirt and slacks, and Jacques in a two-piece suit made of the local printed cloth in the West African fashion. After initial greetings, some general discussion, and my explanation to Jacques's father about my interest in his son's condition, he gave 100 F CFA (about 25 cents) to Jacques, told him to fetch an empty bottle from the house, and go buy some sodabi (a local liquor) from a particular buvette (bar) in the village. While Jacques was gone, his father explained that Jacques's mother joined the local Apostolic church some years ago and attended "mass" quite frequently, even during the week. His own mother was Catholic, but he had not gone to mass since he was a child. As he began to describe all the efforts made to find healing for Jacques, tensions between him and Jacques's mother concerning treatment became apparent. Jacques soon returned with a quarter liter of sodabi and a shot glass. I took the bottle from Jacques and poured a glass to serve his father. This act of hospitality by his visitor, signaling an acknowledgment of the intrusion into their lives, brought a smile, and we both enjoyed a drink and began to relax a little.

Around three weeks before my visit, small reddish bumps began to appear on Jacques's skin, mostly on his torso. Jacques's mother prepared a *mashu*, an herbal treatment both to drink and to be rubbed onto a person's skin. This initial home treatment is common with the Aja as a hastening therapy for possible sickness, most commonly performed by a female head of household. Such initial hastening therapies are not necessarily treatments for specific sicknesses; but some sicknesses, such as *zohwiʒi*, do have specific hastening therapies, such as was given to Jacques by his mother. When sickness reveals itself in some physical manifestation, some bodily change, then it may be treated with a healing or curative therapy—"healing" meaning the sickness has completely left the body. A sickness working its way out of a person's body is a sickness that may be treated and cured. Because of the physical appearance of bumps on Jacques's skin, the hastening therapy used by his mother was specifically for *zohwiʒi*, to help along a process already begun.

Both Jacques's mother and father sought treatment for him, together and individually, over the following three weeks. Soon after the hastening therapy was given to Jacques, his father took him to a *Sakpatanɔ* who lived in their village. While I did not directly observe any of the care given to Jacques, I was able to visit each place and interview those involved in his treatment as well as discuss Jacques's case with other Aja healers. Jacques's skin condition was confirmed to be *zohwiʒi*, as his mother and father suspected, and from this *Sakpatanɔ* Jacques received *mashu* (as described above), other herbs, and was bathed with Sakpata's water—a mix of water, sodabi, and herbs kept in a large clay vessel in Sakpata's shrine house, and was sent home with instructions to return the next day for more treatment.

Any *Sakpata vodunɔ*[2] is considered a healer of *zohwiʒi* since he possesses the knowledge given by *Sakpata*. Older, more experienced *Sakpatashi* (initiates possessed by the deity) may also practice healing. A person need not necessarily be a *vodunɔ* in order to be a healer. The general Aja term for *healer* is *amawatɔ*, and each may specialize in particular sicknesses or conditions.[3] The *Sakpatanɔ* in Jacques's village treated *zohwiʒi* but was not, as he admitted, an *amawatɔ*. Jacques's skin condition spread from his torso to his arms and legs, and the bumps began to emit fluid and group together in high concentrations in various locations on his skin. Jacques received the same treatment for *zohwiʒi* from the *Sakpatanɔ* each day for a week. During this same week, Jacques's mother took him to the Apostolic church near their village each night where prayers were offered specifically for him. After several treatments from the *Sakpatanɔ* and as many nights of prayer, the bumps and blisters on Jacques's skin began to dry, flatten, and lose their reddish color. Jacques interjected that they still greatly itched, even though there was a change. With this change in appearance, Jacques was taken back to the *Sakpatanɔ* who confirmed that the *zohwiʒi* was "cured" but did not know why Jacques's skin appeared the way it did. Jacques's father was not convinced the *zohwiʒi* was cured at that time, and now complained angrily to some other people who were nearby, in earshot of his raised voice. He explained to me, in the same intense voice, how he asked the *Sakpatanɔ* what to do next. "He thinks that the *zohwiʒi* is gone, cured . . . but there is still sickness on his (Jacques's) skin! What am I to do? He told me to find someone else if I think that Jacques is not cured . . . an *amawatɔ*, a *doto* (doctor), or others." Even though this exchange happened almost three weeks before our conversation, the exasperation still showed on the face and in the voice of Jacques's father. Jacques sat quietly and tightly up against his father's side swinging his dangling feet. I asked Jacques if he thought the *Sakpatanɔ* had cured him. He looked down and the gray, dry, raised skin showed from beneath his pant leg as he swung his feet back and forth.

During the week of evening prayers for Jacques at the Apostolic church, the pastor suggested that Jacques be taken to a clinic in the adjacent arrondissement where there was a doctor. After the last visit with the *Sakpatanɔ* by Jacques and his father, his mother decided to take him to this clinic. Jacques's father did not approve of this but did not stop her from going. The clinic recommended by the pastor was approximately 10 kilometers away, and Jacques and his mother took motorcycle taxis there. The clinic was a small concrete block building with a clay tile roof and a covered porch on the front, which served as a waiting area. The day that I visited, there were no people waiting to see the doctor. *UVS-Dekandji* was painted on the front of the building. My friend Julien (language helper, assistant, and guide) accompanied me. Julien entered the building looking for the doctor. *UVS* stood for "Union Villagioses de la Santé" and was originally established by an NGO from Holland, which built several such clinics around southern Benin. However, the NGO ended the project and left Benin in the late 1990s. The current doctor had taken over the building and started his own clinic but kept the same signage and name. The doctor was actually a pastor in the Apostolic church and had some medical training as a nurse but no official certification. He very cordially gave us a short tour and explained the history of the clinic, showing us his consultation room and pharmacy stock with basic medications provided by the church. Julien asked to be excused, and the pastor/doctor pointed to the back door, indicating the latrine. "All consultation is free, and only medications are paid for, if they [patients] are able [to pay]," the pastor/doctor explained sitting behind his desk, white coat and stethoscope hung on the wall behind him.

"People come here because they get well here," he told me with confidence. After providing his cell phone number, he gave us each a Coke before we left.

On our way back to Jacques' village, Julien filled in for me what was missing from our interview. "The real consultation happens out back," Julien said. "All of his real stuff is behind the clinic." "What do you mean? What is back there?" I asked. "Drums. Other instruments, a horn, some clay pots. Kind of looks like *vodun*, but it isn't." This shed some light on Jacques's father's description of this "doctor." He was upset that his wife took Jacques to this clinic: "He's not a real doctor, he's a charlatan. He just makes a lot of noise, shouting and jumping about" was his description. Later I would learn that many *vodunɔ*, healers, and the nurse at the government satellite clinic in this part of Hondjin were in agreement and were concerned with this pastor/doctor for "deceiving" people. However, many others in the community, some from the church and some not, expressed a sentiment similar to the pastor/doctor's: people go there because they get well. I don't know exactly what type of consultation and treatment Jacques received at this clinic, except that he was given paracetamol (acetaminophen), as reported by his father.

At this point Jacques's father took his son to a healer who was not a *vodunɔ* but was described as being knowledgeable in both Aja ways and Western ways. Jacques's father showed me the bottle of medication prescribed for Jacques's skin condition: an older style glass IV bottle with a printed label that still had the rubber stopper where needles were inserted. These bottles are often used to hold roasted peanuts sold in the markets and are readily available. The printed label had the healer's name and village location, a caduceus symbol, a blue border, and the name of the medicine it contained: *zohwiʒi mashu*. As I examined the empty bottle, Jacques's father explained that the medicine was applied to Jacques's skin, not drank. I asked what happened when they used the medicine, and Jacques's father pointed to his own skin (Jacques had run off to join some friends by this point) and said that it made the skin dry and lose all color, meaning the current state of Jacques's skin: dry, gray, slightly raised on much of his torso, arms, and legs.

When I asked Jacques's father if the *zohwiʒi* was cured or if Jacques needed further treatment, he became visibly upset. "I don't know. The *Sakpatanɔ* said the *zohwiʒi* was cured. But he is not—the sickness is not finished. The skin keeps changing, but not healing. What should we do? Jacques! Come here!" When Jacques returned to his father's side, he lifted Jacques's shirt and pointed to different places on his torso. "What is this? I don't know. I don't know what the charlatan (pastor/doctor) said it was. The healer gave his own *mashu*. The *doto* (nurse at satellite clinic) here said go to the *hôpital de zone*, but that is far away. I will try, I will take him there." We had another drink of sodabi, and it was almost dark, so after some general discussion of current events in Benin, I asked the father permission to return later to see how Jacques was doing. We shook hands, Jacques shook my hand, and I returned home. Two weeks later I returned to find that Jacques and his father had left for Lomé, Togo, seeking a physician they had been told about there. I did not learn the final resolution of Jacques's case.

I continued to discuss Jacques's case with various people in the community as well as those sought out for care by his family. The persons who provided therapy for Jacques—the *Sakpatanɔ*, the satellite clinic nurse, the pastor/doctor, the family—often described the variety of therapies and those who provided them in terms of what people knew, or knowledge—*enugɔnmɛsese*, a sense of foundational things (Kennell 2011). While the satellite clinic nurse expressed frustration that many in the community, especially church members, were travelling to see the pastor/doctor who played drums for treatment rather than visiting her right there in their own village, she did describe the pastor/doctor as having knowledge of Western medicine, knowledge of religious healing, and knowledge of Aja ways of healing. She spoke highly of the *Sakpatanɔ* and his knowledge of *zohwiʒi* and ability to heal it, and described their combined efforts to combat it in their village using his knowledge and her vaccinations.

When I discussed Jacques's condition with the *Sakpatanɔ*, he focused on the importance of knowing and being able to divine or diagnose a person's sickness. If hastening therapies are being used, a diagnosis may have not yet been reached. Therapies, hastening or curing, are meant to find healing or health. Whether or not the sickness is yet known, it is still a sickness and is part of an ongoing process of being coaxed into leaving the body, then being treated with curing therapy to complete the process and bring the individual or family back to health. This *Sakpatanɔ* and other *vodunɔ* healers did not distinguish between symptoms and sickness, for the process is ongoing, and therapies are used according to initial events or changes in the presentation of the sickness. The *Sakpatanɔ* explained that therapies may change as the sickness progresses. He had cured Jacques of *zohwiʒi*. The sickness had changed for Jacques, and so treatment should continue to be sought. The ultimate goal, as the *Sakpatanɔ* explained, was to bring the boy to good health—if the sickness changed, then the therapy must change as well. The pastor/doctor, on the other hand, presented himself as someone who possessed various healing abilities and could utilize different forms of knowledge to cure any patient. "I know religious healing and medicine," he said, and explained that while he did not discourage patients from seeking other therapies, they had no need to go anywhere else, since he would heal them. When I asked about the drums (as reported by community members), he smiled and said that sometimes it helps a patient psychologically. While not able to directly interview the herbalist healer who gave Jacques the bottle of *zohwiʒi mashu*, the products of these types of efforts to combine the herbal aspects of local Aja healing (vodun or not) with Western medical materials is common and becoming more prevalent in Aja.

Throughout my fieldwork, I commonly shared cases such as Jacques's with other *Sakpatanɔ* around Hondjin, specifically my mentor, Assa Akpa (see Kennell 2011) and Dekakon Sogadji. I did not ask them to determine diagnoses or to solve a problem, but to explain the narrative, what people meant, why people did what they did. Dekakon, a *Sakpatanɔ* and healer who specializes in psychological issues, offered thoughts that not only illuminate Jacques's case, but the Aja experience of sickness as well. First he talked about suffering and the Aja term *ɖu aya*, which is used often in Aja (including by Jacques's father). Dekakon explained

> It means that there is no satisfaction. How can I explain it. . . . It is like 'to breathe.' . . . But when such problems (sicknesses) exist, there is nothing that can be done. No matter how much effort, no satisfaction is found. You cannot eat the air, you will never be full, there is no substance, no smell, and no matter how much you try, it is futile. The Aja people suffer. Yes, we suffer much. Some of the suffering is brought on to us by ourselves, some is given to us by others. Some suffering exists for all people, even you, regardless of what they do: poverty, illiteracy, bareness, hunger, and disease. . . . We, the Aja, suffer in these ways.

Dekakon also talked about medical knowledge:

> There are different ways and forms to know things; you know one way, I know another. Your knowledge is different than mine, but both are good. . . . I am a healer, I have my knowledge that I learned from my father. I know the chief doctor at the hospital you met. The doctor at the hospital has his knowledge that he learned in a school, maybe in Europe. We both heal people, but we heal in different ways. All healing is good. The doctor does not want to know about how I heal, but I would like to learn how he heals.

The term *ɖu aya* indicates futility, hopelessness, the prospect that there is no solution, that the path leading to resolution is elusive, that healing will not be found. When continuous striving leads to no satisfaction, one is eating the air.

Dekakon and other *vodun* healers generally held the opinion that all medical knowledge is valid and useful; each not being complete but needing to learn from the other. Dekakon spoke of knowledge in two ways: *se gɔnmε* and *se wema*. *Se gɔnmε* and its noun form, *enugɔnmesese*, denote knowledge or understanding. *Se wema*, or *wemasese*, also means knowledge or understanding, but *wema* describes written or printed material: a book, a poster, a letter, a ticket, a doctor's prescription—any paper or like material with writing on it. Dekakon used *se gɔnmε* to refer to his own knowledge and the knowledge he received from his father. What he knew as a healer and a *vodunɔ* fell into the realm of *se gɔnmε*. When speaking of the doctor at the hospital, *se wema* was the term he used.

Jacques's father often elaborated on and spoke with visible frustration about his son's condition and the seeming impossibility of finding complete healing.

He often stated that he did not know what to do, where to go next, who could completely heal his son. Therapies were available; that was not the issue—but which one? Who knew what was wrong and who knew how to heal it? He did not know, and it seems that the more he searched, the more he strove to find satisfaction, the more elusive it became.

Janzen (1978, 1987) describes the *therapy management process* as the negotiation for control of therapeutic resources and the healing process by a therapy management group (all those who play a part in decision making and care seeking for a sick individual). For Jacques and his family, the path leading to healing was determined not only by the apparent changes in Jacques's skin condition, but by what his family knew—and what they did not know. Tension within the family and with therapy providers (over diagnosis and cure), along with the uncertainty of Jacques's condition, also contributed to the elusive path to healing. Medicines were available to Jacques, and his family seemed to be able to pay for them, and they tried several. For Jacques and his family, and for many Aja, from where the therapy comes, from whom, and from what kind of knowledge is not very important when one is on a path where sickness changes, diagnosis is often difficult, and medicines are available but often do not lead to any sign of healing.

A Northern Batonou Family's Suffering: Protection and Healing

In his groundbreaking book, *Quest for Therapy in Lower Zaire*, John Janzen notes, "The sufferer is but a symptom of his family's sickness" (Dr. Denis Bazinga, quoted in Janzen 1978, 114). In the next case, we follow the complex, chronic illness of Moudi, an individual whose life-threatening sickness is potentially a symptom of his family's social malaise, but whose illness also is perceived as putting his family's health at risk.[4] Moudi died in his prime, not older than 35, while enjoying a prosperous career as a member of the Benin military. One of nine children, he was the second-youngest son of his father's first wife. His father, the son of a highly ranked Baatonou[5] chief in the northern region of Benin, eventually inherited the chieftaincy, thus bestowing on his son a certain social standing, as a member of such a prestigious family. In the course of his career as a soldier, Moudi had the opportunity to travel to Europe and to the United States for training programs and moved steadily up the military hierarchy. His promotions enabled him to build an impressive two-story house with electricity and running water in a large town, near the homes of several of his brothers, cousins, and uncles.

Moudi was optimistic that he would achieve the wealth and respect that he merited. He married an equally successful young woman, employed as an administrative assistant by a humanitarian organization based in the primary city, Cotonou, and had four children. Then he was struck by increasingly severe yet vague symptoms. He suffered intermittent fever, loss of appetite, fatigue, and nausea. He consulted physicians and nurses at the military base, as well as at a provincial public hospital. Initially, his symptoms were sufficiently indeterminate that he was variously diagnosed with malaria, an intestinal virus, parasites ("worms"), and the illness known in France and in Francophone Africa as "crise de foie" (liver crisis). As he became increasingly unwell, his symptoms included fever and loss of appetite, and his urine darkened. He occasionally suffered from nausea and vomiting and made repeated visits to the public hospital, and eventually to a respected Italian hospital in the northern town of Tanguieta. There, he was diagnosed with hepatitis B or C (the accounts of his brothers, sisters, and mother varied on this point). After suffering for more than a year, Moudi was diagnosed—again at the Italian hospital—with liver cancer.

Worldwide, the most common risk factor for liver cancer is chronic (long-term) infection with hepatitis B virus (HBV) or hepatitis C virus (HCV). Moudi's diagnosis was therefore not unusual to the biomedical clinicians whom he consulted. In contrast, members of his extended family and his friends had diverse and contested interpretations of his symptoms, in particular the fundamental cause of his illness. After Moudi died in 2013, the discourse surrounding his sickness and death became even more heated. His youngest sister, Mariama, recounted the history of her brother's illness as she cried over coffee in a Paris café. She had come to Europe to visit her husband, a businessman.

I offered condolences and she sobbed; obviously Moudi's death is not "normal." She pointed out that many people suffer from hepatitis but not liver cancer. Surely the liver cancer was a sign that Moudi was afflicted for particular reasons. She went on to observe that her husband's family included Catholics, Methodists, and followers of the regional religion, *vodun*. Her own family was predominantly Muslim, at least nominally. But they also consulted local ritual specialists in the Baatombu community. Her conclusion: *everyone* in both families agreed that Moudi's illness had been "sent"—in other words, he was a victim of sorcery.[6] Echoing Evans-Pritchard's classic account of Azande interpretations of misfortune (1937), she cried "why him, why now?"

There are numerous reasons why Moudi himself suspected his illness was "not normal." His mother, his two brothers, and two sisters, as well as his sister's husband, gave similar (independent) explanations. Two principle causes emerged. First, Moudi had achieved considerable success in his military career. Historically, this had been a matter of some amusement in the family because (as I had occasion to observe), he had been a very stubborn and disobedient yet ingenious child. He once climbed in a locked window high above his head, while his mother was at the market, took a bottle of peanuts, and exited by the front door. His mother said she wondered about his future. Given his personality, he would surely be in the police or the military. She proved to be correct in her prediction.

Following university, he joined the army, and rose rapidly through the ranks. He benefited from several training programs in Europe and the United States and, as noted earlier, built a large concrete house with electricity and running water for his wife and four children, in a provincial capital.

To Moudi's family members, jealousy of his success and prosperity seemed to be the probable cause of his fatal illness. Jealousy about unequal production and consumption or about unequal access to commodities, employment, or a multiplicity of privileges, are well documented by Africanist scholars as associated with witchcraft/sorcery and other occult forces (Moore and Sanders 2001, 15; see also Nyamnjoh's 2001 discussion of how in the Bamenda Grassfields, Cameroon, personal success is thought to come at the expense of others). Moudi, himself, suspected his military comrades. He mulled over their envy of his promotions and his opportunities for international travel, as well as his financial prosperity.

Yet there was another possibility. The prestige and public presence of his father were also implicated in the explanations of Moudi's sickness. Because his father was ritually powerful and seemed well able to protect himself, enemies might have decided to attack one of his children instead. His father, reflecting on Moudi's death, mentioned such enemies as likely suspects in "sending" the illness. Collectively, the interpretation of Moudi's illness and demise began with the diagnosis of hepatitis B/C. Jealousy, either of Moudi or of his powerful father, led this sickness (not thought to be especially dangerous) to evolve into liver cancer, a fate particular to Moudi, because many have hepatitis B but most of these do not have liver cancer. In spite of all the interventions he sought over several years, Moudi could not overcome the assault on his life.

The family remains distraught at the memory of his suffering and the risks to others in the family. Moudi's mother, several months after his death, poignantly described his last hours. She could not forget how he called her name and she went in his room at his older brother's house where he was staying. She stood by his bed for a while, but he couldn't speak (or didn't), and she said well, if you're not speaking, I'll go back to my room. Not fifteen minutes later Moudi's wife called "mother, mother," and she rushed in so fast she fell three times; he was gasping, so she began to pray, "Allah-illah . . ." until he died. To the day of her death, she continued to ruminate on how he called her and what had he wanted to say? Had he intended to name his killer?

Each member of the family with whom I spoke traced Moudi's quest for therapy as his health declined. He visited the Centre National Hospitalier Universitaire, the country's primary public hospital; a hospital in a communal capital; private clinics in the commercial capital; the Italian private hospital in the far northeastern region of the country; and innumerable ritual specialists and herbalists. He contacted ritual specialists and herbalists known for expertise with medicinal plants in his natal community. Some were familiar to him through family connections, but others were recommended by word of mouth as his condition worsened. His mother approved of this multifaceted approach, ranging from biomedicine to ritual healing to herbalism, especially because she was so concerned about sorcery.[7] For a "sent" illness, biomedicine was hardly likely to be effective, whereas an Islamic healer or Baatonu ritual specialist could perhaps intervene successfully. His brothers, both university-educated professionals, relied on biomedicine and local medicines for their own preventive and curative care. For Moudi, they tacitly supported his diverse efforts to find a cure by whatever means.

It was Moudi's father who expressed disapproval of the local practitioners. This was surprising because he was an elderly man who consulted such specialists himself, and one might have expected that he would have confidence in their potential for diagnosis and treatment. However, he expressed the widely shared (see Sargent 1982, 1989) view that healers must be selected with great caution. They have power, but power can be used for good or for evil, depending on the individual character of the specialist. Accordingly, turning to one and then another and yet another healer is dangerous, without sufficient knowledge of each specialist's motivations and political agendas. Moudi's father feared that his own enemies among the population of healers would attack Moudi, rather than seek to heal him. Such enemies might use poison rather than plants designed to heal. Some of Moudi's symptoms, such as swelling of the torso and legs, seemed to him evidence of poisoning.

Two years after Moudi's death, the ramifications of the unresolved explanation of his illness remained significant. All his siblings (same mother, same father) feared that they were also at risk of liver cancer. Some had tested positive for hepatitis B and were searching for preventive medicines to protect against liver cancer. Moudi's mother became increasingly frail. Her knees were swollen and painful, as were her feet. She said her liver was a problem, and the doctor had told her to avoid salt and grease. So she could no longer eat any sauce (she said that I should see her sauce that she prepared for herself: "It's pitiful, a bit of mustard that's all." I did see her eat some fried yams, though). She seemed to focus on sauce as the culprit. Her knees caused her so much pain that she couldn't kneel for old men coming to call on her husband and had to apologize because she felt discourteous.

It was at this point that she left the village in the north and she went to the large southern city of Cotonou for treatment. She lived with her youngest daughter and near her eldest son. Several of her sons and one daughter contributed to her costs at private clinics there. They arranged for her to consult a knee specialist and a rheumatologist, who wanted her to go to Paris for knee replacements. One day she confided that her real question was whether her symptoms were those of "Moudi's sickness," particularly because of the swelling she experienced.

To further investigate this concern, she traveled to the nearby town of Porto Novo, to consult a ritual specialist who also worked with plants and was recommended by a friend of her oldest son. This specialist reassured her that her knee pain and swelling was not "a sickness from which one dies" and gave her medicinal dried plants with which to wash her knees. For a brief period, her knee pain lessened and she felt stronger. But within the year she died suddenly of unknown causes.

During the thirty years that I knew her, I often saw her prepare teas based on medicinal roots, leaves, and other plant preparations. I also watched her use a fumigation treatment, obtained from a village specialist, to protect the interior of our house from evil spirits. Born in a large city, she spent her married life in the village where her husband's parents resided. She prided herself on having adhered to local ideals and having delivered all her nine children at home, alone (see Sargent 1982, 1989). Yet as her children with university educations attempted to educate her about what it means to be "modern," she accepted their advice regarding the efficacy of biomedicine (while continuing to seek advice from herbalists and diviners). At the time of her last illness, she was showering in her youngest son's home in northern Benin. Suddenly, she was unable to move her arm. Her son and daughter-in-law carried her to bed. She could speak and refused to go to the hospital. The following day, when she was unable to move, in spite of her protests, they took her to the provincial capital hospital. She died soon after her arrival there.

Since her death, her children continue to seek ritual counsel and medicinal plant treatments to protect against sorcery-induced liver cancer. They also routinely consult clinicians at private biomedical clinics in the area or in the country's larger cities. On behalf of the youngest daughter, I questioned a prominent specialist in infectious and tropical diseases in Paris. He offered to initiate laboratory work to determine whether, indeed, she had some form of hepatitis and what might be done. To date, the daughter and her husband have not pursued this option.

Moudi's illness, his death, his pursuit of effective therapies, and his family's similar use of a range of therapeutic options exemplify the widespread reliance on diverse healing modalities. These may be used concurrently or alternately over time. Some might see contradictions inherent in a conceptualization of hepatitis that links this condition to both liver cancer and sorcery and considers it potentially responsive to biomedicine as well as local healing rituals and medicinal plant therapies. One might also question whether the lack of public resources for biomedical institutions and the consequent poor quality of care at many hospitals lead patients to consult diverse practitioners. In our experience, however, efficacy and quality of care are not sufficient to explain therapeutic itineraries. The legitimation of a continuum of treatment possibilities indicates that the lived experience of sickness allows for complex, intersecting interpretations of illness etiology and potential resolutions.

An additional case furthers our understanding of thinking through seemingly incompatible realities. At the same provincial hospital where Moudi sought care for his hepatitis, I met with three physicians—one a surgeon—during a conference. As we discussed their difficulties accessing medical journals, finding sufficient quantities of medication, and training adequate personnel, the surgeon's cell phone rang. He looked at the screen and said to his colleagues that the caller was "*him*," the villainous ritual specialist who was trying to kill the surgeon. As the phone continued to ring and no one answered, I offered to take on the role of the surgeon's secretary. I answered the phone and informed the caller that the surgeon could be seen only on the hospital grounds during office hours. The caller declined to leave a message. Subsequent to the call, the three physicians explained to me that the caller had contacted the surgeon previously to tell him that he had been offered a financial contract by an unnamed enemy to kill him. However, this ritual specialist had heard that the surgeon was very competent and would regret killing him. Such an unfortunate fate could be avoided if the surgeon paid the specialist the same sum offered for the contract killing. They asked me if I was afraid, because I had now spoken to the specialist and he might "have my voice" from the cell phone. They promised to let me know the sequel to this intriguing conversation. Months later, I learned from the surgeon that he had identified his enemy as someone opposed to him in a political hospital dispute. When he withdrew from the debate, he concluded that he was no longer at risk and has not received further threats.

In my discussions with the clinicians, we considered the merits of "traditional healers," as they referred to non-biomedical practitioners in the region. One said to me that we could not ever be certain of what powers exist in the universe and how they might be deployed. Describing the psychiatry service at the hospital, he pointed to the shortage of psychiatrists and the lack of interpreters. The local population had no concept of psychiatry and its goals. Occasionally, the psychiatrist would have access to antipsychotics and could help reduce the florid symptoms of a patient. But often there was very little that biomedical psychiatry had to offer. Families prefer traditional healers, he added. Thus "there is the hospital by day and the hospital by night." During the day, doctors and nurses work the wards as best they can. But by night, families bring in ritual specialists to heal their relatives. The psychiatrists are aware of this parallel healing but choose not to address it. In the words of Father Cardot, a Catholic priest long residing in the area, "there are things that are beyond us," a sentiment shared by the physicians with whom I spoke. They are confident that psychopharmacology will eventually lead to confidence in psychiatry among the local population, but they "tolerate" and indeed live with parallel understandings of illness.

These cases suggest that the concept of a therapeutic continuum is more useful than that of more rigidly bounded or discrete medical systems, between which individuals must choose. Rather, it is clear that the sick and those who comprise their therapy management groups (Janzen 1978) find it feasible and meaningful to move along a continuum of therapeutic options. Although some have proposed a link between concepts of illness etiology and choice of treatment, this is overly simplistic. Numerous examples indicate that sufferers may seek biomedical care for symptomatic relief while simultaneously consulting ritual specialists to divine the underlying cause. Causes of illness and sources of cure are often in dispute during a lengthy illness (Rasmussen 2001, 148). Perceptions of efficacy may also be implicated in the process of seeking health care. Both Moudi and his mother consulted herbalists, Islamic healers, Baatombu ritual specialists, nurses, doctors at public hospitals, and clinicians at expensive private clinics. Some consultations followed the failure of a previous treatment to eradicate symptoms. Others were thought of as supplementary or strengthening, preventative of further complications, or likely to enhance an earlier intervention.

Advice from kin often led to a recommendation to consult a particular specialist, not yet in the therapeutic repertoire. In the small community in which Jacques's family lived, they found therapy from a lone nurse with biomedical training who had a positive relationship with a local *Sakpatanɔ* (from whom they also found treatment) as well as a pseudo–religious/biomedical "doctor" who was both admired and scorned in the community. Each turn in Jacques's narrative presented him and his family with a fluid set of options—options that changed depending not only on symptoms but on treatments previously tried, location of possible therapy, familial tensions, alliances/rifts between medical and religious practitioners, and new information or possible therapy not previously available. Competition between medical systems or epistemologies may have played a role in Jacques's therapeutic trajectory, but as his parents sought out a cure for their son, the various epistemological roots of any available therapy were not of great concern. When treatment offered by the local *Sakpatanɔ* moved Jacques's diagnosis from *zohwiʒi* to something outside of his expertise, the change in diagnosis changed the available options for continued treatment. This and other such turns in Jacques's illness narrative show that the individual or familial perspective at a particular moment in the therapy-seeking experience reveal more than comparing or contrasting medical epistemologies.

In seeking to understand suffering as patients follow an elusive path to health, we might benefit from asking "What options when, and why?" "What external forces determine the fluidity of options?" and "What makes a particular option untenable?"

Educational level and expressed religious affiliation notwithstanding, our informants demonstrated different levels of confidence in a rich array of therapeutic options. As Moore and Sanders (2001, 2) argue, "it should not surprise us that education and science, the two most potent symbols and purveyors of progress and modernity, should not eradicate belief in the unseen, in the magical, in powers that transcend ordinary human control and comprehension." Thus the juxtaposition of biomedicine and ritual healing, microbes and sorcery, is not unexpected. The assumptions held regarding available therapies and the knowledge base from which they come are flexible and mixed. The symbols associated with different medical systems (religious, biomedical, local healing) are used in creative ways and draw sufferers based on meanings that are multifaceted. Therapeutic alternatives, drawing on divergent healing modalities, operate in complementarity, as the sick and their supporters strive to alleviate suffering and move towards greater health and well-being.

Notes

1. This section draws on Kennell's research in southern Benin.
2. A priest, the owner of the Sakpata shrine. *Sakpatanɔ* describes a *Sakpata vodunɔ*, and will be the term used from here on to specify Sakpata priests.
3. Many *vodunɔ*, regardless of deity association, are also healers. Not all healers are *vodunɔ*. Many specialize in a particular sickness or condition or even broad areas of health issues. For example, my mentor Assa Akpa specialized in respiratory problems. Dekakon, discussed below, specialized in psychological issues.
4. This section draws on research conducted by Sargent in northern Benin and in the commercial capital, Cotonou.
5. The Baatombu (singular Baatonou, also known as Bariba) are estimated to be the fourth largest ethnic group in the Republic of Benin.
6. I use the term sorcery because the family spoke of "sorcellerie," employing the French term. Geschiere also notes that in Maka villages in Cameroon, villagers now generally translate "witchcraft" as *sorcellerie* (Fisiy and Geschiere 2001, 227). Moore and Sanders (2001, 4) suggest that "occult forces" is more neutral usage than witchcraft or sorcery. However, here I will use the vocabulary of my informants. In the Baatonou language, there are numerous terms for different types of evil-doers (for example, *bii yondo*, witch babies) and for diverse poisons (for example *dobonu*) used to harm others. The family did not refer to these in discussions of Moudi's sickness, relying more generally on the concept of "sorcellerie."
7. Sorcerers may be identified at birth (Sargent 1982, 1989) by means of certain signs, such as breech birth or by appearance of a first tooth in the upper gum. Those who seek to "learn" acts of sorcery may consult a ritual specialist known to have such skills or spend time in certain locales, the village of Bori, for example, known as a site for learning how to use powerful substances for good or evil.

Bibliography

Chary, Anita and Peter Rohloff, eds. 2015. *Privatization and the New Medical Pluralism.* Lanham, MD: Rowman and Littlefield.

Cuellar, Carlos, Andrew Carmona, Andrea Harris, and Piotr Korynski. 2013. *Benin Private Health Sector Assessment: Strengthening Health Outcomes through the Private Sector Project.* Bethesda, MD: ABT Associates Inc.

Fisiy, Cyprian, and Peter Geschiere. 2001. "Witchcraft, Development and Paranoia in Cameroon: Interactions Between Popular, Academic and State Discourse." In *Magical Interpretations, Material Realities: Modernity, Witchcraft and the Occult in Postcolonial Africa,* edited by Henrietta Moore and Todd Sanders, 226–47. London and New York: Routledge.

Janzen, John M. 1978. *The Quest for Therapy in Lower Zaire.* Berkeley: University of California.

———. 1987. "Therapy Management: Concept, Reality, Process." *Medical Anthropology Quarterly* 1: 68–84.

———. 2014. "Imagining the Whole: Local Medicine and Global Health." In *Medical Anthropology in Global Africa,* edited by Kathryn Rhine, John M. Janzen, Glen Adams, Heather Aldersey, 19–27. Lawrence, KS: University of Kansas Publications in Anthropology 26.

Kennell, James Leslie. 2011. *The Senses and Suffering in Aja: Medical Knowledge, Vaccination Programs, and Spirit Possession.* Dissertation manuscript: Southern Methodist University.

———. 2014. "Vaccination Programs and the Sensibilisation of an Aja Community in Benin." In *Medical Anthropology in Global Africa,* edited by Kathryn Rhine, John M. Janzen, Glen Adams, Heather Aldersey, 27–33. Lawrence, KS: University of Kansas Publications in Anthropology 26.

Moore, Henrietta L., and Todd Sanders, eds. 2001. *Magical Interpretations, Material Realities: Modernity, Witchcraft and the Occult in Postcolonial Africa.* New York: Routledge.

Nyamnjoh, Francis. 2001. "Delusions of Development and the Enrichment of Witchcraft Discourses in Cameroon." In *Magical Interpretations, Material Realities: Modernity, Witchcraft and the Occult in Postcolonial Africa,* edited by Henrietta Moore and Todd Sanders, 28–50. New York: Routledge.

Rasmussen, Susan. 2001. "Betrayal or Affirmation? Transformations in Witchcraft Technologies of Power, Danger and Agency among the Tuareg of Niger." In *Magical Interpretations, Material Realities: Modernity, Witchcraft and the Occult in Postcolonial Africa,* edited by Henrietta Moore and Todd Sanders, 136–60. New York: Routledge.

Rhine, Kathryn. 2014. Introduction. In *Medical Anthropology in Global Africa,* edited by Kathryn Rhine, John M. Janzen, Glenn Adams, Heather Aldersey, 3–11. Lawrence, Kansas: University of Kansas Publications in Anthropology 26.

Rhine, Kathryn, John M. Janzen, Glenn Adams, Heather Aldersey. 2014. *Medical Anthropology in Global Africa.* Lawrence, Kansas: University of Kansas Publications in Anthropology 26.

Sargent, Carolyn. 1982. *The Cultural Context of Therapeutic Choice: Obstetrical Care Decisions Among the Bariba of Benin.* Boston: Kluwer.

———. 1989. *Maternity, Medicine, and Power: Reproductive Decisions in Urban Benin.* Berkeley: University of California.

Wendland, Claire. 2014. "The Anthropology of African Biomedicine." In *Medical Anthropology in Global Africa,* edited by Kathryn Rhine, John M. Janzen, Glenn Adams, Heather Aldersey, 45–53. Lawrence, KS: University of Kansas.

12 Legitimate Care, Dangerous Care, and Childbirth in an Urban African Community

Claire Wendland

IN A MILIEU OF THERAPEUTIC pluralism, sources of legitimation are also plural and contested. In this essay, I draw on ethnographic observations and interviews with people who attend women at birth in an urban Malawian community—both in health centers and hospitals, and outside of the spaces labeled medical—to explore the ways in which legitimation of expertise depends upon presumptions about the dangers of care.

Birth attendance is commonly understood in southeastern Africa to be dangerous to the person who provides it. Some forms of it are legally ambiguous. More importantly, according to both nurses and *azamba* (traditional birth attendants, or TBAs, who work outside of biomedical settings), exposure to the blood of childbirth renders caregivers vulnerable to both bloodborne and spirit-borne illnesses. Birth can "kill the eyes" of the attendant and can incite jealousies that erupt into potentially lethal witchcraft accusations.

Care can also be dangerous to the cared-for. Women in labor may be exposed to negligent care, to abuse, to iatrogenic injury. They may learn what they do not want to know, knowledge that is dangerous to them. They are also subject to blame. Maternity workers inside and outside the formal biomedical sector often blame pregnant women themselves—whom they characterize variously as ignorant, fearful, backward, promiscuous, willful, or simply poor—for dangerous birth.

Biomedically trained caregivers, working in places recognized by the state as healthcare facilities, and the informal-sector birth attendants, who work in what is often called "the village" even when it is within city limits, often level blame at one another for the dangers involved in contemporary childbirth. In so doing, each group seeks to bolster its own authority. Contests over authority and legitimation, some waged in the public domain through newspapers and radio announcements or community meetings with traditional authorities, risk exacerbating the maternal health problems they are ostensibly intended to mitigate.

Whose care endangers women, and what is at stake in assigning blame for unsafe care? Tensions over dangerous care, I argue, can make birth all the more dangerous in this community and others like it.

A love note from the TBA

Esme Lifa, twenty years old, came to a large public referral hospital in Malawi (which was also the hospital nearest to her crowded urban neighborhood) reporting fever, abdominal pain, and five months without a menstrual period.[1]

The intern who admitted her did a hasty workup—after all, there were many other women in the long queue, waiting to be seen—and recorded neither a temperature nor a pelvic examination on her medical case file, a few sheets of rumpled paper held together with a bit of string. The short admitting note listed only a tentative diagnosis: "query malaria, query septic abortion." No medications were ordered, no action taken other than assigning the young woman a narrow iron-framed cot on the gynecology ward among fifty-some other patients. More than twenty-four hours later a second intern, the conscientious young Dr. Makano, saw her and decided this was not malaria. He took her to the minor operating theater, carefully dilated her cervix with blunt metal probes, and then scraped out her uterus with a sharp curette.[2] When Dr. Makano found foul-smelling uterine contents and a cervical laceration, he knew he was seeing the aftermath of an attempted abortion. He started antibiotics, but it was too late. Soon after her return from the operating theater to the ward, Esme Lifa died, probably of septic shock caused by an overwhelming infection.

This case was one of several deaths presented at the obstetrics and gynecology department's maternal mortality review, held every two weeks. As Dr. Makano finished the story, a faculty physician began chuckling. "Isn't this the one who came with a love note from the TBA?" The intern leafed through the short file, unearthed a torn piece of lined paper, and read aloud: "I send Miss Lifa to hospital. She is five months. Look like she damaged her pregnancy. She need treatment." Several people giggled at the traditional birth attendant's fractured English.[3] An intern standing next to me, leaning up against the wall in the crowded room, glared down at the floor and muttered "I can't believe this." But the faculty physician laughed again. "A love note! We got a referral from the TBA!" Another doctor broke in: "You may laugh, but it looks to me like the TBA made the right diagnosis and we did not." At that correction, the laughter petered out. But even though another woman died the same week in similar circumstances, no one suggested changes to standard hospital practices to help ensure rapid treatment. Esme Lifa was written off as another disaster from the TBA, her death a consequence of seeking assistance outside the hospital's walls.

Whose labor of care endangers pregnant women, and who cares? How do struggles over whose care is legitimate affect the safety of maternity? This volume considers therapeutic pluralism in contemporary Africa, including the differential valuation and mobilization of care provided by professionals or nonprofessional non-elites. In this chapter, I explore how various experts—people who attend births inside or outside the formal medical sector—speak about dangerous maternity care. Discussions of unsafe care show some commonalities between skilled and unskilled, professional and non-elite birth experts, in addition to revealing the sharp divisions one might expect. Those divisions themselves may exacerbate birth's dangers. Showing how dangerous care gets used rhetorically in a Malawian context to advance some experts' legitimacy at the expense of others, in the course of the chapter I describe how and where care happens, and what the implications are for considering—and perhaps mitigating—the social production of dangerous care.

Rather than writing about dangerous care, I could have chosen to use the term *iatrogenesis*. Etymologically, *iatrogenic* means "brought forth by the physician/healer." Medically trained people use it commonly to describe unintended injuries produced by biomedical interventions. An abdominal abscess that forms around a surgical sponge left in a wound is an iatrogenic injury, for instance. By using *dangerous care* instead of *iatrogenesis*, I am trying to look more broadly at damaging practices: to consider not only those that occur *within* any given medical system, at the encounter between the one charged with healing and the one afflicted, but those that happen in the silences and hostilities *between* medical systems—in a context in which the very existence of a "love note" from the TBA serves as warrant for the superiority of biomedical care and justification to overlook its dangers.

Maternal Mortality in Malawi

Maternal mortality in Malawi, a subject of national and international attention, has been very high for a long time—high even for a region in which maternal death has been a stubborn and refractory problem. The most current reports at the time of writing estimate a girl's lifetime risk of dying from a pregnancy-related complication at one in thirty-four; only fourteen other countries are as bad or worse (Save the Children 2015).[4] Numbers like these put Malawi's maternal death rates in the range of those in deeply troubled post-conflict states like Sierra Leone. It is only fair to add that all numbers, including these, must be taken as highly uncertain estimates. Until very recently Malawi has not mandated any civil registration: given the financial and bureaucratic obstacles entailed in reporting, even now most deaths, like most births, go unreported to any government bureaucracy (see Singogo et al. 2013). Mortality rates like these are estimated rather than counted, a process that—while fascinating—is outside the purview of this chapter.[5]

Despite these limitations and uncertainties, it has been clear to experts and laypersons alike for some decades that Malawi's maternal mortality is bad, even for the region. The national newspapers frequently run front-page reports about maternal mortality and efforts to curtail it. International groups promoting better maternity care, such as Safe Motherhood and the White Ribbon Alliance, have been active in Malawi for decades. The government of Malawi has worked with a host of bilateral and multilateral aid organizations including DFID, EU, JICA, NORAD, UNFPA, UNICEF, USAID, WHO, and the World Bank to improve maternity care in various districts (Ministry of Health 2010). Yet at the time I began conducting fieldwork in Malawi, just after the turn of the millennium, maternal mortality seemed to be getting substantially worse despite all of these efforts (McCoy et al. 2004).

During the decade that followed, maternal mortality was more and more widely spoken about, in part due to well publicized tracking of the Millennium Development Goals, one of which (MDG 5) specifically called for a reduction of maternal deaths by three quarters by 2015. In Malawi, unsafe motherhood got an even higher profile when Joyce Banda, the nation's president from 2012 to early 2014, made a personal and presidential mission of reducing maternal deaths. Banda, a women's rights lawyer, had a long track record as an activist before her selection as vice president in 2009. After the sudden death of the sitting president, she survived an intense succession crisis. In its aftermath, her presidential legitimacy was shaky: she was unelected, she was a woman, and at the time of the president's death, their relationship was so tense that he had been attempting to remove her from her vice presidential position (a move blocked by Malawi's constitution). Reduction of maternal mortality became central to her own political stature as well as an intensely felt personal mission (see discussion in Vaughan 2013). As one key strategy, she devolved responsibility to chiefs, whom she encouraged to try new approaches in their communities—such as, for instance, promoting in-hospital births at community meetings, or developing bicycle ambulance systems. This strategy was a clever one: granting power to the chiefs bolstered Banda's support among the nation's traditional patriarchy. It also ensured that a range of approaches to improving maternal health could be tried out, rather than committing fully to any one strategy that might fail.

Categorizing Births in a Medically Plural Context

For many of the chiefs, the traditional birth attendant was an obvious target for intervention: surely births would become safer if one simply made certain that all births happened in-hospital with trained nurse-midwives and doctors. On closer investigation, however, the category of TBA turns out to be more complex than it initially appears—as does the category of "skilled birth attendant."

Until recently, an estimated half of all births in Malawi happened outside biomedical settings (National Statistical Office 2003). Some of these out-of-hospital births are not attended by anyone: the pregnant woman delivers her own child unassisted. Most births are attended, however, whether by a kinswoman or, more often, by someone who has accrued experience at other births and is known locally as an *mnzamba*.[6] Some *azamba* have delivered hundreds or even thousands of babies. Some have delivered dozens. Some have a little biomedical training from the days in which training them was on the agenda of international safe motherhood programs. Some have none. Some of the *azamba* call themselves TBAs, others leave that label to those who have attended a training program. Some identify as herbalists, spend most of their time administering treatments for infertility, and attend only those rare births for which their treatment is generally considered responsible. The divisions between helpful relatives or neighbors who have attended a few births; *azamba*, who may have attended a few (or many) more; and "traditional birth attendant" are blurry and shifting. For statistical purposes, however, when the National Statistical Office or various nongovernmental groups tally health indicators, essentially anyone who attends an out-of-hospital birth is put in this blanket category of TBA.[7]

Births attended within the formal medical sector turn out to be quite heterogeneous too. The phrase "out-of-hospital birth" may erroneously conjure a hospital—with doctors, ambulances, and operating rooms—as the referent category to which it is Other. Births do happen in the country's two large and two more modest public referral hospitals, its twenty-odd small district hospitals, and its scattered mission and private facilities. Many births also happen in health centers, small outposts often staffed by a single nurse or medical assistant. Health centers do not have surgical capacity (either trained personnel or equipment) and typically lack technologies like oxygen or suction. Maternity care is the sole inpatient service offered.

Just as all these different spaces are covered by the Chichewa word *chipatala*, and all births within them count as "health facility births," so any employee who attends a birth there is likely to get the bureaucratic label "skilled birth attendant."[8] At health centers, most such attendants have two to three years total postsecondary training, most of it spent in general medicine, with a limited time spent on maternity care. These are medical assistants (typically male) or enrolled nurses (typically female). In district hospitals, some have more training—including generalist doctors, or the clinical officers also trained to do surgery, or the trained nurse-midwives who attend most district- and referral-hospital vaginal births. In the referral hospitals, one can find a few obstetricians as well. Some facility births are attended by people who have far *less* training, such as the community health workers called "health surveillance assistants," or HSAs. HSAs are commonly pressed into nursing roles when staff is short; many reported to me that they regularly attend antenatal clinics and occasionally attend births when there is no one else to do so. While health planners are well aware that this kind of stopgap "task shifting" is likely to endanger mothers and newborns, the enormous gap between minimal staffing needed for effective care and actual staffing means it continues to happen (Ministry of Health 2010).[9] Like TBAs, skilled birth attendants are a markedly heterogeneous group in training, skill, and experience.

Since 2001, and more intensively beginning in 2007, I have spoken with many Malawians consulted as experts by childbearing women, about evenly split between people the WHO would designate as skilled birth attendants and people who do not fit that term. These interviews form part of a research project on how people account for maternal deaths in a place of profound diagnostic uncertainty, therapeutic pluralism, and economic scarcity. Roughly a hundred were formal interviews, taped and transcribed; others were informal conversations. I also attended for some of this time as an obstetrician at a large public referral hospital. That position gives me valuable access to some sources. It also entails real limitations: most people who spoke with me, whether in Chichewa on reed mats under a tree or in English on a wooden bench in a health center hallway, knew I was a physician. Their responses were likely shaped by that knowledge. Legal concerns meant that I was prohibited by the two research ethics oversight committees that approved the project from observing births outside the hospital.[10] Because I studied experiences of people who provide maternity care, not those who seek it, I know only a little about what pregnant women and their families understand to be the dangers of care. (I have spoken informally with women who sought care in hospitals and women who avoided them on many occasions, but these conversations were never systematic.) The discussion here focuses, then, on the words of people sought out by members of their communities for antenatal and intrapartum care.

Care Is Dangerous

The experts with whom I spoke included those who had purchased proprietary treatment techniques from other healers, those who had learned as young girls at the side of their *azamba* mothers, those to whom appropriate therapeutic measures were revealed in dreams, and those for whom they were spelled out in handwritten posters curling off a health center wall. They included an herbalist who had apprenticed with a famous healer in South Africa, a doctor who had gone to get obstetrics training there, and many practitioners—whether working in formal or informal medical contexts—who had never left Malawi. When they spoke about care, sometimes it was to describe the good care they provided. Sometimes they spoke about dangerous care.

Dangers to the provider were a frequent topic of discussion. Midwives or doctors in the United States are likely to think of the dangers of medical malpractice litigation. In Malawi too, legal accountability for birth care is a growing concern. Malpractice cases are rare, but a few have been filed and fought in Malawi's judicial system. Negligent care is sometimes also tried in the court of public opinion, including in the newspapers.

Azamba face additional legal dangers. In 2007, Malawi's Ministry of Health made attendance at out-of-hospital birth illegal. Chiefs and traditional authorities were granted enforcement authority. Chiefs instituted bylaws and fines, sometimes for TBAs found attending women in pregnancy, labor, or the aftermath, sometimes also for their clientele, and sometimes for anyone reporting a maternal death outside a health facility. The fines could be substantial: large sums of cash, or several goats. Some *azamba* stopped practicing. Others went underground.

While the ban was repealed three years later, it had substantial lingering effects. Several doctors and nurse-midwives reported that the ban made it possible for them to stop supervising, registering, or training traditional birth attendants—a stoppage that some lamented but most felt was appropriate and that continued even when the ban was over. They contended that the existence of liaison services had legitimized dangerous practices; two also noted that TBA trainings allowed the government to be "doing something" about maternity care at very little expense and without training badly needed additional biomedical personnel. Birth attendance by an *azamba* now lies in something of a legal limbo. The stigma of the ban lingers, the formal relationships with biomedical practitioners have ended, and those who *do* work as *azamba* tend to do so quietly. The typical practice among the *azamba* with whom I have spoken in recent years seems to be to refer women to the health center if they appear to be in early labor, but to make themselves available to attend laboring women too far into the process to make it safely to a formal health facility. Women who prefer to deliver outside the *chipatala* wait until their labor is advanced to make their way to the *azamba*—not a stratagem that is likely to maximize safety. In some communities, chiefs continue to fine anyone attending an out-of-hospital birth, or even found to have had one.

Legality, however, was not the major concern of those providing obstetric care, whether biomedically trained clinicians or *azamba*: exposure to the blood of childbirth was. Many providers, in all settings, worried about HIV. During the period of this research, HIV testing was not available at all in the community setting and not always available at clinics or hospitals when reagents ran out or when people trained to run the tests and provide the designated counseling were unavailable. Even when tests were on offer, however, some women refused to be tested. Clinicians would guess who might be seropositive based on their thin-ness, chronic diarrhea, a characteristic skin rash, or certain infections that were typically opportunistic. One physician frequently canceled operations—even ur-gent ones—for women he suspected of being "chronically ill" based on such clini-cal markers. Given the scarcity of surgeons, this practice converted a perceived danger of care into overtly dangerous care: often enough, there was no one else to do the surgery, and women and infants were put at great risk. This man was an exception, however. Most clinicians did necessary procedures day after day, speaking with resignation—if sometimes also bitterly—about the risks posed by scalpels, needles, and blood splashes.[11]

In villages and urban slums, *azamba* also worried about HIV. In days past, they had sometimes received packets of gloves from the district health office; several asked me to intervene with the office to resume this practice, one of the many that ended with any formal relationship between TBAs and the formal sec-tor. In the meantime, in place of gloves they made do with the ubiquitous thin blue plastic "jumbos" in which sugar and other goods are sold.

Blood could bear dangers other than viruses, however. *Azamba* spoke of spirit-borne illnesses alongside bloodborne infections. Birth work is well known to be spiritually dangerous in the wider region that includes Malawi, and some say that maternity care can "kill the eyes." Nancy Hunt's interlocutors in the Congo used this phrase in the early 1990s; twenty years later it is still common-place in Malawi. *Azamba* and herbalist Mama Agnes Sambani explained that one can go blind from too much looking at the private parts of another's body. Only skilled *azamba* know the protective *mankhwala* to apply to their brows. Ja-net Rose Saikonde, another *azamba* and herbalist, paced herself: "When it is too much I refuse to see them [pregnant women], because as the adage goes, this can kill the eyes. So I kind of take a break and concentrate on the side of traditional healing." Birth work, if undertaken lightly by those without expert knowledge, can have terrible consequences.

Endangered Mothers

The most profound consequences of inexpert or uncaring care are those experi-enced by mothers and infants. Experts in medical spaces typically blame those outside them for dangerous care, while those outside sometimes blame the medi-cal workers. For instance, *azamba* Ruth Welemu explained that pregnancy is safe only as long as people don't rush to the *chipatala* to deliver. Those who filled their minds with fear and went to the hospital for assistance would find trouble there, she warned, but if you stay out of the hospital "so long as you put your mind to the fact that you are pregnant, you will deliver without a problem."[12] Owen

Kamfoloma, a health surveillance assistant at the small *chipatala* in that same neighborhood, believed that birth was dangerous only if one delivered with a TBA. "If [mothers] have got problems, they can easily lose—their baby can easily die, even the mother due to bleeding. Even there are also traditional birth attendants who are not well trained. So if [mothers] go there, they don't give enough care to them: the baby can die, and also the mother." Women could die because they were far from necessary and lifesaving surgical care: as the well-known saying has it, a chance to cut can be a chance to cure.

Rachel Chapman (2010) has shown in Mozambique that simply attending prenatal care at all—whether with a TBA or a nurse—can be dangerous. In making public one's knowledge of pregnancy, one may incite spiritual dangers that arise from the malignant jealousies of others. The Malawians to whom I spoke, in contrast, rarely mentioned the dangers of jealousy. Perhaps the difference is because the people who spoke with me about dangerous care were largely those providing antenatal care rather than those seeking it (or deciding not to seek it); Chapman's work was most intensive with pregnant women themselves. Perhaps the difference is because pregnancy in Malawi, while very much desired, is also feared—an effect, perhaps, of the substantial publicity about Malawi's persistently high maternal death rates conveyed through radio campaigns, politicians' press conferences, safe-motherhood awareness projects and everyday talk. As village counselor Annettie Manyunga said, "In the old days, you used to be jealous of those who beat you to another pregnancy, but nowadays birth is much more a time for fear."

As birth attendants saw it, knowledge, ignorance, inattention, and intervention all pose dangers to pregnant women. In the *chipatala*, sometimes women learned what they did not wish to know. One piece of dangerous knowledge was an HIV diagnosis, which in addition to its psychic burdens was well known to lead to domestic violence, abandonment, or divorce (see, e.g., discussion in Mkandawire-Valhmu, et al. 2013). Nurse Eliza Singano believed the threat of an HIV diagnosis to be the single most important factor driving women away from the clinic. "Most of them are HIV-positive," she said of the women who avoided Malawi's hospitals: they flee to the TBA rather than be forced to opt out of the test or to face their results. For this nurse-midwife and others, going to an *azamba* risked dangerous *ignorance*: women might not learn what they desperately needed to know, whether that be their HIV status or the danger signs of pregnancy complications, drilled into women's minds through posters and songs in the antenatal clinics.

Maternity workers inside and outside the formal sector also blamed one another for dangerous actions, or inaction. Medical personnel reported that TBAs caused obstructed labor by failing to intervene when women labored for days, and that herbalists gave *mankhwala* that effectively induced labor, but gave it in unregulated dosages that were often far too powerful. Some herbalists scoffed at this accusation—or blamed women themselves for incorrect dosing. Mafumu, for instance, explained that "Every time that I am administering medicine, I taste it myself, just to have an idea of the effect of the medicine. We just don't give medicine any which way. . . . I stress on the dosage as well. If they follow what I tell them, then it's fine, but if they mix wrongly, then it becomes poisonous." Others distanced themselves from those who gave such medicines. Kettie Pensulo and Dyna Ng'ong'ola, both *azamba* with over twenty years' experience, ran a spotless little birth center far on the outskirts of the city, accessible only by a long dirt path that wound through fields and gardens. Both of them expressed strong disapproval of the kinds of medications that Mafumu gave. Kettie Pensulo explained: "Some of those herbal concoctions are too strong and they may harm the unborn baby: the baby may be born with blisters, or indeed may die. It is not advisable to use anything to speed up the baby's descent into the birth canal. If you use force you may cause some damage, you [should] let nature take its course." These two *azamba* described cordial relations with the nearest *chipatala* and frequently referred women with complex medical conditions to the nurses there.

Other village healers and *azamba* were not so sanguine about medical care. Some reported that women languished in the *chipatala* waiting for someone to attend to them—or were treated rudely, or sent away because they had neglected to bring along a clean razor blade to cut the umbilical cord, threads to tie it off, or a cloth in which to wrap the newborn.[13] Philippina Macheso, an *azamba*, had delivered her own children in a *chipatala* in days past but did not see much point in doing so now, given the limited supplies there: "Back then we didn't have to bring our own razor blades, we didn't have to bring threads. The hospital used to provide everything." Several charged hospital workers with performing dangerous and unwanted surgeries. These included sterilizations done without consent at a woman's second or third cesarean, once performed, according to unwritten rule, by nearly all obstetrics providers in Malawian hospitals and still widely practiced if now debated.[14] They also included unnecessary cesarean sections, which several informal-sector practitioners reported were especially common among the youngest pregnant women. "Right here in our village there was a young woman who was pregnant, but when her time came she was operated on in the theatre," reported herbalist Dinesi Thomas. "We concluded that it is dangerous to give birth nowadays."

Danger and Blame

While it is not the major focus of this chapter, the evidence suggests that as pressure mounts for *someone* to be held accountable for maternal deaths, many maternity care providers blame women—for not taking care of themselves, for not knowing enough, for being too fearful or not fearful enough, for seeking care late, or not at all, or with the wrong person, or in the wrong place. In this chapter, however, I consider more closely other kinds of work that blame for unsafe motherhood can do.

Providers sometimes stake their own therapeutic legitimacy on the dangerous care of others. The biomedically trained birth workers who spoke about out-of-hospital birth nearly always saw it as a problem. In distancing themselves from the practitioners who worked in that context, speaking of them as dangerous or backward, they positioned themselves as both safe and modern. Out-of-hospital maternity care providers took one of two tacks. While some allied themselves closely with the hospitals, proudly recounting their own earlier training or friendly relations with local healthcare workers and differentiating themselves from the dangerous practices of other informal-sector practitioners, others denigrated the quality and safety of in-hospital care.

Several herbalists and *azamba* boasted of herbal treatments that helped women avoid unnecessary and dangerous surgeries, often claiming that their treatments, unlike the hospital's, never failed. Mama Thokozire, a very old *azamba*, used a mash of cooked wild fruit—applied topically to a woman's vulva and vagina—to open the path for birth in difficult labors. Janet Rose Saikonde administered a medicine locally called *mwanamphepo* (wind that brings the baby) to bring on labor. She had other medicines, revealed to her in dreams, that could straighten out a fetus in an improper position or a fetus that "can't find the birth canal." Women with such pregnancies were advised at the hospital that they needed surgery, she said. But "me knowing my trade, I give her my traditional medicine and before the operation the baby's position changes and the mother has a natural birth."

Meanwhile some physicians claimed that medical control would end the scourge of maternal deaths if out-of-hospital births in general, and *azamba* in particular, were eliminated. Dr. Anderson Muula, a faculty member at the University of Malawi's College of Medicine, wrote in 2010 as follows on an apparent improvement in maternal mortality in Ntcheu and Machinji districts: "What did these districts do? Certainly no randomized controlled trials, no case-control studies, or ecological studies. It is simple. They just banned home deliveries. Traditional leaders formulated a regulation that anyone who delivered or allowed a home delivery will be fined. No excuses; no maternal death has been registered so far" (Muula 2010, 90).

Care happens in relation, Annemarie Mol (2008) reminds us. It is worked out and reworked as particular caregivers and people cared for together use technologies and knowledge to resolve difficulties and address problems. The anthropology of care redirects attention away from amorphous institutions to the intimate practices between people (Stevenson 2014). What can be more intimate than a scalpel incising flesh to expose glistening organs and a waiting fetus, or a hand massaging a vulva with a paste of wild fruits to widen the path for birth? Just like good care, dangerous care also happens between the carer and the cared for: between elite professionals and their patients, or between non-elite *azamba* and their clients. But dangerous care, I am arguing, also happens *between* carers, among those who labor *with* those who labor.

Expert knowledge can be lethal

One last story can show how dangerous care comes about in the silences between health systems, the refusals to anticipate—or even to acknowledge—what is likely to happen in another context of care.

Mercy Kumwenda came to a large Malawi hospital in active labor. Her progress stalled as her contractions diminished. This kind of delay in active labor happens regularly. In practice in the United States, after a careful evaluation, I would typically order an oxytocin drip. Oxytocin, a synthetic version of the hormone that causes labor contractions, is one of the most important and most commonly used medications in obstetrics. One begins with tiny doses and increases slowly, using an intravenous pump to deliver the precise amount ordered. Too little oxytocin, and labor will remain ineffective; too much, and prolonged intense contractions can cause fetal distress or even make the uterine muscle rupture. Uterine rupture is rare but catastrophic. It is more likely when a woman's uterus is worn from many pregnancies or a very prolonged labor.

Even in the central hospitals in Malawi we had no intravenous pumps; they are expensive. Oxytocin must run through a regular IV line. One can make a rough dosage calculation by counting the number of drops that move through the cannula every minute, then adjusting that drip rate using a little roller to wedge the IV line closed for a slower flow or to open it up for a faster rate. But suppose someone bumps the roller? Or suppose the tip of a needle that has been pushed up against the wall of a patient's vein gets jolted free when she moves? Then the drip rate can suddenly increase and she can get a great deal more oxytocin than was planned . . . or is safe. And so, quite understandably, oxytocin is used very cautiously in Malawi. Hospital policy stipulates that anyone who had already had five or more births should not get the drug at all because of the risk of uterine rupture. Mercy Kumwenda was on her ninth delivery. The clinical officer told her she would need a cesarean section. While by all accounts this clinical officer could be brusque and peremptory with patients, I do not know what words he said, or how the conversation went. When the nurses came to the patient's bedside to bring her to the operating theatre for her cesarean, however, she had disappeared.

No one at the hospital knew where Mercy Kumwenda had gone until she was brought back that afternoon dead. Her distraught husband told the labor-ward nurse-midwives that they had gone to a practitioner in the community so that Mrs. Kumwenda could drink *mwanamphepo* to stimulate labor. It worked, as Mafumu and Janet Rose Saikonde and others claimed it always did. The intensity of her contractions increased so much that her uterus ruptured. Her husband bundled her into the minibus in great pain, and she died en route.

Mercy Kumwenda's death, like that of Esme Lifa in the story that began this chapter, is not a simple case of iatrogenesis. It is a fatality produced in the interaction (or failure to interact) of two medical systems that legitimize themselves in opposition. "A chance to cut is a chance to cure," and for that you need a hospital. *Mwanamphepo* never fails to produce contractions, unlike the medicines of those doctors. In this case, the product of two forms of expert knowledge was lethal.

Lisa Stevenson (2014) has recently explored the destruction wrought by anonymous care—that is, the kind of biopolitical projects that simply attempt to keep people alive without recognizing what "living" actually means to them as individuals or communities. In the Canadian Arctic, a tuberculosis epidemic was curtailed at enormous social cost to Inuit families and communities. Anonymous care in the cases I have described here might include protocols intended to apply to every woman who has had more than five children, prescriptions applied to all those heterogenous people lumped into the invented category of TBA, medical and economic policies extended to every low-income country. Perhaps anonymous care has its equivalent in the informal sector too, in practices that "never fail" (unless their failure can in some way be blamed on their users).

The possibility of dangerous care is entailed in the possibility of care: healing and harming are often—perhaps everywhere—two sides of one coin. In rural New Mexico, Angela Garcia (2010) shows us that loving care for a heroin addict may involve procuring the drug that is killing her. In urban Botswana, Julie Livingston (2012) describes the constantly improvised care for cancer that involves poisoning, cutting, and burning under their professional pseudonyms chemotherapy, surgery, and radiotherapy. In a peri-urban Malawian context of therapeutic pluralism, nurses and doctors worry that forging caring or collaborative relationships with *azamba* in the community makes them complicit in dangerous care.

But lack of relationship in this pluralistic world of maternity care may also be complicity. Fractured relations that make listening to one another impossible, indefensible, or professionally threatening bring additional perils to what is already a perilous process for Malawian women. When one person's dangerous care is another person's claim to legitimacy, tensions over dangerous care can further imperil the already fraught process of family and social reproduction in this community and others like it.

Notes

1. All names from fieldnote and interview excerpts in this essay, save one, are pseudonyms: Owen Kamfoloma, a health surveillance assistant, specifically requested that his real name be used.

2. This common procedure is usually known as a dilatation and curettage, or D&C, in North America. It is most often used to reduce bleeding from a miscarriage or to induce abortion, although it can also be used for various diagnostic purposes in non-pregnant women.

3. This referral note was a rarity, as it is quite unusual for a traditional birth attendant to be literate in English. In Malawi, instruction in English begins at grade five and few students achieve English literacy before secondary school. In my study sample, of all peri-urban informal-sector birth attendants interviewed, a third had no formal education at all, most had fewer than three years schooling, and none had gone past primary school.

4. All fourteen are African nations, nearly all of them—unlike Malawi—afflicted by chronic civil conflict or open warfare.

5. See Wendland 2016 for an extended discussion of the statistical modeling process used to estimate mortality rates, and its limits.

6. Because the plural, *azamba*, is also an honorific used in respectful speech to adults, I will use the term *azamba* in the remainder of the chapter whether referring to one or more of these women.

7. Langwick (2012), following Pigg (1995, 1997), explains how TBAs are "made up" through bureaucratic practices of counting and labeling. The invention and homogenization of "the TBA" as third-world Other also renders stable the categories of people to which she is defined in opposition—categories including the "skilled birth attendant."

8. Technically the term "skilled attendant" is reserved for nurses, clinical officers, and doctors. However, any male providing care at a health center is called "doctor" by most patients, as any female is called "nurse" (or "sister"). Given that the statistics on skilled attendance are based on surveys of randomly selected recently delivered women, over-reporting of skilled attendance is a near certainty. The recent push for health facility birth, and the concomitant stigmatization of birth attendance by TBAs, may also be contributing to over-reporting. A comparison of staffing figures in a national assessment of maternity care (Ministry of Health 2010) with estimates of skilled attendance in the Demographic and Health Survey conducted that same year (National Statistical Office 2011) lends further support to the conclusion that many "skilled birth attendants" are probably not people who fit the official criteria.

9. A 2010 survey by the Malawi Ministry of Health confirmed "huge shortfalls in staff": only 40 percent of target positions for enrolled nurses, 47 percent for registered nurses, and 28 percent for clinical officers were filled (Ministry of Health 2010, 20). These shortfalls leave two possibilities: either patients are not treated at all, or they are treated by people with less training than the Ministry of Health deems necessary to the task. Health policy analysts refer to this latter practice as "task shifting."

10. The study of birth attendants was reviewed and approved by the University of Malawi College of Medicine Research Ethics Committee and by the University of Wisconsin-Madison Social and Behavioral Science Institutional Review Board. An earlier study of medical students and doctors, on which I also draw in this chapter, was approved by the University of Malawi College of Medicine Research Ethics Committee.

11. Those risks were not only the dangers of bodily infection; they also included damages to one's reputation. Biomedically trained providers considered not only the possibility of contracting HIV from the blood of childbearing women at delivery, or in surgery, or when setting

up intravenous drips, but also the likelihood that *when* they contracted HIV at work, they would be the subject of gossip about immoral sexual behavior at home. Both blood and rumors made them vulnerable. See the longer discussion in Wendland 2010, ch. 5.

12. As with several other points made by *azamba*, herbalists and counselors, this is my translation of a comment made in Chichewa. It has been checked with a native speaker of the language.

13. These stories from urban contexts fit with the findings of Kumbani and colleagues (2013), who show that stories of bad treatment at health centers circulate widely in rural Malawi. Interviewing women who had attended antenatal care at a clinic but delivered with a TBA, they found numerous reports of bad treatment given to others: cruelty, inattention, rough exams, shouting, even slapping. In almost all cases women reported that they had heard about such care from others but not experienced it themselves. However, these reports were enough to keep them away from the health centers.

14. This practice was intended to eliminate the risk of rupturing the uterine scar in a future pregnancy, a phenomenon that is relatively rare but often devastating when it does occur, especially where prompt medical aid is unlikely. Following the analysis by Denise Roth Allen (2002), based on her work in Tanzania, we might consider unwanted sterilization at repeat Cesarean one of the threats *to* motherhood that are often ignored or discounted by programs invested in reducing threats *of* motherhood.

Bibliography

Chapman, Rachel. 2010. *Family Secrets: Risking Reproduction in Central Mozambique*. Nashville: Vanderbilt University.

Garcia, Angela. 2010. *The Pastoral Clinic: Addiction and Dispossession along the Rio Grande*. Berkeley: University of California.

Hunt, Nancy Rose. 1999. *A Colonial Lexicon of Birth Ritual, Medicalization and Mobility in the Congo*. Durham, NC: Duke University.

Kumbani, Lily, et al. 2013. "Why Some Women Fail to Give Birth at Health Facilities: A Qualitative Study of Women's Perceptions of Perinatal Care from Rural Southern Malawi." *Reproductive Health* 10 (9): 1–12.

Langwick, Stacey. 2012. "The Choreography of Global Subjection: The Traditional Birth Attendant in Contemporary Configurations of World Health." In *Medicine, Mobility and Power in Global Africa: Transnational Health and Healing*, edited by Hansjörg Dilger, Abdoulaye Kane, and Stacey Langwick. Bloomington: Indiana University.

Livingston, Julie. 2012. *Improvising Medicine: An African Oncology Ward in an Emerging Cancer Epidemic*. Durham, NC: Duke University.

McCoy, David, Hannah Ashwood-Smith, Esther Ratsma, et al. 2004. Going from bad to worse: Malawi's maternal mortality. An analysis of the clinical, health systems and underlying reasons, with recommendations for national and international stakeholders. Durban: Health Systems Trust and Global Equity Gauge Alliance.

Ministry of Health, Republic of Malawi. 2010. *Malawi 2010 EmONC Needs Assessment Final Report*. Lilongwe, Malawi: Ministry of Health.

Mkandawire-Valhmu, Lucy, et al. 2013. "Marriage as a Risk Factor for HIV: Learning from the Experiences of HIV-infected Women in Malawi." *Global Public Health* 8 (2): 187–201.

Mol, Annemarie. 2008. *The Logic of Care: Health and the Problem of Patient Choice.* New York: Routledge.

Muula, Adamson S. 2010. "My Africa: What Can Mchinji and Ntcheu Districts in Malawi Tell Maternal Health Pundits Globally?" *Croatian Medical Journal* 51: 89–90.

National Statistical Office. 2003. *Malawi in Figures 2002.* Zomba, Malawi: National Statistical Office.

National Statistical Office and ICF Macro. 2011. *Malawi Demographic and Health Survey 2010.* NSO and ICF Macro.

Pigg, Stacy. 1995. "Acronyms and Effacement: Traditional Medical Practitioners (TMP) in International Health Development." *Social Science & Medicine* 41 (1): 47–68.

———. 1997. "Found in Most Traditional Societies: Traditional Medical Practitioners Between Culture and Development." In *International Development and the Social Sciences: Essays on the History and Politics of Knowledge,* edited by F. Cooper and R. Packard, 259–90. Berkeley: University of California.

Save the Children. 2015. *The Urban Disadvantage: State of the World's Mothers 2015.* Fairfield, CT: Save the Children Foundation, Inc.

Singogo, E., et al. 2013. "Village Registers for Vital Registration in Malawi." *Tropical Medicine & International Health* 18 (8): 1021–24.

Stevenson, Lisa. 2014. *Life Beside Itself: Imagining Care in the Canadian Arctic.* Berkeley: University of California.

Vaughan, Megan. 2013. "Maternal Mortality in Malawi: History and Moral Responsibility." In *Death, Belief and Politics in Central African History,* edited by W. T. Kalusa and M. Vaughan, 293–326. Lusaka, Zambia: Lembani Trust.

Wendland, Claire. 2010. *A Heart for the Work: Journeys Through an African Medical School.* Chicago: University of Chicago.

———. 2016. "Estimating death: A Close Reading of Maternal Mortality Metrics in Malawi." In *Metrics: What Counts in Global Health,* edited by V. Adams, 57–81. Durham, NC: Duke University.

Afterword

Arthur Kleinman

Since the post–world war ii era, anthropologists have studied medical pluralism, and the subject remains salient today as this fine collection of essays demonstrates for Africa. Indeed, that pluralism has become even more complex and influential in Africa as globalization has brought Chinese financial investment, the migration of several million Chinese workers, and the introduction and dissemination of traditional Chinese medicine in virtually every major African urban space and many rural ones. That reality can be encompassed within the overview of salient issues canvassed so effectively in the Introduction.

I seek here to raise additional issues that connect the study of medical pluralism in Africa with the current condition of global health. One longstanding issue that I first ventured to address in my 1980 monograph, *Patients and Healers in the Context of Culture*, but have developed further more recently, is the question of caregiving. Many ethnographic and historical studies reveal the embodied and contextually-embedded processes of caring for others and oneself. There are large cultural differences but also a limited number of existential ways by which people go about addressing the sick and attempting to be of help. In my view, not enough attention has been paid to the actual physical practices of care, including such things as protecting, assisting, feeding, carrying, washing—the hands-on work of ritual and of the most practical acts of accompanying, acknowledging, affirming, and loving.

As anthropologists we (including I) have rightly studied the communicative, explanatory, symbolic, and more broadly moral and political aspects of treatment. We need to complement these crucial aspects with the equally crucial and deeply human acts that represent the bodily work of families, networks, individuals, and culture in order to better document what caregiving is and what is most at stake in it for local communities and individuals. African studies of therapy management teams have long established the key role of families and networks, yet even here more detail is required to really gain an understanding of local differences and translocal similarities and how these relate to global patterns.

Once caregiving acts per se are the focus, the unavoidable question is one of quality. Here there has been a tendency to patronize traditional forms of healing by not addressing the same questions of quality that have become central to how medical anthropologists critically approach biomedical practitioners and their practices. My own assessment is that quality of care is increasingly problematic in all forms of caregiving, including those of families, local folk healers, professionalized traditional medical practitioners and biomedical practitioners. And that is as much due to neoliberal economic consequences as are the negative health effects on disease causation of those injurious international economic conditions. That is to say, neoliberal economic policies and practices are weakening caregiving everywhere in the process of prioritizing cost containment, efficiency, bureaucratic indifference, and one-size-fits-all best-practice guidelines. When it comes to measures of quality, the emphasis in healthcare policy is on preventing errors. While preventing errors is admirable, this emphasis obscures the absence of direct measures of the practical, emotional, and moral processes for high-quality care.

Yet quality of care is more than an issue of neoliberal policies and programs, as influential as they most certainly are. The question of quality forces researchers to try to understand what is locally at stake in treatment for each of the protagonists: healers, patients, families, networks, communities. Of course cultural and social relational factors loom large. Most anthropological work, including mine, has focused on cultural questions; but social, relational, and institutional concerns deserve greater attention. Elsewhere, I have proposed the well-worked-over anthropological model of reciprocal gift exchange as a still-useful way to integrate disparate empirical studies into a more coherent interpretation of how to get at caregiving and the issues of quality. Reciprocity in care is fundamental, and it emerges from a deep reading of social relations and how history, political economy, and culture shape the moral-emotional sentiments, obligations, aspirations, and recriminations that everywhere surround the practices of care. Anthropologists do better here, not surprisingly, on the structural than on the individual aspects of care.

And yet it is impossible to study care in any meaningful way without taking into account the subjectivity of the person suffering, the caregivers and the researchers. This is where studies of caregiving bring anthropology and related interpretive social science up against an unavoidable existential ethical reality that affects all studies in global health and social development. As Iain Wilkinson and I argue in our recent book, *A Passion for Society: How We Think about Human Suffering*, the late-eighteenth-century and early-nineteenth-century founders of systematic social inquiry, such as Adam Smith, who set the foundation for the social sciences, understood that activity to be about not just describing human suffering but using the deep knowledge gained to respond by helping people and reforming society. This idea that social science must, if it is to be ethically

defensible, respond to human problems was transformed during the professionalization of the social sciences to the idea of studying, not just society for its own
sake, but social problems too, for what they tell us about social life—without any
implication that those studies are to be of help with fellow human beings who
are in trouble. The implication for medical anthropological studies is straightforward but profound.

We see the effect in practice in the increasing role of medical anthropologists
in applying their knowledge to make a difference. So too should anthropological
studies of medical pluralism in Africa carry a responsibility to make a difference
with respect to helping people locally and developing policies and programs that
improve human futures. So what is that contribution? In the case of this book,
it is to be found in all the little details that taken together add up to a better understanding and more telling critique of health systems aimed at improving care.
Medical pluralism is the reality of healthcare systems in Africa, and coming to
a better understanding should change and improve those systems. The quality
of services should be improved, as should the planning and delivery of care to
reduce health inequalities and social disparities. But those studies also can be
played back in order to improve care in the United States and other donor nations.

Where medical anthropologists have contributed directly to health services reform—as in the work of MD-PhD medical anthropologists such as Paul
Farmer, Jim Kim, and Salmaan Keshavjee to implement community care for TB
and AIDS among poor populations in Africa and Haiti via accompaniment by local people—this moral mandate is realized. The same can be said about the work
of Anne Becker in Fiji and Haiti on behalf of people with mental health problems.
But even where medical anthropologists don't participate directly in the delivery
of services, they still have an obligation to make the hard-won knowledge they
have built somehow relevant to the experience of real people in need. Again, we
can see in this volume how that might be done either by the applications of researchers themselves or via the development of a translocal social science whose
aim is to create sophisticated applications based on strong ethnographic contributions.

Finally, the empirical studies in this collection call attention to the tasks of
theory building in medical anthropology to build on the existing platform of
detailed empirical research to create more generalizable social theories. Here it
is important to note that we still lack a theory of medical pluralism in Africa and
more broadly that integrates knowledge into a robust social theoretical contribution that can guide further research, demonstrate the comparative advantage
of anthropological knowledge, and frame the intellectual development of this
subject with the aim of developing and improving services. Clearly this volume

shows that this process, incomplete though it be, is now underway. And here Africanists and the African context may hold answers for the greater success of global health implementation in Africa and globally, because when it comes to medical pluralism, the rest of the world has much to learn from the African reality and from those, like the contributors to this book, who have studied that reality and made it part of global knowledge.

Bibliography

Akyeampong, Emmanuel, Allan. G. Hill, and Arthur Kleinman, eds. 2015. *Culture, Mental Illness and Psychiatric Practice in Africa.* Indiana University.

Kleinman, A. 1980. *Patients and Healers in the Context of Culture: An Exploration of the Borderland Between Anthropology, Medicine, and Psychiatry.* Berkeley: University of California.

———. 2006. *What Really Matters: Living a Moral Life Amidst Uncertainty and Danger.* Oxford University Press.

———. 2014. "How We Endure." *The Lancet* 383 (9912): 119–20.

———. 2015. "Care: In Search of a Health Agenda." *The Lancet* 386 (9990): 240–41.

Wilkinson, Iain, and Arthur Kleinman. 2016. *A Passion for Society: How We Think about Human Suffering.* Berkeley: University of California.

Contributors

John M. Janzen, University of Kansas
James Leslie Kennell, Washington University
Arthur Kleinman, Harvard University
Stacey Langwick, Cornell University
Benson A. Mulemi, Catholic University of East Africa
William C. Olsen, Georgetown University
Susan J. Rasmussen, University of Houston
Elisha Renne, University of Michigan
Carolyn Sargent, Washington University
Claire Grundfest Schoepf, Harvard University
Koen Stroeken, Ghent University
Christopher C. Taylor, University of Alabama
Ulrika Trovalla, Nordiska Afrikainstitutet
Claire Wendland, University of Wisconsin–Madison

Index

abortion, 245

African healing systems, 4–6, 23; change in, 111, 160. *See also* traditional healing; therapeutic systems

African medical systems: as open systems, 14–15; professionalization of, 23–24

African Traditional Medicine, 217–218. *See also* traditional healing

Ahmadu Bello University Teaching Hospital, 187, 188, 189–190, 192–194,196, 199

AIDS. *See* HIV/AIDS

Aja, 228, 232, 234,235; causes of disease among, 228, 229

Alma Ata Declaration, 118

alternative therapies, 56, 73; clandestine use of, 208; efficacy of, 116. *See also* medical pluralism

Amen Scientific Herbal Clinic, 23–24

anonymous care, 256

Apostolic Church, 229, 230, 231,

Asante, 9, 13, 18, 57, 58, 59–60, 64; stroke in, 50, 51, 52, 54–56, 62, 63–65; theory of disease, 21

Assa Akpa, 234, 242n3

assisted reproductive technology, 69, 70, 72, 85

asthma, 115, 146, 148

authoritative knowledge, 93

azamba (traditional birth attendant), 244, 245, 247, 248, 249, 250, 251, 253, 254, 256, 257n6

Azande, 82, 91, 151, 236

Baatonou, 235, 236

Banda, Joyce, 247

Bariba, 15, 16. *See also* Baatonou

Batangu Mpesa, E. F., 96, 102, 103–107

Benin, 17; National Health System, 228; traditional healing in, 228–240

biomedicine, 1, 2, 6, 10–12, 16–17, 52–53, 70, 92, 118, 120, 125; attitudes regarding, 62–63, 73–74, 133, 154; culture of, 92; introduction of, 3–4; preference for, 16, 54, 62, 112, 158; prevalence of, 90, 110, 118, 119, 157. *See also* hospitals

birth control pills, 79–80

bogyεsε (witch-catching shrine), 57, 58

bone-setter, 110

cancer, 123; biomedical treatment of, 208, 214–215; community of care and, 219, 220–221; epidemic, 210–211, 223; liver, 236, 238. 239; misdiagnosis of, 211

cancer care, 261, 262, 263; desperation and, 213; dietary supplements and 221–222; traditional Chinese medicine and, 221–222; variation in 214–215

Cartesian dualism, 100, 152, 155, 156, 160

Centre de Recherche Pharmaceutique de Luozi, 96

childbirth, 244–245, 246–247; cesarian section, 253; HIV and, 250–251, 252; uterine rupture in, 255–256, 258n14

childhood illness, 113, 116

childlessness, 70, 71; treatment of, 76, 77–78, 79–81. *See also* infertility

chipatala (health facility), 248, 251, 252, 253

Clastres, Pierre, 178, 180

clinics, 112. *See also* hospitals

collective medicine, 154–155

complementary and alternative therapies, 209; cancer care and, 216–223. *See also* alternative therapies

conception: beliefs about, 70–71

contagion, 2, 70, 72, 73, 86, 125; childlessness and, 71, 77, 80, 86. *See also* pollution

corruption

cosmic panorama, 105–107. *See also* Batangu Mpesa

cosmology, 121, 156; medical, 100, 105, 159; sickness and, 110. *See also* moral frameworks

Csordas, Thomas, 20–21

dangerous care, 246, 249–251, 252, 253–256

decolonization: medical pluralism and, 118

Democratic Republic of the Congo, 17, 20, 121–125, 128; healing paradigms in, 90–108. *See also* Kongo

disability, 92

disease symptoms: social networks and, 51–52, 59

disease: cultural construction of, 92; meaning of, 19–20. *See also* cosmology; illness.

www.ingramcontent.com/pod-product-compliance
Lightning Source LLC
Chambersburg PA
CBHW030730280326
41926CB00086B/995